Adoption Medicine

Caring for Children and Families

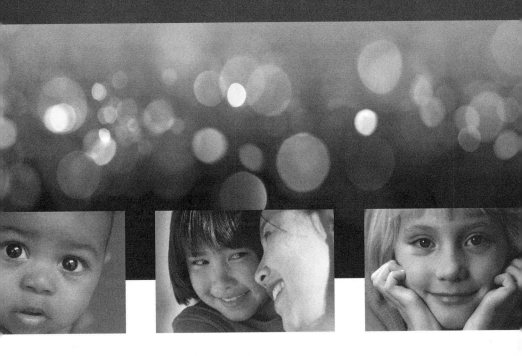

Council on Foster Care, Adoption, and Kinship Care
American Academy of Pediatrics

Editors
Patrick W. Mason, MD, PhD, FAAP
Dana E. Johnson, MD, PhD, FAAP
Lisa Albers Prock, MD, MPH, FAAP

American Academy of Pediatrics
DEDICATED TO THE HEALTH OF ALL CHILDREN™

Library of Congress Control Number: 2013946568
ISBN: 978-1-58110-322-9
eISBN: 978-1-58110-842-2
MA0464

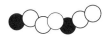

Reviewers/Contributors

Editors

Patrick W. Mason, MD, PhD, FAAP
Dana E. Johnson, MD, PhD, FAAP
Lisa Albers Prock, MD, MPH, FAAP

American Academy of Pediatrics Board of Directors Reviewer

Carole E. Allen, MD, FAAP

American Academy of Pediatrics

Errol R. Alden, MD, FAAP
Executive Director/CEO

Roger F. Suchyta, MD, FAAP
Associate Executive Director

Maureen DeRosa, MPA
Director, Department of Marketing and Publications

Mark Grimes
Director, Division of Product Development

Jeff Mahony
Manager, Digital Strategy and Product Development

Mary Crane, PhD, LSW
Manager, Council on Foster Care, Adoption, and Kinship Care

Kelly Hess, MBA
Division Assistant, Division of Developmental Pediatrics and Preventive Services

Chapter Authors

Susan Branco Alvarado, MAEd, LPC
Licensed Professional Counselor
Doctoral Student
Virginia Tech
Blacksburg, VA
Counselor Education and Supervision
Falls Church, VA

Heather W. Ames, MSW, LICSW
Director of Post-Adoption Services
(retired)
Wide Horizons for Children
Waltham, MA

David M. Brodzinsky, PhD
Research Director
Evan B. Donaldson Adoption Institute
Professor Emeritus, Clinical and
Developmental Psychology
Rutgers University
New Brunswick, NJ

Nicole Ficere Callahan
Research Director
National Council for Adoption
Alexandria, VA

Claire D. Coles, PhD
Professor, Departments of Psychiatry and
Behavioral Science and Pediatrics
Emory University School of Medicine
Atlanta, GA

Katherine P. Deye, MD, FAAP
Assistant Professor, Department of
Pediatrics
George Washington University School of
Medicine and Health Sciences
Pediatrician
Freddie Mac Foundation Child and
Adolescent Protection Center
Children's National Medical Center
Washington, DC

**Madelyn Freundlich, MSW, MPH,
JD, LLM**
Child Welfare Consultant
Excal Consulting Partners
New York, NY

Sharon Glennen, PhD, CCC-SLP
Director, Institute for Well-Being
Professor of Audiology, Speech Language
Pathology & Deaf Studies
Towson University
Towson, MD

Kent P. Hymel, MD, FAAP
Professor of Pediatrics
Geisel School of Medicine at Dartmouth
Hanover, NH
Medical Director, Child Advocacy and
Protection Program
Dartmouth-Hitchcock Medical Center
Lebanon, NH

Chuck Johnson
President and CEO
National Council for Adoption
Alexandria, VA

Dana E. Johnson, MD, PhD, FAAP
Professor of Pediatrics
University of Minnesota
Minneapolis, MN

Paul J. Lee, MD, FAAP
Director, Adoption Program
Winthrop-University Hospital
Mineola, NY
Clinical Associate Professor of Pediatrics
Department of Pediatrics
School of Medicine State University of NY
Stony Brook, NY

Christine Narad Mason, DNP, C-PNP
Children's National Medical Center
Washington, DC

Patrick W. Mason, MD, PhD, FAAP
Division of Endocrinology
Inova Children's Hospital
Falls Church, VA

Laurie C. Miller, MD, FAAP
Professor of Pediatrics
Director, Center for Adoptive Families
Tufts Medical Center
Adjunct Professor of Nutrition
Gerald J. and Dorothy R. Friedman School
    of Nutrition Science and Policy
Tufts University
Boston, MA

Lisa Nalven, MD, MA, FAAP
Director, Developmental Pediatrics &
    Adoption Screening and Evaluation
    Program
Kireker Center for Child Development,
    Valley Hospital
Ridgewood, NJ

**Joyce Maguire Pavao, EdD, MEd,
    LCSW, LMFT**
Lecturer in Psychiatry
Harvard Medical School
Boston, MA

Vicki Peterson, MSW, LICSW
Former CEO
Wide Horizons for Children
Waltham, MA

Jonathan Picker, MBChB, PhD
Assistant Professor of Pediatrics
Division of Genetics and Department of
    Child and Adolescent Psychiatry
Boston Children's Hospital
Boston, MA

Lisa Albers Prock, MD, MPH, FAAP
Assistant Professor
Harvard Medical School
Director, Adoption Program
Boston Children's Hospital
Boston, MA

Linda D. Sagor, MD, MPH, FAAP
Division Director, General Pediatrics
UMass Memorial Health Care
Professor of Clinical Pediatrics
University of Massachusetts Medical
    School
Worcester, MA

Elaine E. Schulte, MD, MPH, FAAP
Chair, Department of General Pediatrics
Professor of Pediatrics, Cleveland Clinic
    Lerner College of Medicine
Cleveland Clinic Children's
Cleveland, OH

Prachi E. Shah, MD, MS
Assistant Professor of Pediatrics
University of Michigan Medical School
Ann Arbor, MI

Sarah H. Springer, MD, FAAP
Medical Director
International Adoption Health Services of
    Western Pennsylvania
Kids Plus Pediatrics
Pittsburgh, PA

Contents

Foreword

The first time you met this family more than 10 years ago, 2 excited but nervous parents sat across the desk, carefully scrutinizing the expression on your face as you examined the documents in your hand. They had been trying for years to have a birth child without success. So after a long, expensive, and intrusive adoption process (exploring international, domestic public, and domestic private adoption), they waited for you to render an opinion about their referral information—only 2 sheets of paper and a picture of a little girl who later became their daughter.

You had concerns about some of what was described, but you knew that within a nurturing family, there is always hope. You wanted to be honest and realistic to ensure the prospective parents were prepared to meet the needs of the child, but the information provided was so limited that accurate health predictions were, of course, impossible.

The second time you met with these parents was for Anna's first pediatric visit after arriving home from South Korea. Over the subsequent years that you've been her pediatrician, she has been quite healthy, yet with some academic ups and downs and emotional concerns, with various diagnoses and suggestions from multiple practitioners. She has also had an adoptive brother and sister join her family. And now—time flies—today is her 12-year well-child check. The family is now considering a trip back to South Korea and wonders if you have any thoughts or suggestions about how to best approach this possible trip with Anna and her siblings.

Health care professionals face scenarios like this on a regular basis. Since the early 1990s, hundreds of thousands of parents have chosen adoption as a way of building their families. While a formal process of adoption can be traced back to the ancient Babylonians (1800 BCE), the field has changed significantly in the past 25 years. Today, adoptions are far more open and come in many varieties, including international, transracial, single parent, same sex couples, and kinship. Gone are the "bad old days" when transracial adoptions were discouraged or prevented and most adoptions were secretive affairs in which a family's greatest concern was if and when to tell a child he or she was adopted. Today, birth parents are often involved, adoptive families and adoptees speak freely and openly about the adoption process, and adopting a child with a different ethnic background or birth country is commonplace. It's hard to go shopping, to church, or to school and not encounter a family built through adoption.

Although adoption has become a much more common way of building a family, the medical community has been slower in appreciating the effect that a child's pre-adoptive life can have on his or her health and development and long-term challenges that adoptive families face in parenting their children. Fortunately, the health care community is now rapidly catching up. More pediatric health care professionals are learning about adoption and its potential short- and long-term effects on the child. A growing literature examines how a child's early life experiences in an orphanage or foster care setting could affect his or her life. Adoption clinics are now a routine part of many children's hospitals, and professionals with interest and expertise in adoption are coming together in meetings to discuss ideas on how to improve care and outcomes for adopted children.

As we developed this book, we recruited a panel of experts to summarize topics pertaining to adoption medicine. Our goal was to present a practical guide with real-life examples that could be used as a resource for anyone working with families affected by adoption. Each author was requested to provide the most current information related to all types of adoption and instructed to write not only for doctors but any professional likely to come in contact with adoptive parents or children, including nurses, therapists, social workers, adoption agencies, and parents. While this process was long and arduous, we are pleased with its outcome.

We have broken this manual down into several sections. Chapter 1, on the history of adoption, is an excellent review of the evolution of adoption, particularly during the past 2 centuries. After that, we have grouped the book loosely into what happens prior to the formal adoption of a child and what may be relevant over time. Lastly, we finish with 2 appendixes that we hope will be useful, including an in-depth discussion of the effect the Hague Convention on intercountry adoption has had on international adoptions (Appendix 1) and resources the reader may find useful (Appendix 2).

In the "pre-adoption" section, we have asked our experts to discuss topics such as the process of adoption and legal issues that families should be aware of as they navigate through the process. Drs Lee and Sagor (Chapter 4) discuss how anyone in the health care field can help a potential parent prepare for an adoption. Details including prenatal exposures (Chapter 5) and the effect of genetics (Chapter 6) are discussed, as well as how these factors can influence a child's risks and hopefully that child's ability to recover (Chapter 7).

Next, we tried to address some of the issues that health care professionals may need to be aware of following the arrival of the new child. Drs Schulte and Springer (Chapter 8) discuss the immediate health issues a child may need evaluated, and Dr Miller reports on developmental and behavioral challenges that may need to be addressed (Chapter 9). Several longer term issues round out the book, including discussions on growth and puberty (Chapter 12), attachment (Chapter 13), language acquisition (Chapter 14), and guides to help families and health care professionals navigate complex long-term issues such as identity, searching for birth parents, working with the school system, and facing complex emotional and behavioral problems (chapters 15–18).

While we tried to group each of these topics in a logical order following a family's adoption journey, not all fit easily into one area or another. Although some of the topics may be more geared to one type of adoption (international) versus another (kinship or domestic), we have tried to make each chapter pertinent to any family's or child's situation. In addition, the field of adoption is constantly changing—countries are constantly opening or closing to adoption by foreigners, bureaucratic procedures change, and forms may be different. As soon as a book such as this is written, parts of it are likely already obsolete. Our goal is to provide readers with information that can be useful despite these changes.

Pediatric health care professionals are the most constant professional contact for adoptive parents and are in an ideal position to advise families as they face the challenges and reap the benefits of parenting adopted children. We hope that the information and knowledge you will learn and can share with families will help to achieve our ultimate goals: to help parents successfully build their family through adoption and support families as they parent their adopted children to competent adulthood.

Patrick W. Mason, MD, PhD, FAAP
Dana E. Johnson, MD, PhD, FAAP
Lisa Albers Prock, MD, MPH, FAAP

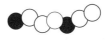

CHAPTER 1

History of Adoption

Dana E. Johnson, MD, PhD, FAAP

Introduction

Since the first human birth, loss of parental nurture and protection through death or abandonment placed a child's survival in immediate jeopardy. Though our religious and literary heritage is replete with stories of children abandoned or orphaned who survived to achieve greatness (eg, Moses, Muhammad), this was certainly not the most common outcome of childhood "exposure." In his exhaustive study of child abandonment in Western Europe from late antiquity to the Renaissance, John Boswell reminds us that only through *The Kindness of Strangers* (the book's title) was death prevented or slavery, lifelong obligatory servitude, or child prostitution avoided.[1] Standing in stark contrast to other options throughout history, ascension of an abandoned child to a position indistinguishable from a birth child within a family through formal or informal adoption was the superior mode of ensuring survival and well-being in a hostile world.

Society has approved of formal transfer of parental obligation and rights since the ancient Babylonians (1800 BCE). Adoption was mentioned in the Hindu Laws of Manu (200 BCE), viewed as a method of insuring progeny in China as early as the fourth century BCE, and established in Roman law and the Napoleonic code.[2–4] Through these legal processes, childless couples could achieve an heir, the adoptee could attain a higher economic or social class, and parents could guarantee themselves economic security in their old age. However, while adoption has been formally sanctioned for millennia, the processes and outcomes were based on the needs and interests of adults and rarely on those of the child. The ambivalent treatment received by orphaned and abandoned children throughout much of recorded history is highlighted in an edict from emperor Constantine in 331 CE.[1]

> *"Anyone who picks up and nourishes at his own expense a little boy or girl cast out of the home of its father or lord with the latter's knowledge and consent may retain the child in the position for which he intended it when he took it in—that is, as child or slave as he prefers."*

While the treatment of abandoned children in the ancient world was generally arbitrary and callous, when a relationship was formalized through adoption, it was viewed as equal to that of a biological child, eg, Julius Caesar and Augustus. The Middle Ages saw an increasing social significance of lineage and birth, which made open adoption problematic and far less desirable. Though parents continued to take children into their homes, it was usually under circumstances in which the parents and child maintained a fictitious biological relationship. With the exception of the lucky few covertly adopted, most at-risk children continued to suffer the usual fates of those lacking parental protection.[1]

Orphanages founded by religious orders originated in Italy in the 13th century and by the 15th century had spread to most major cities in Europe as a method of dealing with the problem of orphaned and abandoned children. One of the earliest and most famous of these institutions was the Ospedale degli Innocenti associated with the church of the same name in Florence. Andrea della Robbia's depiction of Christ as a swaddled infant on the glazed terracotta medallions adorning the portico of this building was adopted in the early 1940s as the insignia of the American Academy of Pediatrics.[5]

Unfortunately, institutional care dealt with abandonment in an even more deadly fashion, particularly in infants. Without a safe and reliable source of nutrition aside from the expensive option of wet-nursing and crowded together in unsanitary conditions, death rates among institutional residents were astronomically high. Between 1772 and 1789, the Hospital for Foundlings in St. Petersburg, Russia, had a mortality rate of 86%. In the Paris Foundling Hospital established by Saint Vincent de Paul in 1638, mortality in infancy between 1840 and 1859 was 56%.[6] Well into the late 19th century, the odds of survival for an institutionalized infant were extremely low. Prior to 1867, mortality in the Randall Island Infant Hospital in New York, NY, for children younger than 1 year ranged between 90% to 95%. A concerted effort to improve conditions by hiring a trained physician and replacing indigent women with paid nurses reduced mortality to 59% by 1870, which was still more than twice as high as the overall infant mortality rate in the city as a whole.[6]

Evolution of Domestic Adoption in the United States

The 19th century saw a dramatic increase in the number of orphaned and abandoned children due to epidemics in large eastern cities, the Civil War, and European immigration. Prior to this time, close family and community relationships were the safety net that provided protection, but as personal and social relationship were strained by urbanization and increasing poverty, orphanages filled the void. The number of orphanages increased from 30 between 1800 and 1830 to more than 200 in 1860.[7] However, by the mid-19th century, unacceptable mortality rates within institutional care settings coupled with an increasing appreciation that children had their own unique developmental needs led reformers of the day to explore other caregiving options. A notable figure of that era was Charles Loring Brace, a Methodist minister who founded The Children's Aid Society in New York in 1853. Brace was appalled by the overcrowding and abject poverty in the city and felt that suffering innocent children of indigent Catholic and Jewish immigrants could be rescued and Americanized if permanently relocated from degenerate urban surroundings and placed with stalwart frontier families. The orphan trains started by his organization were the most famous example of the social experiment of "placing out" abandoned, orphaned, and indigent children. Between 1854 and 1929, as many as 250,000 children from New York and other Eastern cities were sent by train to families in the heartland of the United States, Mexico, and Canada. Families interested in the orphans, many of who still had parents, showed up to choose children who were displayed at the local church or train stations. Those not chosen would get back on the train to be exhibited at the next stop. Placements were made with little investigation or oversight and while some of these children found permanent loving homes, others experienced neglect and abuse.[8–10]

In 1868, the Massachusetts Board of State Charities began paying for children to lodge in the homes of private families. An integral part of this program was an agent paid to visit on a regular basis to insure that a child's living conditions were acceptable. The New York State Charities Aid Association, another pioneer in establishing a specialized child-placement program, embraced this model in 1898. By 1922, homes for more than 3,300 children had been found by this organization.[11] Both were more successful and long-lasting examples of the placing-out movement that evolved into the family foster care programs of today.

This transition from institutional to family care intensified in the first 2 decades of the 20th century, in part through the efforts of James West, who, at the age of 6, had been left by his dying, widowed mother at the Washington City Orphan Asylum.[8] Crippled by tuberculosis of the hip and thus unsuitable to be indentured, as were his peers, West obtained an education and eventually began working on the Child-Rescue Campaign of the *Delineator,* a monthly women's magazine owned by Butterick Publishing Co. In perhaps one of the earliest examples of this genre, the magazine offered subscribers a different selection of homeless children each month, complete with photographs and detailed histories. The public response was overwhelming, influencing West to consider the possibility of placing not only homeless children but children from institutions as well. In 1908 he persuaded his friend, President Theodore Roosevelt, to sponsor a national conference on the care of homeless and neglected children, and on January 25, 1909, the conference convened at the White House. What transpired over the next few days laid the foundation for the child welfare system in the United States and permanently changed the trajectory of care for orphaned and dependent children. The final statement declared that maintenance of the birth family, despite poverty, was in the best interest of the child and that if placement was required for other reasons, children were to be placed in family homes, "the highest and finest product of civilization."[12]

In addition to the evolution in attitudes, the late 18th and early 19th centuries saw major changes in laws governing adoption. In 1851, the Massachusetts Legislature passed "An Act to Provide for the Adoption of Children," the foundation for all subsequent American, Canadian, and British child-centered adoption legislation. This law recognized adoption as a social and legal operation based on child welfare rather than adult interests, directing judges to ensure that adoption decrees were "fit and proper." The law also provided that, for the purposes of inheritance, custody, and all other legal circumstances, the adopted child would be considered the legitimate child of the adoptive parents.[11,13,14] By 1891, Michigan required that "the [judge] shall be satisfied as to the good moral character, and the ability to support and educate such child, and of the suitableness of the home, or the person or persons adopting such child," and in 1917, Minnesota enacted statues mandating social investigation of all adoptions.[11] This era also saw the establishment of the first school for social work, the New York School of Applied Philanthropy (1904), as well as the first private adoption agencies, including Children's Home Society in St. Paul, MN; The Cradle in Evanston, IL; and the Spence Alumni Society, Free Synagogue Child Adoption Committee, and Alice Chapin Nursery in New York.[11,15] By the 1930s, adoption had become a well-established method of building a family in the United States for married couples from a wide range of backgrounds. As we see today, past adoptive parents have included numerous celebrities such as George Burns and Gracie Allen, Bob and Dolores Hope, Pearl and John Buck, and Al Jolson and Ruby Keeler.[16]

Subsequent Trends in US Adoption

Analysis of how many children are adopted and who they are is highly problematic because of the paucity of statistical data on domestic adoption.[17] Prior to 1920, essentially no data were gathered, and what were collected after that time was limited to extremely small geographic areas. A national reporting system for adoption existed between 1945 and 1975, when the US Children's Bureau and the National Center for Social Statistics collected data voluntarily supplied by states and territories. However, from 1976 to 1997, adoption data were not collected systematically, and compilation of statistics required scrutinizing numerous sources. Mandated data collection began again in 1998 under the Adoption and Safe Families Act of 1997, which requires states to report the adoption of children in public foster care.[18] Because visas are required for adoptees entering the United States from abroad, numbers of international adoptees and the countries from which they originate are easily tracked.[19]

From all sources of information, it can be concluded that the number of adoptions (related and unrelated) peaked in 1967 to 1972, then declined abruptly thereafter (Figure 1-1). In 1968, an estimated 86,300 unrelated adoption placements occurred, of which 26,800 were through public agencies, 37,100 were through private agencies, and 22,400 were arranged independently. By 1975, the total number had dropped by 45% to 47,700, with a decrease of 31% through public agencies and 50% in private agencies and independent adoption.[20] This change coincided with an era that saw increasing social tolerance and financial support for unmarried mothers and enhanced reproductive control through reliable contraceptive methods and availability of legal abortion services throughout the United States. The net result was that fewer babies were born to single mothers and fewer were relinquished for adoption. Prior to 1973, the percentage of newborns relinquished for adoption by never-married women younger than 45 years was 8.7%. From 1989 to 1995, the figure was 0.9%.[21] The only area of adoption growth during that era was in inter-country adoption, which more than tripled from 1,612 to 5,663 (Figure 1-2 and Table 1-1).[22]

Over the past 2 decades, adoptions have rebounded somewhat because of increasing numbers from abroad and through the foster care system. Following passage of the Adoption and Safe Families Act of 1997, legislation designed to speed

Figure 1-1.
Adoptions in the United States, 1951 to 1997

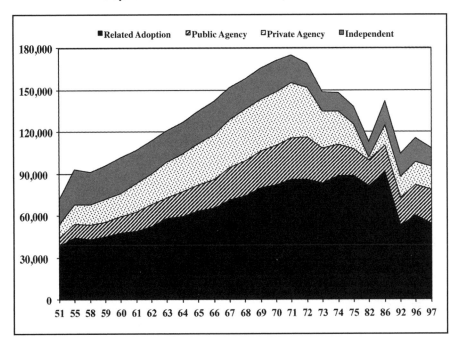

Figure 1-2.
Origins of International Adoptees to the United States, 1963 to 2008

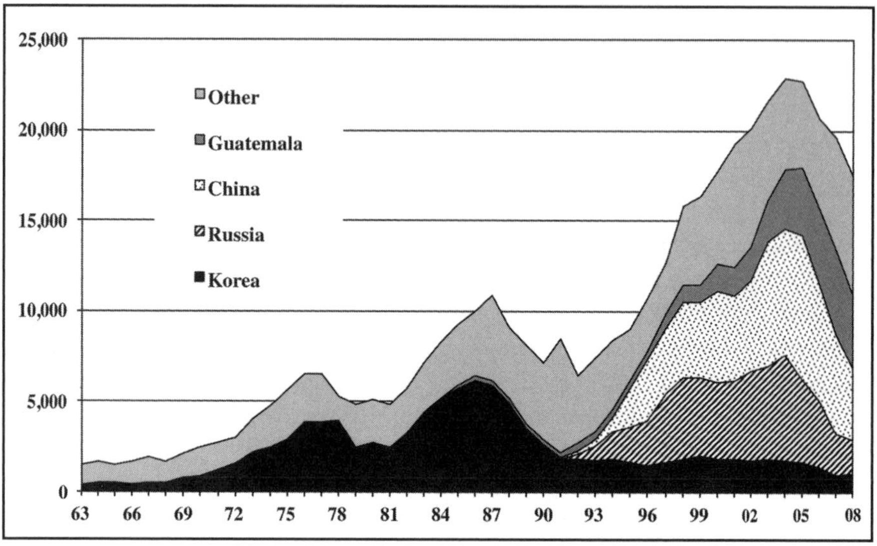

placement of waiting children into permanent homes, the number of adoptions from foster care rose 43% from 37,000 in 1998 to 53,000 in 2002 and has remained at that level since (Figure 1-3).[23] The numbers of children placed through independent adoption (domestic newborns) are much harder to come by, but despite rumors about the difficulty of adopting newborns, estimates range from 25,000 to 30,000 per year.[24,25]

Today, adoption is broadly accepted and part of our shared experience in the United States. The 2002 National Adoption Attitudes Survey revealed that more than 90% of Americans had "very favorable" or "somewhat favorable" opinions about adoption and 64% of respondents reported that a family member or close friend had been adopted.[26] Thirty-nine percent of Americans had very seriously or somewhat seriously considered adopting at some point in their lives, and 86% believed adoptive parents derive the same amount or more satisfaction from raising an adopted child as they derive from raising a birth child.

Evolution of International Adoption in the United States

International adoption is a growing component of adoption in the United States. The 2000 US Census reported 199,136 international adoptees younger than 18 years living with families in the United States (12.5% of adopted children).[27] One common question is why pursue adopting a child from abroad when thousands of children are waiting in domestic foster care for a permanent home? Most

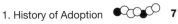

Table 1-1. International Adoptions to the United States, 1948 to 2008

1948 to 1962 (n=19,230)	
Korea	4,162 (22%)
Greece	3,116 (16%)
Japan	2,987 (13%)
Germany	1,845 (10%)
Austria	744 (4%)
1975 (n=5,663)	
Korea	2,913 (52%)
Vietnam	655 (12%)
Colombia	379 (7%)
Philippines	244 (4%)
Mexico	162 (3%)
1986 (n=9,945)	
Korea	6,118 (62%)
Philippines	634 (10%)
India	588 (9%)
Guatemala	228 (4%)
El Salvador	147 (2%)
1991 (n=8,481)	
Romania	2,594 (31%)
Korea	1,818 (21%)
Peru	705 (8%)
Colombia	521 (6%)
India	445 (5%)
2003 (n=21,616)	
China	6,859 (32%)
Russia	5,209 (24%)
Guatemala	2,328 (11%)
Korea	1,790 (8%)
Kazakhstan	825 (4%)
2008 (n=17,438)	
Guatemala	4,123 (24%)
China	3,909 (22%)
Russia	2,310 (13%)
Ethiopia	1,725 (10%)
Korea	1,065 (6%)

Figure 1-3.
Numbers of Children in the US Foster Care System Adopted and Available for Adoption (Waiting), 1998 to 2007

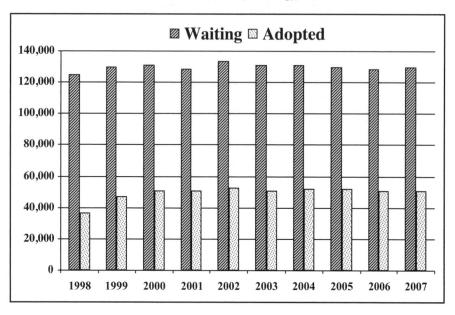

individuals who pursue international adoption desire the entire spectrum of the parenting experience and therefore pursue as young a child as possible. In fiscal year (FY) 2005, only 3% of children adopted from foster care through public agencies were younger than 1 year and 55% older than 5 years, compared with 40% and 16% of international adoptees, respectively.[28] Adoptive parents also choose international adoption because of concerns about the child's relationship with her or his birth parents and potential health issues in fostered children. In the 2002 National Adoption Attitudes Survey, 84% of respondents stated that if they were thinking about adopting, a major concern would be making sure that birth parents could not take the child back.[26] Other families were concerned about open adoption and wished to avoid ongoing interactions with their child's birth parent(s). Medical problems (53%) and mental health issues (63%) also were major worries when adopting from foster care.[26] International adoption does provide some degree of security that birth parents will not contact or reclaim their adopted child, but excluding domestic adoption in hopes of avoiding medical or behavioral problems is flawed reasoning because the children currently available for adoption from abroad share many of the same risk factors and medical and behavioral problems as children in domestic foster care.[29–33]

Other factors aside from biological and social drives for progeny compel individuals to adopt internationally. Religious beliefs play a powerful, central role in many people's decisions. Judeo-Christian tradition holds individuals who adopt in high esteem, and in Islam taking custody of a foundling is deemed an act of piety.[34] Rescuing children from humanitarian disaster triggers resolve in many people, as was evident following the media's depiction of the plight of children in Romanian orphanages in 1990 and 1991.[35] Family origins in the sending country or an affinity with the sending country's culture may also weigh heavily in this choice. Finally, some families seek children with correctible handicaps who would otherwise not be treated, or parents may wish to share skills they acquired dealing with long-term disabilities in children with similar problems, eg, blindness, deafness.

History of International Adoption

International adoption is rooted in conflict and grew out of the humanitarian tragedies of World War II.[22,36,37] Following the war, thousands of children previously orphaned, abandoned by their soldier-fathers, or uprooted and separated from parents were in need of homes. Military personnel occupying these countries were the first to step forward to adopt these children. Between 1948 and 1962, American families adopted 1,845 German, 744 Austrian, and 2,987 Japanese children (Table 1-1).[22,36] Additional waves of adoptees arrived in the United States following the Greek Civil War (3,116 from 1948–1962), the Korean War (4,162 from 1953–1962), the Vietnam War (3,267 between 1963 and 1973), and the war in El Salvador (2,083 between 1980 and 1990) (Table 1-1).[22,36]

These adoptions were not only international but predominately interracial as well. The arrival of the first wave of international adoptees during the late 1940s and early 1950s coincided with a heightened appreciation of racial issues in US society.[22,36] This era saw progress in reversing many of the more deliberate racist practices of the day, a fact that is highlighted by the Supreme Court's decision to end school segregation in *Brown v Board of Education* (1954).[38] Many families of that period saw international adoption not only as a way to build a family but to do so in a way that clearly displayed the values that directed their lives.

The "One-Family United Nations" of Helen Doss and her Methodist-minister husband Carl that graced the pages of *Reader's Digest* and the cover of *Life* in the mid-20th century was the first international adoption "poster family."[39–41] Infertile but desiring to have children, the Doss family ultimately adopted 12 children, some with special needs, who were considered unadoptable because of their mixed-race parentage. The children represented Korea, Japan, the Philippines, Spain, France, Malaysia, Burma, Mexico, Hawaii, and 3 Native American tribes—Chippewa, Blackfoot, and Cheyenne. Two of the most prominent figures in the early history of international adoption in the United States, Bertha and Harry Holt, shared the same roots and motivations.[42] Already birth parents of 6, the Holts eventually made the decision to adopt 8 Korean orphans, and in 1955 a special act of Congress permitted the Holts to adopt the children they sought.[42] This legislation permanently transformed adoption in the United States, establishing Korea as the principal source of international adoptees to the United States for the next 35 years.

From 1963 to 1969, the annual number of international adoptees arriving in the United States remained stable at between 1,450 and 2,100 children per year.[22] However, due to the growing shortfall of adoptable babies in the United States, there was a consistent annual rise in the number of children placed, beginning in 1968 (Figure 1-2). As the list of countries placing children in the United States grew, the number of international adoptees steadily increased over the next decade. Children from Central and South America, India, and the Philippines, as well as an increasing number of children from Korea, boosted the total number of international adoptees to 9,945 in 1986.[22] However, Korea began to limit the number of international adoptions after facing increased international criticism about adoption practices, particularly during the 1988 Summer Olympics in Seoul, South Korea.[22] From a high of 6,188 in 1986, the number of Korean placements in the United States dropped precipitously to 1,818 by 1991 and 1,065 by 2008 (Figure 1-3 and Table 1-1).[19,22]

During 1990 to 1995, the fall of Communism in Eastern Europe, the dissolution of the Union of Soviet Socialist Republics, and the liberalization of the Chinese adoption policy in response to population control initiatives ushered in the next era of international adoption. While rates of adoption from Romania flared briefly in 1991 (Figure 1-2 and Table 1-1), the number of children adopted from Russia and China steadily climbed during the ensuing decade. By 1995, Korea had been supplanted as the top placing country, and in FY 2003, China and Russia accounted for 56% of international adoption placements in the United States (Figure 1-2 and Table 1-1).

During the past decade, the increasing number of available children coincided with a rising demand to adopt internationally. By 2000, the average American woman had her first baby at 25 years of age, 3.6 years later than in 1970.[43] Delayed childbearing brings about an increase in involuntary infertility. The probability of conceiving decreases for women in their 30s, particularly after the age of 35.[44] For the first time since the end of World War II, a significant number of white children from Eastern Europe were available for adoption. Countries also were more willing to permit adoption by single parents. In 2004, a record number of 22,884 orphan visas were issued in the United States, up 353% from the 1992 nadir (Figure 1-2 and Table 1-1).[19] This phenomenon was observed in many countries, including Canada, where intercountry adoptions increased from 232 (1988) to 2,181 (2003), an 8-fold increase.[45]

This increase in adoptions heralded not only a change in countries of origin but also a very different population of children than had been previously placed through international adoption. In the mid-1980s, most international adoptees were from Korea. These children were relinquished by healthy women stigmatized by single parenthood, raised in foster families, provided a high level of medical care, and adopted as infants. In comparison, international adoptees today are far more likely to be abandoned by mothers who are poorly nourished and destitute and who have abused alcohol or intravenous drugs, be cared for within institutional care settings, receive inadequate medical care, and join their adoptive families as toddlers or older children.[46,47]

Since 2004, international adoptions have fallen and are projected to return to levels seen in the mid-1990s within the next few years. The reasons behind this decline are complex but relate to factors such as implementation by the United States of the Hague Convention on Protection of Children and Co-operation in Respect of Intercountry Adoption, economic downturn of 2008 and 2009, development of successful programs of domestic adoption in many sending countries, and ongoing controversy about whether intercountry adoption is in the best interest of children. As we proceed forward, medical issues in international adoptees are likely to become more significant with time. The success of incipient domestic adoption programs in many sending countries relies on placing normal, healthy infants. In such locales, the children available for adoption abroad are those who are older and have clear medical or surgical diagnoses or known cognitive or behavioral issues. In other words, international adoptees have become essentially indistinguishable from children within the domestic foster care system. Therefore, the involvement of health care professionals in adoption is likely to be greater and more necessary in the future.

Controversies and Conflicts in Adoption: A Rights-Based Historical Perspective

The desire to parent and the subsequent bond between child and family evolves into one of life's most treasured relationships. In addition, because the family is the cornerstone of society, determining who are appropriate parents is a subject that engenders strong emotions. Because adoption challenges traditional ideas of the parent-child relationship as well as the concept of the "family," it is not surprising that controversy has been a constant companion through the years.

Personal and Cultural Identity

While a joyful event in many respects, for some members of the adoption triad (child, birth family, and adoptive family), this is perhaps the most poignant human tragedy—severance of the bond between birth parents and child. Once placed, adoptees are at risk of losing not only contact with their birth parents but their birth culture as well. This justifiable focus on the importance of each child's lineage and cultural heritage is articulated in the United Nations Convention on the Rights of the Child (UNCRC).[48] Of note, the United States has signed but not officially ratified this treaty.

Article 7
1. The child shall be registered immediately after birth and shall have the right from birth to a name, the right to acquire a nationality and, as far as possible, the right to know and be cared for by his or her parents.

Article 8
1. States Parties undertake to respect the right of the child to preserve his or her identity, including nationality, name and family relations as recognized by law without unlawful interference.
2. Where a child is illegally deprived of some or all of the elements of his or her identity, States Parties shall provide appropriate assistance and protection, with a view to speedily re-establishing his or her identity.

Personal Identity

Before World War II, US adoption records were open to adoptees, birth parents, and adoptive parents. However, during the next 3 decades, legislation was enacted to deny easy access to birth records by birth parents and then by adopted adults.[49–51] The reasons behind this change centered on the perceived benefits of confidentiality for members of the triad. Though probably well intended, the effect of this change enabled perpetuation of attitudes and myths about adoption that were prevalent at the time—that birth outside of marriage was shameful and should be hidden, that parents need not confront the fact that adoptive families are inherently different, and that contact with other members of the adoption triad would inevitably lead to emotional trauma. In response to this change, adoptees banded together and attempted to influence policy on sealed records through organizations such as the Life History and Study Center and Orphan Voyage founded by Jean Paton in 1953, Adoptees' Liberty Movement Association founded by Florence Fisher in 1971, and the American Adoption Congress founded by Jean Paton in 1978. Though these groups had little success overturning confidentiality laws in state and federal courts, their arguments did persuade social work professionals, agencies, and state legislatures to pass statutes and alter policy to enabled searches that maintained privacy of triad members through such instruments as mutual-consent voluntary adoption registries and confidential intermediaries.[51]

However, for many adoptees, access to information on parentage and culture was as stated in the UNCRC—a fundamental human right. For these individuals, any strategy short of free access to information was unacceptable. Bastard Nation, a far more confrontational adoption activist organization founded in 1996, has achieved some success in restoring the rights of adopted persons to receive their original birth certificate. While at least 5 states—Alabama, Alaska, Kansas, New Hampshire, and Oregon—permit unconditional access, court orders are still required in most states.[51,52] To further complicate this field, the issue of open records has entered the maelstrom of the abortion debate. As stated by the National Council For Adoption, a group that has strongly opposed open records,

> "For understandable and legitimate reasons, some women facing an unplanned pregnancy prefer the option of confidential adoption. They should have the right to choose this option. Removing the option of privacy in adoption would mean that any woman facing an unplanned pregnancy, who wanted to protect her privacy, would have no private choice but abortion."[53]

While the trend appears to be moving toward more transparency, the polarization of this debate will make resolution of the issue of open records in the United States more difficult.

Concerns about this loss of personal identity are being addressed through the growing phenomenon of open adoptions, in which birth parents, adoptive parents, and the child remain in contact. While studies are limited, several indicate improved outcomes for children when avenues of communication remain open among adoption triad members.[54-57] Concurrent with the growing desire to identify and contact birth parents, a growing cadre of amateur and professional identity investigators and the Internet permit many adopted individuals access to their birth histories.[58] These developments have been a boon for those whose feelings of birth family loss are greatest, permitting contact or closure in situations in which resolution was once thought impossible.

Racial and Cultural Identity

Because of the traditional stringent racial boundaries in the United State, the first recorded adoption of an African American child, by a white family in Minnesota, did not take place until 1948.[59] Organized activity in North America to promote transracial adoption dates to 1960 when the Open Door Society in Montreal, Quebec, attempted to place black children in same-race homes but recruited white families if this effort failed. A similar organization, Parents to Adopt Minority Youngsters, was founded in Minnesota in 1961. Because children of color have always been disproportionately represented in foster care, additional agencies began transracial placement in situations in which same-race homes were unavailable.[60]

Breakdown of racial barriers during the 1960s increased interest in transracial adoption, and during 1971, 2,574 African American children were adopted by white families in the United States.[60] In 1972, concerned about a child's loss of racial and cultural identity, the National Association of Black Social Workers issued a strongly worded response to this growing trend of transracial adoption.

"The National Association of Black Social Workers has taken a vehement stand against the placement of black children in white homes for any reason. We affirm the inviolable position of black children in black families where they belong physically, psychologically and culturally in order that they receive the total sense of themselves and develop a sound projection of their future.

"Ethnicity is a way of life in these United States, and the world at large; a viable, sensitive, meaningful and legitimate societal construct. This is no less true nor legitimate for black people than for other ethnic groups…

"The socialization process for every child begins at birth and includes his cultural heritage as an important segment of the process. In our society, the developmental needs of black children are significantly different from those of white children. Black children are taught, from an early age, highly sophisticated coping techniques to deal with racist practices perpetrated by individuals and institutions. These coping techniques become successfully integrated into ego functions and can be incorporated only through the process of developing positive identification with significant black others. Only a black family can transmit the emotional and sensitive subtleties of perception and reaction essential for a black child's survival in a racist society. Our society is distinctly black or white and characterized by white racism at every level. We repudiate the fallacious and fantasized reasoning of some that whites adopting black children will alter that basic character."[61]

This organized opposition immediately decreased the number of transracial adoptions of black children by white families to about 1,000 in 1973, down 71% from 1971.[60] However, the trend was to change again in the 1990s when Congress enacted 2 pieces of legislation. The first, the Multiethnic Placement Act of 1994 as amended by the Interethnic Provisions of 1996, is a federal civil rights law enacted to speed placement of children in foster care into permanent homes.[62] This legislation prohibits using race, color or national origin for decisions delaying or denying a child in foster care of adoptive placement or denying individuals the opportunity to become a foster or an adoptive parent. States must also be diligent in recruiting foster and adoptive parents who reflect the racial and ethnic diversity of the children who need homes. The Adoption and Safe Families Act of 1997 was designed to accelerate permanent placement of children who resided in foster care.[17] In addition to establishing an incentive program for states to increase the number of children adopted from the public foster care system, the legislation required states to initiate procedures to free children for adoption if they had been in foster care for 15 of the previous 22 months. Following passage, the number of children placed for adoption from the foster care system increased and remained substantially higher than previous years (Figure 1-3).

Concerns about the loss of racial and cultural identity were also raised about adoption of Native American children by white families. In 1958, the federal government and Child Welfare League of America, working together with the Bureau of Indian Affairs, began the Indian Adoption Project, an initiative designed to address what was perceived as neglect and suffering of Native American children on US reservations. Native American families were not encouraged to adopt, and children were placed primarily in white families.[63,64] While the program was modest in size, placing only 395 children, this organized attempt by the federal government was viewed by most tribes as yet another example of cultural genocide and a direct challenge to the sovereignty of tribal governments. In 1978, with passage of the Indian Child Welfare Act, tribes were given jurisdiction over custody proceedings involving Native American children living on reservations. This made it much more difficult for non–Native Americans to adopt Native American children and to remove children from their families.

Within the realm of international adoption, individuals and organizations that focus on perpetuating family identity find fault with the definition of an orphan under US immigration law, where the term is defined not only as "a child…who is an orphan because of the death or disappearance of, abandonment or desertion by, or separation or loss from both parents," but also "for whom the sole or surviving parent is incapable of providing the proper care and has in writing irrevocably released the child for emigration and adoption."[63,64] The Joint United Nations Programme on HIV/AIDS, United Nations Children's Fund, and US Agency for International Development publication *Children on the Brink 2002* reported that almost 108 million children younger than 15 years in 88 African, Asian, and Latin American countries had lost at least one parent. However, fewer than 10% had lost both.[65] The point made by opponents of international adoption is that making children with surviving parents eligible for international adoption diminishes emphasis and diverts resources from strengthening the family and social structure in the country of origin in favor of building families in wealthy Western countries. Irrespective of altruism, any appearance of exploiting the financial and social misfortune of others opens the door to charges of colonialism. International concern about this loss of cultural identity cannot be overemphasized. While international adoptees have many opportunities to celebrate their heritage through, for example, food, secular and religious celebrations, playmates, and language studies, many continue to view international adoption as an irrevocable loss of a cultural birthright.

Adoption policy in the sending countries often centers on this issue. Some governments extend preferential treatment to families who have cultural ties to their country, and some countries preclude adoption by individuals who are unlikely to raise the child in the same religious or cultural tradition. Islamic countries generally forbid adoption by non-Muslims, not only because Islam explicitly forbids establishing a fictive relationship of descent between the child and father, as happens under Western secular adoption law,[34] but also because there is absolutely no guarantee that a child's rich faith and cultural heritage will be respected or even acknowledged in Western countries where Islam is poorly understood and underappreciated. Concern and even outright anger at this loss of identity and culture emerge as international adoptees traverse the difficult years of adolescence, searching for self and their place in the world.[34] Passionate accounts posted on online message boards communicate the raw emotions at play in individual lives.

Integrity of the Adoption Process: Prevention of Exploitation and Profiteering and the Hague Convention on Intercountry Adoption

As we are reminded all too frequently in headlines reporting children trafficked for sex, labor, or armed combat, some adults have always been willing to exploit children for personal gain. The field of adoption has never been free from the taint of commercialism and outright exploitation. Children are desired and therefore of value, and through the centuries profiteers have been willing to commodify children, placing their economic value ahead of their intrinsic dignity and worth as human beings. Frank exploitation of single unwed mothers and their children was common in the 19th and early 20th century in "baby farms" in Britain and the United States.[66,67] Imprisoned by the sexual mores of the day, a pregnant unwed mother had few choices and often paid a baby farmer to "adopt" her infant. If the child survived, which was doubtful, the baby farmer made additional money placing the child in another family. In Ireland, well into the mid-20th century, single pregnant women endured harsh servitude in the Magdalene Laundries while awaiting the birth of their babies, after which the children were placed by Catholic religious orders into families oversees.[68]

Safeguarding the rights of children as well as birth parents during adoption is specifically addressed in the UNCRC.[48]

Article 21

State Parties that recognize and/or permit the system of adoption shall ensure that the best interests of the child shall be the paramount consideration and they shall:

a) Ensure that the adoption of a child is authorized only by competent authorities who determine, in accordance with applicable law and procedures and on the basis of all pertinent and reliable information, that the adoption is permissible in view of the child's status concerning parents, relatives and legal guardians and that, if required, the persons concerned have given their informed consent to the adoption on the basis of such counseling as may be necessary;

Informed consent is one of the key elements in this section of the UNCRC, and understanding the controversy surrounding this issue begins by acknowledging the asymmetries involved, particularly in the process of international adoption. In virtually all situations, birth mothers are destitute, stigmatized by their pregnancy, and rarely able to share with the birth father the burden of childbearing and rearing. They are often members of an exploited racial or ethnic minority and politically impotent. Protections afforded women and their children in these situations may be minimal. In contrast, adoptive parents are well-to-do members of a politically powerful majority in the most economically advantaged countries on Earth. In many ways, the history of US adoption is recapitulating the early and mid-20th century history of adoption in the United States, with well-to-do parents taking advantage of the shame of unwed motherhood and poverty.

In some countries, it is a social norm to temporarily place a child in an institution or with another family with the expectation of future unification. The recent history of adoption in the Marshall Islands illustrates how critical social context is to the issue of informed consent. Within the Marshallese community, all adoptions are considered "open" and the child is commonly expected to return to the birth family at a later date. As opposed to the perspective of US parents, who view adoption as a severance of ties, more than 80% of 73 Marshallese birth mothers surveyed believed at the time of placement that their child would be returned to them after the child reached adulthood.[69] When drastically different cultural perspectives on adoption are part of the equation, tragic outcomes are likely for one or more of the adoption triad members.

Article 21 (continued)

b) Recognize that inter-country adoption may be considered as an
alternative means of child's care, if the child cannot be placed in a
foster or an adoptive family or cannot in any suitable manner be
cared for in the child's country of origin;

c) Ensure that the child concerned by inter-country adoption enjoys
safeguards and standards equivalent to those existing in the case
of national adoption;

d) Take all appropriate measures to ensure that, in inter-country
adoption, the placement does not result in improper financial
gain for those involved in it;

Despite the enthusiasm of potential adoptive parents and the positive outcomes
reported for children,[47] international adoption has been viewed by the world community as the least desirable option, aside from institutional care, for children
deprived of parental care. Unfortunately, the focus on the primacy of the biological
family makes it difficult for many to understand how a child could be adequately
cared for by anyone other than a birth parent or relative. This view helps perpetuate notions that adoptive parents have ulterior motives for seeking to adopt an
unrelated child. The home study process makes families adopting internationally the
most scrutinized parents in the world, yet the rare reports of abuse and even murder
of international adoptees in the United States only reinforce the false concept that
families who adopt are not fit parents.[70,71] When paired with the sums of money
that change hands during the adoption process, which are easily equivalent to a
decade or more of income for an average family in a sending country, it is under-
standable why international adoption may not be viewed as a humanitarian gesture
but as child trafficking for economic gain.[72]

Contemporary articles on international adoption inevitably highlight the large
dollar amounts involved. Irrespective of this hyperbole, the actual or perceived
possibility that money could corrupt every point in the process and every level of
bureaucracy must be acknowledged. While financial indiscretions most commonly
are "gifts" to insure that the adoption process goes smoothly,[73] other examples
include the alleged selling of children in countries without well-developed adoption safeguards (eg, Cambodia, Guatemala, India, Kenya, Vietnam, Romania) and
preferential placement of children for lucrative international (rather than domestic)
adoption.[72–74] The belief that financial motives drive international adoption is so
strong that outlandish rumors about child exploitation are easily perpetuated. At
the far end of this spectrum are horrifying reports that international adoptees are
being butchered to use their body parts for transplantation.[74]

Protecting the Integrity of the Adoption Process

The final portion of Article 21 of the UNCRC mandates the following[48]:

> e) Promote, where appropriate, the objectives of the present article by concluding bilateral or multilateral arrangements or agreements, and endeavor, within this framework, to ensure that the placement of the child in another country is carried out by competent authorities or organs.

This challenge was taken up by the Hague Conference on Private International Law, an intergovernmental organization founded in 1893 that focuses on unifying the rule of private international law.[75] Drafted in consultation with principal placing and accepting countries, the conference presented to its member countries a draft convention on international adoption in 1993,[76] which, as of February 2009, is in force in 81 countries, including the United States, and is awaiting ratification by another 3.[77]

Fundamental tenants of the Hague Convention on intercountry adoption parallel the UNCRC in many respects, but in other areas the draft convention places international adoption in a more favorable context.[76,78,79] In brief, the major advantages of the Hague Convention are

- It provides formal international and intergovernmental recognition of international adoption.
- As opposed to the UNCRC, the convention states that intercountry adoption is acceptable if a "suitable family" cannot be found in the child's home state, thus endorsing international adoption as a viable alternative to domestic placement for many children and not as the least desirable option.
- It establishes a set of minimum requirements and procedures that apply when a child moves from one convention country to another.
- It establishes a system of cooperation among states to prevent the trafficking of children, and it requires that states amend their national adoption laws to conform to the convention principles and guidelines, which require the sending and receiving countries to clean up corrupt adoption networks, crack down on child trafficking, and certify that children are in fact legally adoptable.
- It requires that each convention country establish a central authority (eg, US Department of State) to oversee the adoption process (accredits agencies involved in Hague adoptions) in its own territory, including the implementation of convention directives through new domestic legislation and coordination of adoption procedures with other states.
- For more on the Hague Convention, see Appendix 1 on page 411.

Since the Hague Convention has been implemented in the United States, significant improvements have been made in transparency, professionalism, and protection of the adoption triad, though much more needs to be done to assure critics of international adoptions that the world's largest placement country is truly interested in the protection of children's rights as articulated in the UNCRC.

The matched need of a family for the well-being of a child and the fulfillment of adults is fundamental to survival of the species and society. Toward that goal we have seen a positive trajectory in adoption over the past 2 centuries, transitioning from viewing a child as property to the perspective that a child is a unique individual with needs and deserving protection. Though the number of children needing permanent homes continues to outstrip their availability, practice barriers that once seemed immutable are now accommodated with evidence-based practices. Most adoptions from foster care and abroad have become transracial, open adoption is the norm, and families of diverse and nontraditional composition and sexual orientation are viewed as being conducive to normal child development. All of these developments bode well for providing additional families for children deprived of parental care. Out of calamity and loss, children recover and progress to become functionally and emotionally competent adults. As stated by the distinguished adoption researcher Richard Barth,[80]

> "Adoption is a time-honored and successful service for children and parents. The outcomes of adoption are more favorable for children than any social program that I know. My own research and that of my colleagues indicates that the modest difficulties experienced by children who are adopted are far outweighed by the significant benefits that they receive from having a permanent family."

References

1. Boswell J. *The Kindness of Strangers: The Abandonment of Children in Western Europe from Late Antiquity to the Renaissance*. New York, NY: Pantheon; 1988
2. Adamec C, Pierce WL. *The Encyclopedia of Adoption*. New York, NY: Facts On File; 1991
3. Bullough VL. Ancient Babylonia and adoption. In: Shepperd Stolley K, Bullough VL, eds. *The Praeger Handbook of Adoption*. Westport, CT: Praeger; 2006:72
4. Bullough VL. Ancient China and adoption. In: Shepperd Stolley K, Bullough VL, eds. *The Praeger Handbook of Adoption*. Westport, CT: Praeger; 2006:73–74
5. AAP insignia dates back to Middle Ages. *AAP News*. 1985;1:22
6. Brace CL. *The Dangerous Classes of New York and Twenty Years Working Among Them*. New York, NY: Wynkoop and Hallenbeck; 1872
7. Hacsi TA. Orphanages. In: Shepperd Stolley K, Bullough VL, eds. *The Praeger Handbook of Adoption*. Westport, CT: Praeger; 2006:449–452
8. Crenson MA. *Building the Invisible Orphanage: A Prehistory of the American Welfare System*. Cambridge, MA: Harvard University Press; 1988
9. Bullough VL. Orphan trains. In: Shepperd Stolley K, Bullough VL, eds. *The Praeger Handbook of Adoption*. Westport, CT: Praeger; 2006:459–460
10. Herman E. Orphan trains. In: *The Adoption History Project*. University of Oregon. http://darkwing.uoregon.edu/~adoption/topics/orphan.html. Accessed February 11, 2014

11. Herman E. Timeline of adoption history. In: *The Adoption History Project*. University of Oregon. http://darkwing.uoregon.edu/~adoption/timeline.html. Accessed February 11, 2014

12. First White House conference on the care of dependent children. http://www.libertynet.org/edcivic/whoukids.html. Accessed February 11, 2014

13. Herman E. Massachusetts Adoption of Children Act, 1851. In: *The Adoption History Project*. University of Oregon. http://www.uoregon.edu/~adoption/archive/MassACA.htm. Accessed February 11, 2014

14. Carp EW. Massachusetts Adoption Act (1851). In: Shepperd Stolley K, Bullough VL, eds. *The Praeger Handbook of Adoption*. Westport, CT: Praeger; 2006:393

15. Herman E. First specialized adoption agencies. In: *The Adoption History Project*. University of Oregon. Available at: http://www.uoregon.edu/~adoption/topics/firstspecial.html. Accessed February 11, 2014

16. History of the Cradle. http://www.cradle.org/history. Accessed February 11, 2014

17. Herman E. Adoption statistics. In: *The Adoption History Project*. University of Oregon. Available at: http://www.uoregon.edu/~adoption/topics/adoptionstatistics.htm. Accessed February 11, 2014

18. Child Welfare League of America. Summary of the Adoption and Safe Families Act of 1997. http://library.adoption.com/articles/summary-of-the-adoption-and-safe-families-act-of-1997.html. Accessed February 11, 2014

19. US Department of State Bureau of Consular Affairs. Intercountry adoption. About us. Statistics. http://adoption.state.gov/about_us/statistics.php Accessed February 11, 2014

20. Placek PJ. National adoption data. In: Marshner C, Pierce WL, eds. *Adoption Factbook III*. Alexandria, VA: National Council for Adoption; 1999:24–68

21. Miller BC, Coyl DD. Adolescent pregnancy and childbearing in relation to infant adoption in the United States. *Adoption Q*. 2000;4:3–25

22. Alstein H, Simon RJ. Introduction. In: Alstein H, Simon RJ, eds. *Intercountry Adoption: A Multinational Perspective*. New York, NY: Praeger; 1991:1–13

23. US Department of Health and Human Services Administration for Children and Families. Statistics & research. http://www.acf.hhs.gov/programs/cb/stats_research/index.htm. Accessed February 11, 2014

24. Domestic newborn adoption. http://www.adoptivefamilies.com/domestic. Accessed February 11, 2014

25. Carney EN. The truth about domestic adoption. *Adoptive Families*. http://www.adoptivefamilies.com/articles.php?aid=522. Accessed February 11, 2014

26. Evan B. Donaldson Adoption Institute. 2002 National Adoption Attitudes Survey. http://www.adoptioninstitute.org/survey/survey_intro.html. Accessed February 11, 2014

27. US Census Bureau. Adopted children and stepchildren: 2000. http://www.census.gov/population/www/cen2000/briefs/phc-t21/index.html. Accessed February 11, 2014

28. Child Welfare League of America. International adoption: trends and issues. *National Data Analysis System Issue Brief*. November 2007. http://www.ccainstitute.org/pdf/international_adoption/International%20Adoption%20Trends%20and%20Issues.pdf. Accessed February 11, 2014

29. Chernoff R, Combs-Orme T, Risley-Curtiss C, Heisler A. Assessing the health status of children entering foster care. *Pediatrics*. 1994;93:594–601

30. Garwood MM, Close W. Identifying the psychological needs of foster children. *Child Psychiatry Hum Dev*. 2001;32:125–135

31. Halfon N, Mendonca A, Berkowitz G. Health status of children in foster care. The experience of the Center for the Vulnerable Child. *Arch Pediatr Adolesc Med*. 1995;149:386–392

32. Simms MD, Dubowitz H, Szilagyi MA. Health care needs of children in the foster care system. *Pediatrics*. 2000;106:909–918

33. Takayama JI, Wolfe E, Coulter KP. Relationship between reason for placement and medical findings among children in foster care. *Pediatrics.* 1998;101(2):201–207

34. Pollack D, Bleich M, Reid CJ, Fadel MH. Classical religious perspectives of adoption law. *Notre Dame Law Rev.* 2004;79:693–753

35. Hunt K. The Romanian baby bazaar. *N Y Times Mag.* 1991;140:24–53

36. Herman E. International adoptions. In: *The Adoption History Project.* University of Oregon. http://www.uoregon.edu/~adoption/topics/internationaladoption.htm. Accessed February 11, 2014

37. Evan B. Donaldson Adoption Institute. International adoption facts. http://www.adoptioninstitute.org/FactOverview/international.html. Accessed February 11, 2014

38. US Supreme Court. *Brown v Board of Education.* 347 US 483 (1954). http://www.nationalcenter.org/brown.html. Accessed February 11, 2014

39. Herman E. *The Family Nobody Wanted,* 1954. In: *The Adoption History Project.* University of Oregon. http://www.uoregon.edu/~adoption/topics/familynobodywanted.htm. Accessed February 11, 2014

40. Doss H. Our international family. *Read Dig.* 1949:58–59

41. Doss H. *The Family Nobody Wanted.* Boston, MA: Little Brown and Co; 1954

42. Herman E. Bertha and Harry Holt. In: *The Adoption History Project.* University of Oregon. http://www.uoregon.edu/~adoption/people/holt.htm. Accessed February 11, 2014

43. Centers for Disease Control and Prevention, National Center for Health Statistics. American women are waiting to begin families [press release]. Atlanta, GA: Centers for Disease Control and Prevention; 2002. http://www.cdc.gov/nchs/pressroom/02news/ameriwomen.htm. Accessed February 11, 2014

44. American Society for Reproductive Medicine. Age and fertility: a guide for patients. http://www.asrm.org/uploadedFiles/ASRM_Content/Resources/Patient_Resources/Fact_Sheets_and_Info_Booklets/agefertility.pdf. Accessed February 11, 2014

45. Selman P. The demographic history of intercountry adoption. In: Selman P, ed. *Intercountry Adoption: Development, Trends and Perspectives.* London, United Kingdom: British Agency for Adoption and Fostering; 2000:15–37

46. Johnson DE. Medical and developmental sequlae of early childhood institutionalization in international adoptees from Romania and the Russian Federation. In: Nelson C, ed. *The Effects of Early Adversity on Neurobehavioral Development.* Mahwah, NJ: Lawrence Erlbaum Associates; 2000:113–162

47. Johnson DE. Adoption and the effect on children's development. *Early Hum Dev.* 2002;68:39–54

48. United Nations. Convention on the Rights of the Child. 1989. http://www.ohchr.org/en/professionalinterest/pages/crc.aspx. Accessed February 11, 2014

49. Herman E. Confidentiality and sealed records. In: *The Adoption History Project.* University of Oregon. http://www.uoregon.edu/~adoption/topics/confidentiality.htm. Accessed February 11, 2014

50. Norris BL. Closed adoption. In: Stolley KS, Bullough VL, eds. *The Praeger Handbook of Adoption.* Westport, CT: Praeger; 2006:161–165

51. Carp EW. Adoption search movement. In: Shepperd Stolley K, Bullough VL, eds. *The Praeger Handbook of Adoption.* Westport, CT: Praeger; 2006:41–43

52. Carp EW. Bastard nation. In: Stolley KS, Bullough VL, eds. *The Praeger Handbook of Adoption.* Westport, CT: Praeger; 2006:98

53. Herman E. National Council for Adoption, "Protecting the option of privacy in adoption." In: *The Adoption History Project.* University of Oregon. http://www.uoregon.edu/~adoption/archive/NCFAPOPA.htm. Accessed February 11, 2014

54. Barth RP, Berry M. *Adoption and Disruption.* Hawthorne, NY: Aldine de Gruyter; 1988

55. Berry M. The practice of open adoption. *Child Youth Serv Rev.* 1991;13:379–395

56. Grotevant HD. Coming to terms with adoption: the construction of identity fron adolescence to adulthood. *Adoption Q.* 1997;1:1–27

57. Grotevant HD, McRoy RG. *Openness in Adoption.* Thousand Oaks, CA: Sage Publications; 1998
58. Pertman A. *Adoption Nation.* New York, NY: Basic Books; 2000
59. Herman E. Transracial adoption. In: *The Adoption History Project.* University of Oregon. http://www. uoregon.edu/~adoption/topics/transracialadoption.htm. Accessed February 11, 2014
60. Simon RJ. Transracial adoption. In: Stolley KS, Bullough VL, eds. *The Praeger Handbook of Adoption.* Westport, CT: Praeger; 2006:632–640
61. Herman E. National Association of Black Social Workers, "Position statement on trans-racial adoption," September 1972. In: *The Adoption History Project.* University of Oregon. http://www. uoregon.edu/~adoption/archive/NabswTRA.htm. Accessed February 11, 2014
62. Hollinger JH, American Bar Association Center on Children and Law. *A Guide to the Multiethnic Placement Act of 1994 as Amended by the Interethnic Adoption Provisions of 1996.* Washington, DC: American Bar Association Center on Children and Law; 1998. http://www.americanbar.org/ content/dam/aba/administrative/child_law/GuidetoMultiethnicPlacementAct.authcheckdam.pdf. Accessed February 11, 2014
63. Miller D. The Indian adoption project and the Indian Child Welfare Act of 1978. In: Stolley KS, Bullough VL, eds. *The Praeger Handbook of Adoption.* Westport, CT: Praeger; 2006
64. Herman E. Indian Child Welfare Act (ICWA). In: *The Adoption History Project.* University of Oregon. http://pages.uoregon.edu/adoption/topics/ICWA.html. Accessed February 11, 2014
65. US Agency for International Development, United Nations Children's Fund, Joint United Nations Programme on HIV/AIDS. *Children on the Brink 2002: A Joint Report on Orphan Estimates and Program Strategies.* Washington, DC: TvT Associates; 2002. http://data.unaids.org/Topics/ Young-People/childrenonthebrink_en.pdf. Accessed February 11, 2014
66. Ferguson CP. Baby farming. In: Stolley KS, Bullough VL, eds. *The Praeger Handbook of Adoption.* Westport, CT: Praeger; 2006:87–88
67. Herman E. Baby farming. In: *The Adoption History Project.* University of Oregon. http://www. uoregon.edu/~adoption/topics/babyfarming.html. Accessed February 11, 2014
68. Feng V. The Magdalene laundry. CBS News, February 11, 2009. http://www.cbsnews.com/ stories/2003/08/08/sunday/main567365.shtml. Accessed February 11, 2014
69. Roby J, Matsumura S. If I give you my child aren't we family? A study of birthmothers participating in Marshall Island-U.S. adoptions. *Adoption Q.* 2002;5:7–31
70. Man charged in son's 2005 Iowa City murder. *The Gazette* (Cedar Rapids, IA). 2008. http:// thegazette.com. Accessed August 26, 2013
71. Greiner M. The Russian adopted dead: a review of killers and sentences. The Daily Bastardette [blog]. December 21, 2008. http://bastardette.blogspot.com/2008/12/russian-adopted-dead-review-of-killers.html. Accessed February 11, 2014
72. Graff EJ. The lie we love. *Foreign Policy.* November 1, 2008. http://www.foreignpolicy.com/ articles/2008/10/15/the_lie_we_love. Accessed February 11, 2014
73. Wheeler C. Babies-for-sale trade faces a global crack-down. *The Observer* (UK). November 20, 2004. http://www.guardian.co.uk/society/2004/nov/21/adoptionandfostering.adoption. Accessed February 11, 2014
74. Johnson DE. International adoption: what is fact, what is fiction, and what is the future? *Pediatr Clin North Am.* 2005;52:1221–1246
75. Dillon S. Making legal regimens for intercountry adoption reflect human rights principles: transforming the United Nations Convention on the Rights of the the Child with the Hague Convention on Intercountry Adoption. *Boston Univ Int Law J.* 2003;21:179–257
76. Convention of 29 May 1993 on Protection of Children and Co-operation in Respect of Intercountry Adoption. http://www.hcch.net/index_en.php?act=conventions.text&cid=69. Accessed February 11, 2014

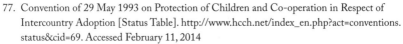
77. Convention of 29 May 1993 on Protection of Children and Co-operation in Respect of Intercountry Adoption [Status Table]. http://www.hcch.net/index_en.php?act=conventions. status&cid=69. Accessed February 11, 2014

78. US Department of State Bureau of Consular Affairs. Intercountry adoption. Understanding the Hague Convention. http://adoption.state.gov/hague_convention/overview.php. Accessed February 11, 2014

79. Kapstein EB. The baby trade. *Foreign Affairs*. November/December 2003. http://www.foreignaffairs.com/articles/59373/ethan-b-kapstein/the-baby-trade. Accessed February 11, 2014

80. Duke MD. Groups seeking to eliminate adoption. In: Marshner C, Pierce WL, eds. *Adoption Factbook III*. Washington, DC: National Council for Adoption; 1999:219–222

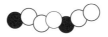

CHAPTER 2

The Process of Adoption in the United States

Vicki Peterson, MSW, LICSW, and Heather W. Ames, MSW, LICSW

Looking Back: The Early Years and Shifts in Attitudes

Adoption has been part of US culture since the mid-1800s, when "orphan trains" first began to bring orphaned and homeless children from industrialized East Coast cities to farm families who needed child laborers. Arrangements were informal—some children were treated like family but never legally recognized as such, while other were treated as indentured servants. Over time, this began to change as society started to be concerned about the protection of children's rights. The concept of legal adoption evolved in the early 1900s with each state eventually passing legislation to legitimize and protect the adoptive family.

By the middle of the 1900s, adoption was sought by infertile couples but conducted with great secrecy. Birth and adoption records were sealed by courts. Social workers felt that any information about background would interfere with a child's ability to bond with his or her adoptive parents. Relinquishing birth parents were encouraged to forget about the child they were giving up and move on with their lives. Most adopted children were not told of their adoption until later in life, if at all.

Over time, those working in the field of child welfare came to understand that the secrecy of adoption was not healthy for anyone. During the next 50 years, there were enormous changes in the acceptance of adoption. In 1976, Governor Michael Dukakis proclaimed a week in May as Adoption Week for Massachusetts. Many states followed, expanding this celebration to an Adoption Awareness week or month. President Gerald Ford announced that Adoption Week would be celebrated nationally in November 1976; President Ronald Reagan proclaimed the first National Adoption Week in 1984, followed by President Bill Clinton (who was adopted himself) proclaiming November as National Adoption Month in 1995. During this same period, there was a boom in the publication of books covering a variety of adoption-related topics. Legitimized, well accepted, and now celebrated, adoption was ripe for expansion abroad.

Contributing Factors to International Adoptions

Melting Pot

As the "melting pot" of diversity, the United States was fertile soil for intercultural and interracial adoption, which first began in the 1950s after the Korean War. Many babies fathered by American soldiers were not accepted in Korean society, leading birth mothers to abandon their children or bring them to orphanages. Americans received cooperation from both governments in arranging for the adoption of interracial children by US citizens. This was the first significant international program of adoption by citizens of one country arranging for the adoption of children from a different one.

Twenty years later, during the war in Vietnam, many children of mixed race were born of liaisons between young Asian women and American soldiers. Like the interracial children that resulted from the Korean War, many of these children were rejected by their culture and brought to the United States for adoption. It was during this period, the mid-1970s, when many private US agencies were formed and began doing the work of international adoptions.

Increased Options for Adoption

Over the next 30 years, international adoption agencies multiplied and began to operate all over the United States. The option of adopting a child from abroad became more comfortable for prospective parents when they saw others doing it successfully. The need for more parents was expanding as international adoption programs were opened in a variety of countries in Asia and Latin America. Faster and more predictable adoptions from abroad became an attractive option.

Media Focus on Domestic Problems

There was another phenomenon that also began to take place in the 1980s and 1990s that boosted interest in adopting from abroad. Rare but heartbreaking, well-publicized court battles over the legal custody of US-born children attracted great media attention. Front-page stories showed haunting photos of children being ripped from the arms of their adoptive parents and returned to the birth parents, who were now strangers. Many prospective parents began to worry about the legal risks of adopting from within the United States.

Political Factors

Many issues in other countries contributed to increased interest in adoptions from abroad. In the early 1990s, political changes around the world had a major effect on the needs of children from many countries. Attention by the media to the conditions of children in other countries made foreign adoption appealing for those who wanted to help a child while also bringing a son or daughter into their lives. International adoptions allowed prospective parents to have many choices and feel that the children they adopted would have opportunities they would not have had in their country of birth.

China opened its doors to adoptions by Westerners in 1991. Its 1-child policy led to a high rate of infanticide and abandonment of baby girls. These practices resulted from a cultural phenomenon that is a long-standing tradition in China in which a married daughter is expected to care for her in-laws but a son holds the responsibility for the eventual care of his parents. Thus, Chinese parents have a strong preference for a male child who would take care of them when they grew old. As a result, in the 1990s, orphanages were filled with baby girls. Chinese citizens who already had a child were not allowed to adopt, and the few who did adopt wanted a son.

At the same time, the breakup of the former Soviet Union strongly affected the need for parents in many Eastern European countries. There was much poverty, unemployment, and family instability in these newly independent countries. In other countries, cultural barriers against single parenthood continued to drive the growth of international adoptions.

More Americans Traveling Abroad

Another shift for Americans over the past generation was an increase in foreign travel that made the world seem smaller and other cultures more familiar. This phenomenon made the idea of adopting from other countries more comfortable for many people than it would have been in years past. As an example, for the past 15 years, American and Chinese travel agencies have offered a variety of tours for Americans who want to visit China; the same is true in Eastern Europe. It is no longer considered unusual for Americans to travel to these places, and it is often a requirement of the adoption process. The same is true in many other non-Western countries where Americans rarely traveled in the past.

Current Trends in International Adoption

Recent Reductions in Numbers

Fifteen years ago, the requirements from most countries were quite flexible, and applicants had a wide variety of choices of international adoption program options. Over the past few years, this has changed significantly as the need for families has started to decrease. This has resulted in adoptive parents waiting progressively longer to have a healthy, young child placed with them. Since 2008, the US government has shown a marked decrease each year in the number of orphan visas issued for children coming from other countries for adoption.

Changes of Economies and Attitudes

The economies of many placing countries have improved over time, and many governments are now strongly promoting domestic adoption for their citizens. China, for example, places more than 3 times as many children with Chinese citizens as the number of children annually adopted abroad. In South Korea, where adoptions were always very secretive, the government now offers a $1,000 monthly subsidy to parents who adopt a child. In addition, there are newly formed adoptive parent organizations in Korea, where parents meet openly. Bloodline is becoming less of a barrier to adoption than it was previously.

Citizens from South Korea, India, and Eastern European countries are given the choice of adopting the youngest and healthiest babies before children are allowed to be considered for international adoption. In Russia, adoptive or foster parents are given a substantial financial incentive to help meet the needs of a child. The government of India strongly promotes domestic adoption by limiting the number of children placed abroad to no more than 50% of all adoptions. Most Indian agencies attempt to make 70% of their placements in-country, and an increasing number of children allowed to be adopted abroad are school age.

Who Are the Children Needing Families?

While adoption is still a popular way to build or add to a family, there are fewer young children in need of a family than ever before. Once children reach age 4 years, this begins to change. Older youngsters are still in great need of a family, with far fewer interested applicants than available children. Agencies try to keep large sibling groups together, and it is also more difficult to find homes for these youngsters. The same is true of children who have a higher health risk or special needs. Because of this, it is likely that in the United States, adoption agencies in the future will focus on the placement of older children and those with special needs.

More Country Restrictions

Each placing country has restrictions on the parents that it will accept to adopt a child. Many countries have become more rigid in their policies and requirements for prospective parents. The recent changes have significantly reduced options for single people. In particular, country restrictions now almost universally bar gay and lesbian applicants from foreign adoption. In addition, tighter regulations have limited possibilities for those who have been treated for serious health issues and who are divorced or have any history of arrest.

Most adoption agencies respect and abide by requirements of foreign countries, but some are less accepting of these restrictions and the right of governments to make decisions about who can adopt a child. This is a controversial issue now that adoptions from abroad are on the decline and there are fewer options for prospective parents.

Growth of African Adoptions

In the past few years more Americans have taken a personal interest in the orphaned and needy children of many African nations. The adoption of African children by a few celebrities has focused media attention on the plight of these children. The idea of pursuing such an adoption becomes less formidable for average prospective parents when they see others who have done so successfully. The government of Ethiopia has established a well-organized adoption program that ranked second in placements to US families in 2011. Other African countries where programs are growing include Nigeria, Ghana, Congo-Kinshasa, and Uganda.

Requirements at Home and Abroad for International Adoption

Internal Requirements

The US government has strict requirements on children who come into the country for the purpose of adoption. Each child must be granted an orphan visa to enter the United States. Specific regulations govern eligibility for this visa. It is the government's way of insuring that children are not being taken illegally from their birth family and that birth parents are not being financially compensated for a child. In addition, the government wants to insure that the adopting parents have good motives for adoption and can meet the child's long-term needs. These issues and assurances are verified by required legal documentation from the birth country and, on this end, from information in a home study report.

Adopting parents are required to have a positive recommendation for adoption in the home study evaluation. Social workers and agencies have the responsibility to make a professional evaluation for each applicant and not recommend anyone who does not meet the criteria for adoption. Making such a determination requires a psychosocial history, background information, criminal record investigation, letters of reference, medical reports, and supporting documentation on finances, health, and marital history. If an agency believes that prospective parents cannot meet basic requirements, they are counseled not to continue with the adoption process.

On rare occasions, the US Citizenship and Immigration Services (USCIS) may question the eligibility of particular clients for international adoption based on information in the home study report. Most often, the US government relies on the recommendation of the licensed agency.

External Requirements

Clients must meet regulations and requirements from the country in which they expect to adopt a child. All countries have requirements for the age and marital status of applicants. Some countries have other requirements as well, such as health factors or the number of children already in the family. In most cases, the clients' credentials are reviewed soon after the application is received.

International Adoption: The Step-by-step Process

- Research agencies.
- Apply to full-service or home study agency.
- Choose country for placement.
- Complete home study.
- Apply to US government for initial visa approval.
- Receive child's referral.
- Prepare for child's arrival.
- Travel to birth country as required or receive child via escort.
- If applicable, legalize child's adoption abroad.
- Work with agency through post-placement period.
- If applicable, legalize adoption in United States.
- United States citizenship received by child at time of adoption.

Domestic Adoption: Options and Shifts

There are many more domestic adoptions in the United States each year than adoptions from abroad. Unfortunately, statistics on domestic adoptions are much less precise than those of international adoptions. Federal law governs and maintains information on orphan visas for all children who are foreign born, but there is no national mechanism for keeping statistics on domestic placements, which are governed by state law. Although attempts are made to track adoption statistics through the US Census Bureau, this has been unreliable in part because domestic adoptions also include kinship placement in which a stepparent or relative adopts a related child. Domestic adoption records do not separate these adoptions from adoptions arranged through the private or public system.

There are many older children and non-white children available for adoption despite the widely held belief that there are fewer children available for domestic adoption. While accurate statistics are difficult to find, the major decrease over the past 30 years is with the number of healthy white infants being placed for adoption. One of the major reasons for this decrease is the changing attitude and acceptance of unmarried parenting. Before 1973, never-married white women placed 19.3% of their children for adoption, whereas between 1989 and 1995, the relinquishment rate was 1.7%. Of never-married African American women, the relinquishment rates have ranged from 0.2% to 1.5%.[1] Other important factors in the decrease of available infants are the widespread use of contraception and the legalization of abortion in 1973, resulting in fewer unplanned pregnancies and more terminations of unplanned pregnancies.

Domestic Options: Public or Private

Public Domestic Adoption

Child welfare advocates support a system in which the best interest of each child is paramount. Each US state government has a social service department providing oversight for child welfare issues, including adoption and foster care. Specific regulations vary from state to state. Most children who come into state care have been involuntarily removed from their parent(s) because of issues of abuse or neglect. Usually, when children are removed from the care of their parents, the primary goal is reunification. In general, most states and judges ultimately favor returning children to their biological parents. In most cases, the state department of welfare develops a plan that will enable parents to regain custody of their children. Kinship care with extended family may be planned as a temporary or permanent alternative to reunification with parents.

Unless parents have voluntarily terminated their parental rights, the only way that children in the foster care system can be adopted is through an involuntary termination of parental rights. This is usually the final recourse and can be a lengthy process. Thus, many thousands of children spend their childhood in foster care, growing up in the public welfare system.

Private Domestic Adoption

Voluntary adoption has become a more open process in the past 30 years. Expectant parents who are considering an adoption plan actively participate in decisions made about the placement of their child. Children become identified for adoption through private adoption agencies, placing agencies, hospitals and clinics, medical personnel, adoption professionals, or prospective parents. Expectant parents may select adoptive parents and expect ongoing contact during the child's life. Contact after relinquishment may be as little as a letter from the adoptive parents once a year or as much as regular visits between birth parents and the adoptive family. Multicultural and multiethnic adoptive families have become more widespread, and matching of characteristics of parent and child is no longer of primary significance.

Because of extensive media attention to a small number of controversial domestic adoption cases, many people have the mistaken impression that domestic adoption is quite risky. The reality is that once a child is placed with a family, most domestic adoptions are secure and successful. However, prior to the time that a final relinquishment is given, many expectant parents change their minds and end up making a decision to raise their newborn. With the support of their counselors during pregnancy, expectant parents carefully consider all of their options and the implications of each choice. Once they learn about available support services and subsidy programs for young or single parents, they often choose to raise their child. This means that couples who have been matched with an expectant mother may be greatly disappointed; this is very difficult and a reason why good pre-adoption counseling is essential in preparing clients for all possible outcomes.

Mental health and child welfare professionals generally believe it is preferable for children to be raised by their biological parents. Therefore, while the decision to keep a child may be disappointing for prospective adoptive parents, it is usually a very good decision for the child, whose best interest is the focus of the adoption process.

Most birth parents choose adoption because their circumstances make it difficult for them to provide a safe and nurturing home for their child. It is a complex, difficult decision, and professional counseling is very important for anyone considering adoption. For many expectant parents, the option to meet the adoptive family and have ongoing information about their child enables them to choose adoption and be reassured about their choice.

Agency-Identified Domestic Placement

An agency-identified placement matches expectant parents with prospective adoptive parents. The adoption agency provides impartial counseling to help them consider all options and the implications of each decision. Should they decide to make an adoption plan, most agencies present birth parents with a choice of profiles of potential adoptive parents that reflect the type of family that they want for their child. Expectant parents select a profile and a match is made.

Parent-Identified Domestic Placement

Sometimes prospective adoptive parents learn of a woman who is considering an adoption plan for her unborn child through their own private contacts. They may enter into an informal plan to adopt this baby. These connections may take place through networking with friends and acquaintances, the Internet, newspaper advertising, or working with adoption attorneys or facilitators. Depending on state laws, coordination of the process may be done with the assistance of an adoption agency, adoption attorneys, or other adoption professionals. Not all states allow advertising or facilitated assisted adoptions.

Interagency-Assisted Domestic Placement

An interagency-assisted placement is one in which prospective adoptive parents work with a local agency or adoption professional for their home study and are matched with expectant parents through the services of another agency, adoption attorney, or other adoption professional. Requirements for all states involved in this plan must be met.

Shifts in Practice

Increased Openness in US Adoption

While it was once common for birth parents to "disappear" after a baby was placed for adoption, it is now a widespread practice to have some level of contact, referred to as *openness,* between adoptive families and birth parents. Many adoptions that began as closed are being opened before the adoptee becomes an adult. While adoptive parents once feared contact with birth parents, many parents now realize that a level of openness may be helpful and answer many questions for their child.

In private adoptions, the current practice is for expectant parents to select adoptive parents for their child. Studies show that an large number of "birth mothers have met the adoptive parents of their children—probably 90% or more—and almost all the remaining birth mothers helped to choose the new parents through profiles."[2] Most agencies request that adoptive parents send a minimum of one letter with accompanying photos to the agency each year to be passed on to the birth parents. According to the Evan B. Donaldson Adoption Institute, "Research on birth parents in the era of confidential adoptions suggests a significant proportion struggled—and continue to struggle—with chronic unresolved grief. The primary factor bringing peace of mind is knowledge about their children's well-being. Current research on birth mothers concludes that being able to choose the adoptive family and having ongoing contact and/or knowledge results in lower levels of grief and greater peace of mind with their adoption decisions."[3]

For some, there is a one-time meeting between expectant and adoptive parents prior to the birth of a child with only first names exchanged. For others, there may be regular ongoing visits with full disclosure of identifying information. Open agreements may be legal contracts or informal understandings. As of 2011, approximately 26 states and the District of Columbia have laws to enforce post-adoption contract agreements in infant adoptions.[3] The degree of openness varies with the parties involved, but the most effective agreements take into consideration the best interest of the child and provide for flexibility as the child matures.

Domestic Birth Father Rights

Birth fathers have become increasingly aware of their constitutional rights concerning their birth children, and some have expressed interest in participating in their upbringing. Whether the birth father is still in a relationship with the birth mother or even if a birth mother is unsure of the identity of the birth father, his rights cannot be ignored. The rights of a putative father (alleged father of a child born out of wedlock) are determined by state law. If an expectant father comes forward when an adoption plan is being made, he can be involved in making adoption-related choices. If he opposes the adoption plan, a court may need to determine his rights. This may put the adoption plan in jeopardy because an expectant mother may decide she would rather parent the child herself than allow the birth father to be given custody. Almost universally, a putative father is entitled to notice of termination of parental rights or adoption proceedings. In many states, he may try to protect his parental rights by registering on a putative father registry.

Step-by-step Domestic Process for Prospective Adoptive Parents

- Completion of home study.
- Preparation of a non-identifying family profile, including a letter and photos for expectant parents.
- Match with an expectant mother.
- Possible contact with expectant parents, if requested.
- Attend or be informed of baby's birth.
- If legal rights of birth parents are relinquished, take physical custody of baby.*
- Complete post-placement services.
- Legalize adoption in probate court.

Step-by-step Process for Domestic Expectant Parents

- Arrange for counseling at an agency or service provider.
- Review profiles of prospective adoptive parents.
- If desired, meet with prospective adoptive parents.
- After baby's birth, make final decision about relinquishment.
- Sign legal surrenders or take custody of baby.
- When appropriate, terminate parental rights.
- Continue counseling as needed.
- In cases of open adoption, continue agreed-on contact.

Decisions for Prospective Parents

Choosing an Agency

At the outset of the adoption process, prospective parents are faced with making important decisions about the type of agency they should work with on this life-changing process. Before commitments are made, researching types of adoptions and agencies can save adopting parents significant time, disappointment, and money.

---

*Foster care may be utilized prior to relinquishment if extended time is needed by expectant parents for a final decision on relinquishment.

With the help of the Internet, gathering preliminary information about adoption is significantly easier than it used to be. This is a great asset to those who are starting their search for the right agency. When possible to do so, parents should attend one or more introductory meetings at different agencies. It is common practice among adoption agencies to offer such meetings free of charge. Many people use an agency that has been highly recommended by someone they know. It is always a good idea to speak to others who have worked with an agency that is being considered.

It is not unusual for applicants to work with one agency on the home study evaluation and another on the placement of a child. The other option is for people to work with a full-service agency that is capable of handling the entire adoption, from beginning to end.

Working With a Full-service Agency

Full-service agencies provide home study evaluations, placement programs, and post-placement and post-adoption services. These will usually include counseling on adoption-related issues such as search and support. Other services commonly offered are educational and cultural programs as well as referrals for more specialized or long-term therapy needs. A well-organized full-service agency will be helpful to an adoptive family for long-term adoption-related issues.

Most full-service agencies offer placement options from different countries. Some agencies may focus their placement work in one country or one part of the world. Then there are agencies that offer adoption programs on different continents and many countries. For some people, having many choices will be very helpful; for others, the choices may seem overwhelming. In reality, most people will not meet the requirements set forth by every country.

Working With a Home Study Agency

Prospective adopting parents may work with a state-licensed agency that does only the home study evaluation and post-placement service. Because these agencies offer fewer services, they tend to be smaller than full-service agencies. The home study agency may partner with placement agencies that have adoption programs in other countries or may require clients to find a placement agency on their own. With the advent of search engines on the Internet, this is not nearly as daunting a project as it might seem.

Choosing a Placement Agency

A few agencies offer only placement services. All clients working with a placement-only agency will need to have their home study and post-placement work done by a different licensed agency located in their state of residence.

Most full-service agencies provide placement services to clients who have had their home study done through another agency. Exceptions to this are agencies that have a catchment area and will only provide placement services to their full-service clients and those who live outside their area. An agency may make exceptions to this on a case-by-case basis.

For the adoption of children from particular countries, many US agencies arrange group trips so that the needs of many families can be met efficiently. Depending on the country, parents return from their adoption trip with a child and a new appreciation for the history, sights, and culture of their child's birth country.

Differences Between International and Domestic Adoptions

Availability of Background Information: Domestic Adoption

One of the major differences between domestic and international adoption is the medical and family history information that is available for each child. Although there are exceptions, most US-born children will have extensive background information, while much less information is available when a child comes from another country.

Information available on domestic children may include a thorough family history for both birth parents, an educational assessment for older children, and a complete medical history.

Availability of Information: International Adoption

Children coming from other countries are likely to have only current medical information and little or no educational or family medical history. Assessments of development may be made by caregivers rather than medical personnel. There may be large gaps in information about the birth family or child's history. Older children referred for international adoption seldom have any access to psychological counseling.

All internationally adopted children have at least one medical examination, and while some children may come with more information, parents cannot expect more than one report. There may be some general information about a birth mother, but other family history is seldom known. Depending on the birth country, children may be seen regularly by a doctor in the months leading up to adoption, but little if any information may be known prior to that child coming into state or orphanage care.

With the growth of international adoption has come the development of international adoption clinics across the country. Some pediatricians have developed expertise in reviewing medical information that prospective parents have received with a child's referral. They look for abnormalities, developmental delays, and congenital/

genetic syndromes and then are able to discuss the information objectively with prospective parents. When prospective parents receive no information regarding the child prior to traveling, a clinic can give them guidance on what to observe in interactions with the child. A clinical physician is usually available for support and consultation while adopting parents are meeting or visiting with a child. These services can be very helpful and reassuring to parents.

Surrender or Termination of Parental Rights

Domestic Adoption

Legal doctrine addressing consent to relinquish parental rights varies greatly from state to state. In general, state law requires a waiting time after the birth of a child to allow biological parents to spend time with the newborn, have more counseling, and make a final decision about relinquishment. In a few states, expectant parents may consent to relinquish their rights as soon as the day of birth, while in other states, this may not be done until 30 days after a child's birth. In some states, the consent to terminate parental rights may be reversed up until the time an adoption is finalized in court. It is not unusual for expectant parents to need or request more time to make a final decision. When this happens, a baby is usually placed in private foster care for a limited period.

Unmarried expectant fathers have the right to notice of the birth of a baby and the right to petition the court for legal custody. Each state addresses this right in its laws. Some states have a simpler process, while others states have a lengthy judicial process to determine or terminate a biological father's rights. In some states, these rights are automatically terminated at the time an adoption is finalized.

Anyone can petition a court to overturn a ruling for reasons of fraud, coercion, or duress. However, a court is not obliged to hear a case or grant a petition. Expectant mothers are usually counseled to identify the birth father early in the process so that he may be part of the adoption plan and avoid an adversarial legal process after the baby is placed with an adoptive family. Many prospective adoptive parents choose to adopt internationally rather than deal with the legal uncertainties of domestic adoption.

International Adoption

Although some expectant parents may receive counseling prior to relinquishing a child, in most countries, very little counseling is available. Even when available, in many cultures those expecting a baby do not seek or accept counseling because the benefits of this kind of support are not understood or are felt to be unnecessary.

United States federal law does not permit the international adoption of a child by US citizens if that child has 2 living, identified birth parents. However, adoption by a US citizen may be possible if the foreign government has determined that the legal rights of at least one parent have been terminated or the child has been declared abandoned by at least one parent. Eligibility to obtain an orphan visa for that child to enter the United States for the purpose of adoption requires proof of the death of one or both parents, proof of the termination of legal rights of one or both parents, or a court certificate of abandonment by one or both parents.

American citizens who reside overseas and adopt a child under the laws of a foreign country may be able to obtain a US visa for a child who has lived with them for an extended period.

Openness in Adoption

Domestic Adoption

Contact, or openness, between birth and adoptive parents has become very common in domestic adoption, as previously discussed. It may be done with total openness and ongoing direct contact between all parties or through a mediated process in which contact is maintained through an agency.

International Adoption

In general, international adoption usually provides little if any contact between adoptive and birth parents. Even in cases in which birth parents or relatives have initial contact at the time of placement, it seldom results in an ongoing relationship. Adoption information may not even be fully shared with the partnering US agency. Some adoptive parents choose international adoption with the belief that it would be impossible for birth parents to be reunited with their child. However, there are signs of a change toward a movement of more openness in international adoption. This varies from country to country, depending on the culture and reasons for children being relinquished or abandoned.

In the same way that attitudes have changed around adoption and secrecy in the United States, several countries are now allowing more openness and sharing of information. A small but increasing number of Korean birth mothers are asking to meet adoptive parents and exchange letters as their child grows up. During the past decade, more Korean adoptees have successfully searched for and been reunited with birth and foster parents. This is a major change from the first 50 years of international adoption. Guatemala is unique in that many adoptive parents have met the birth mother at the time of relinquishment, but most do not maintain contact. In other Latin American countries, young adult adoptees are now searching for more information about their birth families with limited success. In general, there is still not much support in place for those who wish to get more information or search for birth parents, but over time this is likely to change as adoptees become more assertive about finding more information.

More international adoptions are happening in African countries where the advent of international adoption is newer. In these countries, typically, children are placed for adoption because of illness and poverty. HIV and AIDS have had an enormous effect on the establishment of international adoption programs for children who have lost both parents.

Although many Ethiopian children are truly orphaned, it is very common for surviving birth family members to desire ongoing contact with adoptees. In Ethiopia, it is common for adopting parents to meet birth relatives when they travel to adopt their child. Frequently, adoptive families maintain direct contact with extended members of the birth family. It is not uncommon for older adoptees to write letters to birth relatives or even occasionally have phone conversations. Adoptive parents are now counseled ahead of time so that they will understand and support this ongoing contact.

Finally, because of cultural traditions in the Marshall Islands, all international adoptions are legally open with the expectation that the birth family, adoptive family, and child will have a lifelong relationship. As adoption programs mature and communication modalities improve, the expectation is that openness in international adoption will gain the support it has in domestic adoption.

Matching of Child With Adoptive Parents

Domestic Adoption

Adoption specialists will tell prospective parents that the more flexible they can be, the easier it will be to match a child with them. Parents who can accept a child of any race or with some special needs are likely to be matched more quickly than those who have little flexibility in these areas. Gender flexibility is also important in the speed of a placement.

Prospective parents who are flexible may be matched with a child within months of completing their home study evaluation. Those adopting an older child through the public system are likely to have the opportunity to get information about many children before making a decision about which child they are interested in adopting. Also, in most states, single parents are more able to adopt from the United States than abroad if they are flexible about the race or age of a child.

International Adoption

Flexibility is also a great advantage in adopting from abroad. In most cases, prospective parents who wish to adopt a baby must be willing to adopt a child up to a minimum of 1 year old and sometimes much older. In general, those adopting from another country are expected to be fully accepting of a child of a race and nationality that is different from their own. Matching is not done by characteristics other than age, health, and sometimes gender.

Even those who want to adopt a healthy child are prepared for the possibility that a child may initially be somewhat delayed with respect to his or her development. Also, prospective parents need to expect little, if any, background information on a child. In general, there is more risk of unknown medical conditions in younger children and children from countries in which health care is substandard.

Interstate Compact

The Interstate Compact on the Placement of Children (ICPC) is an agreement among all 50 states and the District of Columbia to oversee the movement of children across state lines for purposes of adoption or foster care. When a child is adopted internationally, the compact applies to cases in which a private agency holds legal custody of the child on entry into the United States. Since US adoption law falls under the jurisdiction of each state, the ICPC protects each child by ensuring that the laws of every state involved are followed. Thus, the laws of the child's original state of residence as well at the state of the adoptive or foster family are met. Approval by the authorities in both states must be given before a child is relocated.

Post-placement

Domestic Adoption

During the period after placement of a child, there are visits with a social worker and reports written about the child's and family's adjustment. One or more health reports are required by most states during this period. It is expected that the social worker will give the family support and advice about parenting, as needed. When appropriate, referrals may be made for specialized services. The post-placement period may sometimes be extended in the case of older child adoptions or a difficult adjustment.

In most cases, the final post-placement report will conclude with a recommendation for legalization of the adoption in probate court. In most cases, an attorney is present at the legalization of the adoption, but this can vary depending on state law. Once an adoption is legalized in a US court, the adoptive parents retain full legal custody of the child.

International Adoption

Depending on the country, the post-placement period may start when a child is adopted abroad or when he or she arrives in the United States. In most cases, the post-placement period lasts for 6 months or until re-legalization of the adoption in the United States. During this period, a social worker usually has several meetings with the family and reports are written about the initial adjustment of all family members. These reports are sent back to the child's birth country so the country will know of the child's progress. The social worker is expected to provide support and advice on parenting as well as cultural issues. The post-placement time frame may be extended in cases in which more service is required. Health reports from physicians are also required during this period. When appropriate, referrals are made for specialized services.

In some countries, children are legally adopted in their country of birth before arrival in the United States. In other countries, children come to the United States in legal guardianship of a state-approved private adoption agency. That agency then holds legal guardianship until the end of the post-placement period when the child is adopted in a US court.

Post-adoption Services

It is universally accepted that adoption is a lifelong process that changes with time. While it was once thought best for parents not to discuss the subject of adoption and to raise their child as if he or she was a biological offspring, it is now believed that a child who learns about his or her adoption story can form a better sense of self, even if the story is a painful one. Along with the change to greater openness in adoption has come greater support for all members of the adoption triad. Post-adoption services are growing and are offered by many adoption agencies as well as nonprofit organizations created specifically for this purpose.

Adoption Triad

For adopted children, learning about adoption and their birth family heritage is a developmental process. At each stage, a child integrates a greater understanding of adoption that contributes to forming an identity.

For adoptive parents, adoption is a learning process that begins before a child enters the family. Most agencies offer pre-adoption classes for perspective parents. Parents are often challenged by their children's need for information and complicated questions. They can best support their children by being open and honest in answering questions, providing age-appropriate information, anticipating difficult situations, being sensitive to their children's concerns, and finding support when needed.

Birth parents have often felt disempowered and shied away from talking about the children they placed for adoption, feeling that it only complicates their lives. This is changing with more open adoptions and birth parents connecting through support organizations and online chat groups.

Support Groups, Mentorship Programs, and Counseling

Support groups allow individuals to share their experiences and feel less isolated in their experience. Adoptive family gatherings organized around the type of adoption or the country from which a child was adopted offer opportunities for families to connect and share experience. Adoption agencies or family support groups sponsor culture camps so that adoptees can learn about their birth culture.

As adoptees have become adults, many have formed their own support organizations to share their experience. Likewise, birth parents have joined together to support each other and help navigate ongoing relationships with their children.

Mentorship programs have been developed by some adult adoptee groups and college student organizations as a way to provide role models for younger adopted children. Some provide one-on-one relationships while others offer group activities.

Individual and family counseling is offered by some full-service adoption agencies, a few nonprofit organizations specializing in adoption support, and individual therapists who are trained in adoption.

Homeland Visits

Often adoptees have said they feel as if their lives began when they were adopted. If adopted when young, they have no memories of their lives in their birth country. Their story of adoption doesn't seem real to them. Homeland tours and other opportunities to visit a birth country have become a valuable way for internationally adopted children and their families to learn more about the child's birth country and feel emotionally connected to that culture. Sometimes adoptees visit orphanages and meet caregivers or foster parents who remember them and are able to share memories of their early life. Sometimes memories are recovered by experiencing sights, sounds, smells, and tastes that have been absent since they left their country of birth. Homeland visits can bring a better understanding of the reasons for adoption and help adoptees develop a pride in their birth heritage. It can also help adoptees better appreciate their current life circumstances compared with possible alternatives if they had been raised in their country of birth.

Search

Just as more domestic adoptees are interested in searching, more internationally adopted youngsters and young adults are voicing a desire to learn more about their lives before adoption or search for their birth families. To the frustration of adoptees, many countries are not in favor of searching, nor do they have staff or accurate records to assist in searches. This is changing in some countries, but it will take time, just as it has in the United States. Importantly, the process of searching for one's birth family is not the same as reunion with one's birth family—the 2 processes may occur sequentially or with many years of separation.

Summary

The experience of adoptive families and birth parents over the last 50 years has led to a greater understanding of the typical issues of all members of the triad throughout the adoption process, with a resulting greater opportunity for all members of the triad to ask questions and explore their relationships with one another. Ultimately, the goal for each triad member is to achieve a better understanding of the ways in which adoption affects his or her life. This enables each person to make thoughtful choices that are respectful of everyone to whom he or she is connected.

References

1. Evan B. Donaldson Adoption Institute. Research: adoption facts. http://www.adoptioninstitute.org/research/adoptionfacts.php. Accessed February 11, 2014
2. Smith S. Safeguarding the rights and well-being of birthparents in the adoption process. http://www.adoptioninstitute.org/research/2006_11_birthparent_wellbeing.php. Accessed February 11, 2014
3. Child Welfare Information Gateway. *Postadoption Contract Agreements Between Birth and Adoptive Families.* Washington, DC: US Department of Health and Human Services, Children's Bureau; 2011. http://www.childwelfare.gov/systemwide/laws_policies/statutes/cooperative.pdf. Accessed February 11, 2014

Resources

Web Sites

- US Department of State: http://adoption.state.gov/about_us/statistics.php
- Center for Adoption Support and Education: http://adoptionsupport.org
- Child Welfare Information Gateway: www.childwelfare.gov
- Child Welfare League of America: www.cwla.org/programs/adoption
- Evan B. Donaldson Adoption Institute: http://adoptioninstitute.org
- North American Council on Adoptable Children: www.nacac.org

Books

- Davenport D. *The Complete Book of International Adoption: A Step by Step Guide to Finding Your Child.* New York, NY: Three Rivers Press; 2006
- Gritter J. *The Spirit of Open Adoption.* Washington, DC: Child Welfare League of America Press; 1997
- Melina LR. *The Open Adoption Experience—A Complete Guide for Adoptive and Birth Families.* New York, NY: William Morrow Paperbacks; 1993
- Pavao JM. *The Family of Adoption.* Boston, MA: Beacon Press; 2005
- Pertman A. *Adoption Nation: How the Adoption Revolution is Transforming Our Families—and America.* Cambridge, MA: Harvard Common Press; 2011
- Schooler JE. *The Whole Life Adoption Book.* Colorado Springs, CO: Pinon Press; 1993
- Silber K, Dorner PM. *Children of Open Adoption.* San Antonio, TX: Corona Publishing Co; 1989

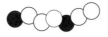

CHAPTER 3

Legal Considerations in Adoption

*Madelyn Freundlich, MSW, MPH, JD, LLM**

Adoption is a legal and social process. The legal process associated with adoption in the United States has evolved over time from largely informal to one that is now regulated by states and the federal government and which internationally is regulated by the Hague Convention on Protection of Children and Co-operation in Respect of Intercountry Adoption. Domestically and internationally, there have been significant developments in adoption law over the past decades. This chapter briefly reviews the history of adoption law in the United States; describes the legal issues that are relevant to 3 major types of adoption—adoption of infants in the United States, international adoption of children by US citizens, and adoption of children from the US foster care system; and concludes with a review of some of the overarching legal issues in adoption. See Box 3-1 for frequent questions that a pediatrician may face concerning patients during the adoption process.

A Brief History of Adoption Law

Adoption laws in the United States may be seen as having stronger roots in Roman law antecedents than in English common law principles.[1] Under English common law, adoption was not formally recognized, whereas under Roman law, adoption was used for inheritance purposes. Under Roman law, families that lacked a male offspring were permitted to bring male strangers, typically adults, into their households and designate these individuals as their lawful heirs.[2] These adopted individuals then became members of their new families with no ties to their birth families. The goal of adoption in Roman society was to continue family lines, thereby principally serving the interests of the adoptive families.[3] English common law, by contrast, did not embrace adoption, largely owing to the strong English commitment to blood lineage as the basis for differentiating class and social status.[4]

*The author wishes to acknowledge the research assistance of John Rhee, who was obtaining his undergraduate degree at Cornell University during the preparation of this chapter.

Box 3-1. Frequent Questions Health Care Professionals May Have During the Adoption Process

1. **Who has medical decision-making rights while an adoption is pending or during the mandatory period when the birth mother can revoke consent to the adoption?**
   Birth parents retain all decision-making rights unless they have voluntarily relinquished their parental rights, their parental rights have been involuntarily terminated, or they have assigned guardianship to another individual. When an adoption is planned, typically a birth mother (or birth parents) relinquishes custody to an attorney or an agency or social worker in the postnatal period. If a child enters custody of a public child welfare agency as a result of prenatal exposure to substance abuse or other imminent risks to the child, the public child welfare agency makes decisions on behalf of the child. Policies, however, vary from one jurisdiction to another. In these situations, the health care professional should verify with the custodial agency who has the authority to make medical decisions for the child.

2. **Who is allowed to have physical access to a newborn in the delivery room and nursery when the plan is adoption?**
   Prior to birth, a child's mother (and father, when involved) has decision-making capacity about who will be present in the delivery room within the constraints of local hospital policies. The mother and father (when present) have the right to determine who will have physical access to the baby following birth. Until parental rights have been transferred to an attorney, adoption or child welfare agency, or adoptive parents, the child's birth mother (and father, if present) may delegate authority to others within the constraints of local hospital policies.

3. **What kind of legal documentation do hospitals require prior to discharging a neonate who is leaving the hospital to an adoptive family?**
   Local policies vary. Typically, however, hospitals require evidence of voluntary relinquishment by the birth parent(s), evidence of the involuntary termination of parental rights, or a signed consent confirming that an agency, attorney, or prospective adoptive parent has legal custody of the child.

4. **Who should manage the baby's hospital discharge, solely the hospital social worker or the hospital's attorney?**
   Typically, a hospital social worker, working with adoption agency staff and members of the medical team, manages the discharge without involving a hospital attorney. If questions arise, however, about legal or physical custody, legal consultation should be sought.

5. **What medical information about the birth, newborn, and mother and father is the health care professional allowed to share with prospective adoptive parents before the adoption is finalized?**
   A health care professional may share information about the birth, newborn, and parents with consent of the parent who retains legal custody or another individual or entity that has legal custody of the child, such as an adoption agency, child welfare agency, or legal guardian.

However, English courts did recognize quasi-adoption arrangements that later influenced the development of adoption law in the United States—arrangements that included wardships and guardianships designed to protect or provide support for orphaned children.[1]

As the social climate in the United States differed significantly from that of England, US adoption law developed quite differently. In the mid-1800s, religious and moral concerns about the welfare of children and economic interests merged in the United States, and efforts were initiated to find ways to support dependent children beyond almshouses or apprenticeships for learning a trade.[5] During this period, the first state statutes appeared that legitimated the many informal transfers of parental rights that had been occurring since the colonial era.[1]

The adoption statutes that appeared in the 1850s and 1860s in the United States did not establish adoption as a legal relationship but simply recognized the informal transfers of children to relatives or strangers by poor parents or institutions that had assumed responsibility for the care of children.[1] These arrangements typically involved agreements that the child would provide farm or domestic services for the family while the family supported and educated the child and included the child as an heir to the family's property. Several states enacted adoption statutes during this period, including Mississippi (1846), Texas (1850), and Massachusetts (1851). The Massachusetts statute recognized the principle of judicial oversight of adoption and is considered the first modern adoption statute. The Massachusetts statute provided that an individual adopted through judicial proceedings was a child of the adoptive parents "to all intents and purposes," and it provided that the child was entitled to parental support until he reached the age of majority and to a share of the parent's estate.[4] Later, California (1872) and New York (1873) enacted adoption statutes that contained similar provisions. These laws, although not specifically grounded on the needs and interests of the child, set the stage for the later development of the principle of "best interest of the child."[6,7]

Formal adoptions began to take place in the late 1800s, although in a social and economic climate that differed greatly from the current adoption environment. During this era, many of the children who were adopted lived in publicly supported institutions that had the authority to "bind out" indigent children to unrelated families through indenture or "adoption."[8,9] During this period, state statutes broadly incorporated certain concepts that more fully characterize adoption law and practice today—the concept of parental consent to adoption, recognition of the principle of "best interest of the child," the relationship between the child and biological family post-adoption, the status of adoption records, and the nature of adoptive relationships.[5,6]

The adoption statutes during this period recognized the need for parental consent for a birth child's adoption but did not specify when consent should be given or how. There were few procedures in place to ensure that parental consent was informed and voluntary, and parents were rarely represented by attorneys. When children were born to single mothers, only the mothers were required to consent to the adoption. Unmarried fathers played no role in adoption unless they were themselves adopting the child or, in a very rare case, they formally legitimated the child. Procedures for review of parental consent were even more minimal when institutions placed children for adoption. Negative societal views of poor parents who placed their children in institutions as morally and personally lacking enabled institutions to elude judicial scrutiny of the adoption arrangements for children placed in these facilities.[9] During this period, state statutes did not address the rights of birth parents to revoke consent to adoption or reclaim their children from the institutions in which they had placed their children. Few parents attempted to do so, as most parents lacked the resources or knowledge to regain custody of their children.[7]

With regard to the concept of "best interest of the child," statutes enacted during this period generally required that adoptive parents be determined to be suitable and that the "moral and temporal" interests of the child be served through adoption.[2] These requirements typically existed more in form than substance. Suitability of the adoptive parents, if addressed at all, largely was a question of the prospective adoptive family's financial means, and the "best interest" of the child was principally viewed in economic terms. The one noneconomic criterion that factored into placement decision-making was the religion of the child and adoptive family.[2] The religion of many children, however, was not known, and consequently, the preference for same-religion adoptive parents usually translated into an institution's or agency's preference for families of the same religion as the religious affiliation of the institution or agency.[2] During this period, judicial oversight of the suitability of adoptive parents was largely ministerial rather than judicial, with the proceedings simply validating an already accomplished transfer of the child to the family.[10] In the case of institutions and other child-placing agencies, the routine placement of children with families continued with little judicial oversight.

The latitude of child-placing agencies during this era is illustrated by the freedom with which Charles Loring Brace of the Children's Aid Society gathered up children he described as "street Arabs" from the streets of New York, NY, and dispatched them via "orphan trains" to the Midwest and West to provide agricultural and other labor for families who took in the children.[9] These children were rarely formally adopted by their "adoptive" families, and there was little, if any, court oversight of this practice.[2] In the early 1900s, social reformers such as Julia Lathrop (who became the first director of the US Children's Bureau) attacked the orphan train movement and the failure of the Children's Aid Society to screen the families with whom children were placed and monitor the welfare of these children after families took in these children.[11] As criticisms mounted, efforts intensified to create the forerunner of modern foster care—the practice of *boarding out*—and the orphan train practice eventually came to a close.[11]

Although statutes during this period allowed children to be adopted by families selected by birth parents or child-placing agencies, they did not prohibit the practice of placing children for profit or without a judicial proceeding; nor did they address the activities of unlicensed agencies in placing children for adoption.[2] Baby-selling scams, as well as questionable placements of children with families as laborers, were well known, but the law did not punish the individuals and agencies engaging in these practices or attempt to prevent such activities in the future.[2]

Through the mid-1900s, there was continuing ambiguity about the nature of the ongoing relationship between the child and his or her biological family. The concept of *exclusivity,* meaning that adoption ends all ties between the birth family and child and the adoptive family becomes the child's family, was not fully embraced. Under the law, for example, adopted children could inherit from their birth parents if the birth parents died intestate. There continued to be disputes as to whether a child was the child of the adoptive family "for all intent and purposes" in connection with distribution of the adoptive parent's property at time of death. Similarly, courts were divided as to whether, if the adoptive family became destitute, the birth parents could be required to support the child whom they had placed for adoption. As late as the 1930s, in about half of the states, there was uncertainty about child-support obligations of birth parents under these circumstances.[2]

Through the early 1900s, adoption records were not treated as confidential. Adopted persons could readily obtain their original birth certificates if they existed. To the extent that information about an adoption was protected, barriers to information access were designed to maintain the privacy of the arrangement from the public, not to shield adoption information from the parties to the adoption.[12] If information was not shared among the parties to the adoption, it was usually the result of incomplete records. By the 1930s, however, confidentiality provisions had begun to be included in some state adoption statutes.[12] States began to provide new birth certificates for children, substituting the adoptive parents' names for birth parents' names.[13] Paralleling this legal development were changes in the practice of some child-placing agencies, reputable and not reputable, with regard to information access. For example, with increasing frequency, it was reported that agencies threatened single pregnant women that privacy regarding their pregnancies would not be honored unless they placed their babies for adoption.[2] At the same time, it was reported that agencies promised prospective adoptive parents that their identities would be withheld to attract families to child-placement agencies and away from direct placement of children by their birth parents.[2] These practices, though of concern, did not trigger a legal response.

Beginning in the 1930s, adoption law began to emerge in fuller form on a state-by-state basis. By this time, adoption of a child had become a more broadly accepted form of family formation, and courts and social workers had come to recognize the need to work cooperatively to ensure that adoptions were properly arranged.[2] The concept of "best interest of the child" broadened beyond economic well-being to include social and psychological well-being, and with this fuller concept of best interest, a number of key changes occurred in adoption law and practice.

One key legal development after 1930 was the inclusion in state statutes of provisions designed to ensure greater oversight of the entities that placed children with adoptive families. States began to enact legislation that required state licensing of child-placing agencies and maintenance of records of the children who were placed for adoption. State legislatures also began to enact laws that required formal home studies of prospective adoptive parents that extended beyond an inquiry into financial solvency. State laws incorporated stronger procedures for parental consent for adoption.[14] Courts began to interpret existing statutes to ensure that the interests of children were met.

After 1930, state statutes were enacted to require the sealing of adoption records beyond the earlier dictates designed to protect adoptions from public scrutiny. These new laws prevented the disclosure of adoption information among the parties themselves, with records to be opened only on a showing to the court of good cause. By the 1960s, court records of adoptions were closed to all persons in all states but Kansas and Alaska, which did not, at any point, close adoption records to the parties to the adoption.[13]

As in previous eras, reports of baby-selling schemes continued to be periodically exposed with resulting public outrage. In 1955, Senator Estes Kefauver conducted a congressional investigation that denounced baby selling as a national disgrace and revealed a number of egregious cases of intrastate and interstate trafficking in children.[15] It was only in the 1950s that state statutes were enacted to penalize the illegal procurement of children and illegal advertising of children.[2] The efficacy of these statutes, however, remained highly questionable, an issue that has persisted to the current day.

By the 1940s and 1950s, the general statutory framework for adoption laws had been set, although specifics varied significantly from state to state. State statutes embodied common themes and, in some cases, utilized the same legal approach to certain issues, but state adoption laws generally lacked uniformity and court interpretation of state laws did not necessarily coincide. This lack of uniformity continues to the present day. State statutes vary considerably in how they govern the relinquishment of children for adoption, the assessment of prospective adoptive parents, who may place children for adoption (and who may not), fees and expenses for adoption, the circumstances under which an adoption can be overturned, and the procedures for finalizing adoptions.

Since the 1950s, there have been several efforts to achieve greater uniformity in state laws that govern adoption, but each effort has failed. Two Uniform Adoption acts (UAAs) were proposed by the National Conference of Commissioners on Uniform State Laws, one in 1951 and another in 1994.[16] The more recently proposed UAA incorporated a range of provisions governing legal protections of children, birth parents, and adoptive parents, some of which met with broad support and others, such as the sealing of adoption records for 99 years, which became the subject of bitter debate.[16] As of the writing of this chapter, no state has embraced the proposed 1994 UAA in full form. Similarly unsuccessful were 2 other efforts in the 1980s to bring uniformity to state adoption laws, one on the part of the US Department of Health and Human Services (then the Department of Health, Education, and Welfare) to develop a comprehensive model state adoption statute, and the second, an effort on the part of the American Bar Association Section of Family Law to draft a model adoption act.[16]

Contemporary Adoption Law in the United States

Adoption in the United States currently occurs in a variety of contexts—intra-family adoptions in which children are adopted by stepparents or other relatives, the domestic adoption of infants, the international adoption of children, and the adoption of children in the US foster care system. Intra-family adoptions by stepparents and other relatives represent more than half of the children who are adopted in the United States each year.[16] Typically, these adoptions legally recognize children's existing custodial relationships with family members. Intra-family adoptions are the least well regulated of all types of adoptions, and as a result, they are not the focus of this chapter. Instead, the discussion considers private domestic adoptions of babies, international adoptions, and the adoption of children from the US foster care system.

Legal Issues Common to All Domestic Adoptions

Certain legal issues are common to all domestic adoptions, whether privately arranged or arranged by public agencies on behalf of children in the foster care system. For any adoption to take place, a person available to be adopted must be placed in the home of a person or persons eligible to adopt. All states have laws that specify which persons can be adopted, which persons are eligible to adopt, which persons or entities have the authority to make an adoptive placement, and the adoption placement process for children. Also common to all domestically arranged adoptions is the process for finalizing the adoption.

Who May be Adopted

State laws vary as to who may be adopted (see an example in Box 3-2). All states permit the adoption of a child. Many states and the District of Columbia allow the adoption of any person, regardless of age. In several states, the law allows the adoption of an individual older than 18 years

> **Box 3-2. An Example of State Law: California Law on Who May Be Adopted**
>
> Under California law, the following adoptions are permitted:
> - An unmarried minor may be adopted by an adult.
> - An adult, including a stepparent, may adopt another adult who is younger, except for the spouse of the prospective adoptive parent.
> - A married minor who is legally separated or whose spouse has given consent to the adoption may be adopted.
> - An adult who is developmentally disabled may be adopted.[17]

only under certain conditions. Some permit the adoption of a young adult older than 18 but younger than 21 years. A few states specify that the adult to be adopted must be younger than the adoptive parent. A few other states limit the adoption of adults to persons who are permanently and completely physically or mentally disabled.[18]

Who May Adopt

Laws that regulate who may adopt also vary from state to state. Some statutes disqualify unmarried or single individuals. Some states have eligibility requirements based on age. Some, for example, require that a prospective adoptive parent be 18, 21, or 25 years or older. In a few states, adoptive parents are required to be a specified number of years older than the person to be adopted, with the required number of years varying from 10 to 15.[18] Some states have imposed "reputability requirements," under which individuals with criminal histories or employment instability do not qualify as suitable adoptive parents. A few states, including Utah and Mississippi, have restricted gays and lesbians from adopting children. Other jurisdictions allow the consideration of a prospective adoptive parent's sexual orientation as one factor when considering an adult's eligibility to adopt.[19] It should be noted that the American Academy of Pediatrics is unequivocally supportive of adoption by qualified individuals irrespective of their sexual orientation.[20–22] In addition, some states have residency requirements that adoptive parents must meet. These states require that a prospective adoptive parent be a state resident for a specified period, ranging from 60 days to 1 year.[18]

An individual cannot petition a court to adopt a child unless the court makes an official finding that the individual is "acceptable" as an adoptive parent. Before an adoption becomes legally recognized, the court must review and accept the prospective adoptive parent's home study prepared by a social worker. The adoption home study generally includes the following information, some of which may be required by state law:

- Autobiography/family background
- Neighborhood/community/schools
- Physical health
- Financial ability to raise a child
- Criminal clearances
- References
- Interviews with the prospective adoptive parent(s)

All states legally require criminal record and child abuse record checks on prospective adoptive parents. Felony convictions for crimes involving children or illegal substances generally are disqualifiers.

There is no legal right to adopt. An adult may desire and attempt to adopt, but no one has an absolute right to adopt unless and until he or she complies with all of the requirements that are necessary for the adoption to take place, including obtaining an approved home study.

Some state laws also require that prospective adoptive parents complete adoption training through a licensed child placement agency. Once prospective adoptive parents have obtained an approved home study and completed any required training, they are eligible to adopt.

Who May Place a Child for Adoption

State laws are uniform in providing that any person or entity that has the right to make decisions about a child's care and custody may place that child for adoption. Individuals who may place a child for adoption include the birth parents or the child's legal guardian or guardian ad litem; legal entities include state departments of social services or child-placing agencies. All states specifically designate which persons or entities hold the authority to make adoptive placements. A few states require that all adoptive placements be made by the state department of social services or child-placing agencies that are licensed by the state or meet certain standards. Most states, however, allow "non-agency" placements of children for adoption, often referred to as *private* or *independent* adoption. One type of private adoption that most states allow is the direct placement of a child by the birth parent with an adoptive family. Generally, states that allow these types of placements have detailed statutory regulations that must be followed to protect the interests of the child, birth parents, and adoptive parents.[18]

Placement of Child With Prospective Adoptive Family

A match between prospective adoptive parents and a child may be made by a licensed agency, an attorney, or an unpaid or paid adoption facilitator or through personal advertising through which prospective adoptive and birth parents find one another. Following the match, the child is placed with the prospective adoptive parents. State laws vary with respect to the period that a child must be in the home of the prospective adoptive parent prior to the legal finalization of the adoption; the most common period is 6 months.

Finalizing Domestic Adoptions

Only state courts and, in some instances, tribal courts are authorized to grant adoptions of children in the United States. The *finalization hearing* is the court hearing at which adoption becomes final. If the court is satisfied that all legal requirements have been met and the adoption would be in the best interests of the child, a decree of adoption is issued and signed, finalizing the adoption. A judicial decree of adoption ends the legal relationship between a child and the child's birth parents and causes the children to become "for all purposes" the child of the adoptive parents.[16] A certificate of adoption is signed and transmitted to the state department of vital records, which issues an amended birth certificate that contains the names of the adoptive parents as the child's parents. This process may vary for international adoptions.

Adoption of Babies in the United States: Legal Considerations

There are certain legal issues that are unique to the domestic adoptions of babies in the United States. These issues include the law governing birth parents' consent to the adoption, the use of adoption facilitators and personal advertising in connection with matching prospective adoptive and birth parents, and adoptive parents' payment of expenses related to the adoption. With respect to private adoptions of infants in the United States, state law governs these considerations.

Birth Parents' Consent to Adoption

Consent is the agreement by a parent or person or agency acting in place of a parent to relinquish a child for adoption and release all parental rights and duties with respect to that child. In most states, the consent must be in writing and witnessed and notarized or executed before a judge or other designated official.[23] The legal requirements for giving consent are designed to protect children from unnecessary and traumatic separations from their families; prevent uninformed, hurried, or coerced decisions by birth parents; and alleviate adoptive parents' possible anxiety about the legality of the adoption process.

In all states, the birth mother and father (Box 3-3), if he has properly established paternity, have the right to consent to adoption of their child unless a court has

---

Box 3-3. Working With Birth Fathers in the Adoption Planning Process

Reputable agencies and attorneys follow certain procedures to locate birth fathers if they are not already part of the adoption planning and ensure that a birth father, if located, is aware of the adoption plans and knows his rights. In cases of adoption in which a birth father cannot be located, there is a degree of risk with that child's adoption because the birth father may later appear and claim his parental rights to the child. To legally protect prospective adoptive parents in these situations, agencies and attorneys do the following:

- **Inform the birth father of the adoption plan:** The adoption is less likely to be challenged if the birth father cooperates and participates in the planning. Even if the father does not agree to the adoption, he should be kept well informed of the events. Otherwise, he may return later and claim that the adoption took place without his knowledge.
- **Try to locate missing birth fathers:** The best possible outcome is that the legal father or anyone presumed to be the biological father is informed and involved with the adoption plans. These steps cannot take place if the birth father is not present. To address this issue, agencies and attorneys search putative (alleged) father registries and publish notices in newspapers in locales where it is possible that the birth father may be. Many state laws require that these procedures be followed.
- **Counsel prospective adoptive parents about the birth father's attitude, cooperation level, and involvement in the adoption plan and explain the risks involved.**

determined that they no longer hold this right. How consent is executed varies considerably from state to state. In many states, consent may be executed through a written statement witnessed or notarized by a notary public. Some states, however, require an appearance before a judge or the filing of a petition of relinquishment. Some states require that the parent be provided with counseling, have his or her rights and the legal effect of relinquishment explained to him or her, or be provided with legal counsel prior to giving consent.[23]

Most states specify in statute at what point in time a birth parent may consent to adoption. Usually, birth fathers can give consent at any time. Birth mothers, on the other hand, generally cannot consent to an adoption until after the child is born. Sixteen states and the Northern Mariana Islands allow birth parents to consent at any time after the birth of the child. Thirty states and the District of Columbia require a waiting period before consent can be executed. The shortest waiting periods are 12 and 24 hours, and the longest are 10 and 15 days. The most common waiting period, required in 15 states and the District of Columbia, is 72 hours (3 days). Only 2 states (Alabama and Hawaii) allow the birth mother to consent before the birth of her child; however, the decision to consent must be reaffirmed after the child's birth.[24]

The process of adoption is intended to create a permanent and stable family for a child. As a result, a validly executed relinquishment and consent to adopt is designed to be final and irrevocable, and the right of a birth parent to revoke consent is strictly limited. In most states, the law provides that consent may be revoked prior to the entry of the final adoption decree under specific circumstances (Box 3-4) or within specified time limits. Consent becomes final and irrevocable once the court issues a final decree of adoption.

Adoption Facilitators and Personal Advertising

Adoption facilitators are individuals who are not licensed as adoption agencies or attorneys who are engaged in the matching of prospective birth parents with prospective adoptive parents. The use of an unpaid adoption facilitator such as a doctor, minister, nurse, rabbi, family member, or friend who assists in matching a baby with a prospective adoptive family without compensation for services is allowed

---

Box 3-4. Circumstances Under Which Withdrawal of Parental Consent May Be Permitted

- The consent was obtained by fraud, duress, or coercion.
- The court finds that withdrawal of consent is in the best interests of the child.
- The birth and adoptive parents mutually agree to the withdrawal of consent.
- An adoptive placement is not finalized with a specific family or within a specified period.

in virtually every state in the United States. Legal issues can arise, however, when adoption facilitators require payment for the matching services they provide..

In a few states, including California and Pennsylvania, the law authorizes adoption facilitators to charge for their services in adoption matching if the services fall within specific parameters.[25] These state statutes detail the activities that adoption facilitators are permitted to offer or must offer. Except for these few states, the laws of most states do not allow adoption facilitators to charge for adoption matching services within the state at all, or adoption facilitators are prohibited by law from charging for any services that they perform within that state.[25] In these states, it is illegal for these persons or agencies to receive any payment for placement of the child.[26] The use of a paid adoption facilitator in those states can negatively affect the finalization of an adoption; as a result, care should be taken in using these services.

> **Practice Tip:** Professionals should advise adoptive parents to be cautious when considering use of the services of paid adoption facilitators. Adoptive parents should discuss the matter fully with the adoption attorney who will finalize the adoption.

Legal considerations may affect prospective adoptive parents' attempts to address challenges to adoption, including locating a child who is appropriate for the family or finding birth parents willing to place their child for adoption. Some parents choose to advertise their interest in adopting. About half of the states have laws that in some way limit or regulate the use of advertising in adoptive placement. States that permit adoption advertising may limit who may advertise. Some allow birth parents and prospective adoptive parents to advertise; others limit advertising to agencies only.[26] The Internet has brought new challenges to adoption advertising regulation.[27]

> **Definition of Advertising for Adoption Placement Purposes:** *Advertising* is generally defined as the publication in any public medium, print or electronic, of an interest in adopting a child or the availability of a specific child for adoption. Advertising venues include newspapers, radio, television, the Internet, billboards, or print flyers.

Regulation of Adoption Expenses

Unlike adoption of a child from foster care through a public agency, which involves fairly minimal costs, the private adoption of infants often involves significant adoption fees paid to the entity or individual who arranges the adoption as well as payment of expenses on behalf of the birth mother. In private adoptions of infants, adoptive parents may pay some of the birth mother's expenses, particularly in the case of a pregnant woman planning to place her newborn for adoption. Almost all states have laws that regulate the fees and expenses that adoptive parents may be expected to pay when arranging a private placement or independent domestic adoption (Box 3-5). These laws specify the type of birth parent expenses a prospective

---

Box 3-5. Types of Adoption Expenses Most Commonly Allowed by State Statute

- Maternity-related medical and hospital costs
- Temporary living expenses of the mother during pregnancy
- Counseling fees
- Attorney and legal fees and guardian ad litem fees
- Travel costs, meals, and lodging when necessary for court appearances or accessing services
- Foster care for the child, when necessary

---

adoptive family is allowed to pay and generally address the level of payment, typically by using the standard "reasonable and customary."

Some state laws explicitly prohibit adoptive parents from paying certain types of expenses. Prohibited expenses often include educational expenses, vehicles, vacations, permanent housing, or any other payment for the monetary gain of the birth parent. State laws often set time limits for these payments, which range from as few as 30 days to as long as 6 months after the child's birth or placement.[28]

Adoption of Children in Foster Care in the United States

Each year, approximately 50,000 children are adopted from the US foster care system.[29] The law governing these adoptions is a mix of federal and state statutes. At the federal level, 5 key statutes govern public child welfare agencies in planning and providing adoption services for children in foster care (Table 3-1). With respect to the adoption of children in foster care, these statutes, taken together, require state child welfare agencies to recruit adoptive families for children in foster care who are waiting for adoptive families, expedite the adoptions of children who cannot be safely reunited with their birth families, and provide services and supports to children and their adoptive families.

Supplementing the federal statues, state laws also play an important role in the adoption of children in foster care. These laws govern the involuntary termination of parental rights and the provision of post-adoption support to families who adopt children from foster care.

Termination of Parental Rights

For children in foster care who cannot be safely reunited with their birth parents, state law provides a process for involuntarily termination of the rights of their parents, freeing the child for adoption when parents do not voluntarily relinquish their rights. Most states require that courts considering the involuntary termination of parental rights determine by clear and convincing evidence that the parent is unfit and whether severing the parent-child relationship is in the child's best interest.

Table 3-1. Federal Statutes Regulating the Adoption of Children in Foster Care

Federal Statute	General Description	Key Provisions
Indian Child Welfare Act of 1978	Designed to protect the interests of American Indian children, families, and tribes	• Recognized tribal jurisdiction over American Indian and Alaska Native (AI/AN) children resident or domiciled on reservations • Established higher evidentiary standards for removing AI/AN children from their families and for termination of the rights of their parents • Established a hierarchy for decisions regarding foster care and adoption placements, giving preferences to AI/AN families
Adoption Assistance and Child Welfare Act of 1980	Established the federal foster care program and a new federally funded adoption assistance program	• Emphasized permanency planning for children in foster care • Required states to have a case plan for each child under state care and to make the plan available to the parents • Required states to make reasonable efforts to prevent a child from entering foster care and to reunite child and parents when a child must enter foster care • Provided federal funds for assistance to families who adopted children in foster care with special needs
Multiethnic Placement Act of 1994, as amended by Interethnic Provisions of 1996	Aimed at removing the barriers to adoption for children of color in foster care	• Prohibited states and other entities that are involved in foster care or adoption placements and receive federal child welfare financial assistance from delaying or denying a child's foster care or adoptive placement on the basis of the child's or the prospective parent's race, color, or national origin • Prohibited these states and entities from denying to any individual the opportunity to become a foster or adoptive parent on the basis of the prospective parent's or the child's race, color, or national origin • Required that states diligently recruit foster and adoptive parents who reflect the racial and ethnic diversity of the children in the state who need foster and adoptive homes

Table 3-1. Federal Statutes Regulating the Adoption of Children in Foster Care, continued

Federal Statute	General Description	Key Provisions
Adoption and Safe Families Act of 1997	Established unequivocal national goals for children in foster care—safety, permanency, and well-being	• Reaffirmed the need for a collaborative approach to providing services for children and families • Clarified the importance of removing barriers to moving children waiting in foster care to permanent families • Shortened judicial time frames and the time frames for initiating termination of parental rights proceedings • Clarified reasonable efforts requirements to avoid foster care placement
Fostering Connections to Success and Increasing Adoptions Act of 2008	Designed to achieve greater permanence and improve the well-being of children served by public child welfare agencies, particularly children in foster care, those who leave foster care in their late teens, and AI/AN children	• Permitted states to claim an open-ended federal reimbursement for a part of eligible state costs related to providing kinship guardianship assistance • Authorized direct access for tribes to open-ended federal reimbursement for the costs of operating a foster care, adoption assistance, and kinship guardianship program on behalf of children under tribal authority • Expanded federal support for adoption assistance by de-linking, over time, eligibility for that program from income and other criteria that were a part of the Aid to Families with Dependent Children program

With respect to the judicial determination of "parental unfitness," some state statutes specify factors that constitute grounds for termination of parental rights; other states use general language. The most common state statutory grounds for involuntary termination of parental rights are

- Severe or chronic abuse or neglect
- Abuse or neglect of other children in the household
- Abandonment
- Long-term mental illness or deficiency of the parent(s)
- Long-term alcohol or drug-induced incapacity of the parent(s)
- Failure to support or maintain contact with the child[30]

Many state statutes specify that an additional ground for termination of parental rights is the felony conviction of the parent for a crime of violence against the child or other family member, or a conviction for any felony when the term of conviction is such a length as to have a negative effect on the child and the only available provision of care for the child is foster care.[30]

With respect to the judicial determination of the best interests of the child, some state statutes use general language mandating that the child's health and safety be paramount in all proceedings. Other state laws specify factors that must be considered, including the child's age; physical, mental, emotional, and moral well-being; cultural and attachment issues; and reasonable preferences about adoption.[30]

The federal Adoption and Safe Families Act of 1997 (ASFA) requires state child welfare agencies to file a petition to terminate parental rights under certain conditions (Box 3-6).

In response to ASFA, many states specified limits to the maximum period that a child can spend in foster care before termination of parental rights proceedings must be initiated. Typically, states have adopted the ASFA standard of 15 out of the most recent 22 months in care. Some states, however, specify shorter time limits, particularly for very young children.[30]

Box 3-6. Termination of Parental Right Requirements Under Federal Adoption and Safe Families Act of 1997

Federal law requires that a petition be filed to terminate parental rights when
- A child has been in foster care for 15 of the most recent 22 months *or*
- A court has determined
  — The child to be an abandoned infant *or*
  — The parent has committed murder or voluntary manslaughter of another child of the parent; aided, abetted, attempted, conspired, or solicited to commit such a murder or voluntary manslaughter; or committed a felony assault that has resulted in serious bodily injury to the child or another child of the parent.

Adoption Assistance and Post-adoption Services and Support

Adoption assistance in the form of monthly subsidies is available for most children who are adopted from the foster care system. Adoption assistance is provided in each state through 2 programs.

- A federally supported adoption assistance program for certain children adopted from foster care (established under federal law)
- A state-funded adoption assistance program for other children adopted from foster care (established under state law)

States generally first determine whether a child is eligible for the federally supported adoption assistance program. Criteria for this program are a mix of federal and state requirements. Under federal law, the child must be determined to be a child with special needs as defined in the state where the child resides (Box 3-7). If a child is not eligible for the federally supported adoption assistance program, the state will determine the child's eligibility for the state-funded program. Most children adopted from foster care qualify for an adoption subsidy. In fiscal year 2011, 90% of the children adopted from the foster care system received an adoption subsidy of some type.[32]

Each state also statutorily defines criteria that a child must meet to be eligible for state-funded adoption assistance. Typically, the child must have one or more special needs to qualify. Examples of state laws defining special needs are provided in Box 3-8.

Box 3-7. Federal Eligibility for Federally Supported Adoption Assistance: Special Needs Determination

Special Needs Determination[31]

The child must be determined to have special needs, which include *all 3 requirements* as follows:

1. The child cannot or should not be returned home to his or her parent(s).

AND

2. The child has a "factor or condition" (uniquely defined by each state) that qualifies him or her as having special needs. Depending on the state, this factor or condition may consider a child's
   - Ethnic background
   - Age
   - Membership in a sibling group
   - Medical, physical, or emotional condition or handicap

   The factor or condition must prompt the conclusion that the child cannot be placed without providing adoption or medical assistance.

AND

3. An attempt to place the child without adoption assistance was made but was unsuccessful except where it would be against the best interests of the child.

Box 3-8. Examples of State Definitions of Special Needs for Purposes of Adoption Assistance[33]

Florida

A child with special needs is defined as a child who has at least one of the following needs or circumstances that may be a barrier to placement or adoption without financial assistance:

- Eight years or older
- African American or racially mixed parentage
- Member of a sibling group of any age, provided 2 or more members remain together for purposes of adoption
- Mentally handicapped
- Physically handicapped
- Emotionally handicapped
- Significant emotional ties with foster parent(s)

Illinois

A child with special needs is defined as a child who has at least one of the following needs or circumstances that may be a barrier to placement or adoption without financial assistance:

- One year or older
- Member of a sibling group being adopted together in which at least one child meets one of the other criteria listed here
- Being adopted by adoptive parents who have previously adopted, with adoption assistance, another child born of the same mother or father
- Irreversible or non-correctable physical, mental, or emotional disability
- Physical, mental, or emotional disability correctable through surgery, treatment, or other specialized services

Maryland

A child with special needs is defined as a child that has at least one of the following needs or circumstances that may be a barrier to placement or adoption without financial assistance:

- Six years or older and younger than 18 years
- Race or ethnic background (considered in addition to other special needs)
- Member of a sibling group of 2 or more children placed in the same family
- Physical, mental, or emotional disability or disease
- High risk of physical or mental disability or disease
- Emotional disturbance

A few states have enacted laws that require that post-adoption services and supports be provided to children adopted from foster care and their adoptive families. These statutes contain provisions such as the following:

- Requirements for the state to establish a program of specialized training and supportive services to families adopting court-dependent children who are HIV positive or prenatally exposed to alcohol or a controlled substance (California)[34]

- Authorization to provide counseling and referral services after adoption to adoptees and adoptive families for whom the state provided such services before the adoption with a requirement that post-adoption services include mentoring, post-licensure training, support groups, behavioral management counseling, therapeutic respite care, referrals to community providers, a telephone help line, and training for public and private mental health professionals in post-adoption issues (Connecticut)[35]
- Requirement that the commissioner of human services establish a post-adoption service grant program to be administered by local social service agencies to preserve and strengthen adoptive families (Minnesota)[36]
- Requirement of a comprehensive strategic plan to assist "created families," including families formed through adoption of children from state custody (Oklahoma)[37]
- Authorization of the provision of post-adoption services to children and adoptive families for whom the state provided services before the adoption directly by the state child welfare agency or through contract (Texas)[38]

International Adoption: Legal Considerations

Key legal considerations in international adoption involve the mandates of the Hague Convention on Protection of Children and Co-operation in Respect of Intercountry Adoption and the treaty's implementing law and regulations in the United States, the requirements in these laws addressing who may be adopted and who may adopt, and the process for finalizing an international adoption.

Governing Law: The Hague Convention and the Intercountry Adoption Act of 2000

International adoptions by United States citizens are regulated by the Hague Convention on intercountry adoption and the Intercountry Adoption Act of 2000 (IAA). In 1993, 66 countries, including the United States, signed the Hague Convention, which built directly on the United Nations Convention on the Rights of the Child and seeks to protect all parties to international adoptions and prevent international traffic in children. The Hague Convention regulates how international adoptions are to take place and the respective responsibilities of the child's and adoptive parents' countries of origin. After signing the Hague Convention, the United States enacted federal legislation to implement the convention requirements. The IAA addressed these issues, including the designation of a central authority for international adoptions as required by the Hague Convention. The IAA assigned to the US Department of State the primary responsibility for implementing the convention. Subsequently, the Department of State made the Office of Children's Issues in the Bureau of Consular Affairs responsible for the day-to-day implementation of the convention. The IAA required the Department of State to develop regulations for accreditation of adoption agencies arranging international adoptions. With these regulations in place, the Hague Convention entered into force for the United States on April 1, 2008. The convention applies to adoptions between the United States and all other countries that have become part of the convention.

Hague Convention Adoptions: Requirements Addressing Who May Be Adopted and Who May Adopt Internationally

The Hague Convention states that a child may be adopted internationally if the authorities of the child's country of origin have established that the child is adoptable and have decided that intercountry adoption is in the child's best interests. Countries that receive children through international adoption also are free to set forth requirements for children's immigration for purposes of adoption. In the United States, the legal requirements addressing who may be adopted depend on whether the adoption is taking place with another country that has signed the Hague Convention (a convention adoption) or a country that has not (a non-convention adoption). Box 3-9 outlines the legal requirements in the United States addressing who may be adopted internationally.

Finalizing an International Adoption

International adoptions may be finalized abroad or domestically. International adoptions are governed primarily by state law once an adopted child arrives into the state of residence of the adoptive parent(s). States regulate international adoptions finalized abroad in 1 of 3 ways.
- Most states grant full effect and recognition to foreign adoption decrees issued abroad.
- A few states grant full effect and recognition to foreign adoption decrees only after validation of the decrees by a state court or re-adoption of the adopted child in a state court.
- The remaining states do not grant any effect or recognition to foreign adoption decrees and require validation or re-adoption under state law or, alternatively, may not grant full effect and recognition to foreign adoption decrees under certain circumstances.[41]

Under US Citizenship and Immigration Services regulations, children who were not seen by all relevant parents prior to their overseas adoptions are not considered to have full and final adoptions. They must be readopted in the state where they will reside even in cases in which the child's country of origin considers such adoptions final. Under these US regulations, children who are not seen by all relevant parents prior to their overseas adoptions cannot be considered automatic citizens until re-adoption occurs.[42] *Re-adoption* is a process by which a US state court in the

Box 3-9. Who May Be Adopted Internationally: US Legal Requirements[39]

Convention Adoptions

In addition to other possible requirements, all of the following must be true for a child to be adopted through a convention adoption:

- The child is younger than 16 years, is unmarried, and lives in a convention country.
- The child will be adopted by a married US citizen and spouse jointly or by an unmarried US citizen at least 25 years of age, habitually resident in the United States, who has been found to be suitable and eligible to adopt with the intent of creating a legal parent-child relationship.
- The child's birth parents (or parent if the child has a sole or surviving parent) or other legal custodian, individuals, or entities whose consent is necessary for adoption freely give their written irrevocable consent to the termination of their legal relationship with the child and to the child's emigration and adoption.
- If the child had 2 living birth parents who were the last legal custodians who signed the irrevocable consent to adoption, they are determined to be incapable of providing proper care for the child.
- The child has been or will be adopted in the United States or in the convention country in accordance with the rules and procedures in the Hague Convention and the Intercountry Adoption Act of 2000 (IAA).

Non-convention Adoptions

Children who are adopted from non-convention countries must meet the definition of *orphan* as defined in the Immigration and Nationality Act before they can be considered for US permanent residence or citizenship. When a child is adopted from a non-convention country, the child is issued an IR-3 visa when the adoptive parents physically see the child prior to or during the adoption proceedings or an IR-4 visa when the child was not seen by the parent(s) prior to or during the adoption. When children enter the United States with an IR-3 visa, they automatically acquire citizenship and automatically receive a Certificate of Citizenship. When children enter the United States with an IR-4 visa, citizenship is not automatically conferred. Instead, they become Permanent Residents and receive a permanent resident card (green card). They become citizens of the United States when their adoption is finalized in the United States before the child's 18th birthday.[40] An important difference in this process is that parents must apply for a Certificate of Citizenship rather than expecting it to be sent automatically. Pediatricians should encourage parents to follow through with this application process because their child may be deprived of certain federal benefits without documentation of citizenship.

Three sets of law govern US citizens' ability to adopt internationally—the Hague Convention as implemented by the IAA, the laws of the child's country of origin, and the laws of the individual's home US state. The Hague Convention and IAA require that prospective adoptive parents receive 10 hours of training on issues specific to international adoption. The IAA requires that prospective adoptive parents be fingerprinted for purpose of a required US Federal Bureau of Investigation criminal background check. Children's countries of origin have different requirements for eligibility to adopt, such as requirements related to age, health, marital status, and sexual orientation. State laws, as discussed earlier, govern the nature and scope of the home study process and finalization of adoptions.

state of the parents' or sole parent's residence reviews the details of the adoption abroad along with additional information that it deems necessary and then issues a new adoption decree. The new adoption decree is independent from the foreign decree and states that the child has been adopted in conformity with the adoption law of the applicable state. Requirements regarding re-adoption vary from state to state.[43]

> **Practice Tips on Re-adoption:** Parents may obtain information about re-adoption from their state court system or through their home study or placement agency. Families should recognize that some states have re-adoption requirements such as post-placement visits or the updating of some documents, such as child abuse and police clearances.

Many families choose to readopt their child even when it is not legally required. There are several advantages of re-adoption, including 2 key legal benefits. First, a state court adoption decree issued as a result of a re-adoption is fully independent of the foreign decree. As a state court decree, it is entitled to full faith and credit by other states, as required by the US Constitution. A US state adoption decree ensures that every state in the United States will recognize the decree and makes it unnecessary to rely solely on the validity of a decree issued under the law of another country. Second, federal laws can be based on a state's underlying law on adoption and inheritance. In certain circumstances, a US state-issued adoption decree is required for an adopted child to be entitled to Social Security benefits through his or her parent(s).[43]

Overarching Legal Issues in Adoption

The concluding section of this chapter discusses 3 overarching legal issues in adoption—interstate adoptions involving the placement of infants or children in foster care across state lines, adoption dissolution, and legal issues related to information sharing and ongoing contact between birth and adoptive families.

Interstate Adoptions

The placement of infants or children in foster care with adoptive families in other states brings into play the Interstate Compact on the Placement of Children (ICPC). The ICPC is a contract among and between states that is designed to ensure that children placed across state lines for adoption (as well as for foster care) receive adequate protection and support services. The ICPC has jurisdiction over any placement that is made prior to an adoption, including placement with parents and relatives in another state when a parent or relative is not making the placement. The legal framework of the ICPC ensures that

- The child is placed in a suitable environment.
- The state that will receive the child (where the adoptive parent[s] lives) has the opportunity to assess the proposed placement.

- The state that is sending the child (the state where the child lives) obtains enough information to evaluate the placement.
- The care of the child is supervised and appropriate jurisdictional arrangements are made.

The ICPC has been enacted into law by all 50 states and the District of Columbia.[44]

A second compact applies when children are adopted from foster care and their adoptive parents reside in another state or the adoptive family moves to another state after the adoption is finalized. The Interstate Compact on Adoption and Medical Assistance (ICAMA) was established in 1986 to safeguard and protect the interests of children covered by adoption assistance agreements when they move or are adopted across state lines. It enables states to coordinate the provision of medical benefits and services to children receiving adoption assistance in interstate cases by providing a framework for uniformity and consistency in administrative procedures. Currently, 49 states and Washington, DC, have adopted ICAMA through legislation.[45]

Dissolution of Adoption

Adoption *dissolution* refers to a reversal or voiding of an adoption after its legal finalization. State laws vary regarding the conditions under which an adoption may be dissolved. Idaho's statute, for example, states the following:

> An adoption may be dissolved, upon petition, with the agreement of both the adoptee and the adopting parent, when the adopting parent was the spouse of a natural parent, and the marriage of the natural parent and adoptive parent was terminated. If the petition for dissolution occurs after the death of the adoptive parent, the court shall, in the finding of dissolution, specify the effect upon rights of inheritance. The court must determine that avoidance of statutory care is not the purpose of the dissolution, unless the court finds grounds to waive this finding. An action to obtain a decree of dissolution of adoption may be commenced at any time after the adoptee reaches twenty-one (21) years of age.[46]

Information Sharing and Ongoing Contact Between Adoptive and Birth Families

State laws govern the sharing of non-identifying and identifying information between birth and adoptive families. In many states, laws also provide mechanisms through which birth and adoptive families can develop legally enforceable plans to have ongoing contact following the finalization of the adoption.

Sharing of Non-identifying and Identifying Information

In nearly all states, adoption records are sealed and withheld from public inspection after the adoption is finalized. Most states have developed procedures by which the parties to an adoption—adoptive parents, adopted persons, and birth parents—may obtain non-identifying and identifying information from an adoption record while protecting the interests of all parties.

Non-identifying information refers to descriptive details about an adopted person and the adopted person's birth relatives. This information is generally provided to the adopting parents at the time of the adoption. Non-identifying information may include the following:

- Date and place of the adopted person's birth
- Age of the birth parents and general physical description, such as eye and hair color
- Race, ethnicity, religion, and medical history of the birth parents
- Educational level of the birth parents and their occupation at the time of the adoption
- Reason for placing the child for adoption
- Existence of other children born to each birth parent

All states allow adoptive parents or the guardian of an adopted person who is a minor to access non-identifying information. States also allow the adopted person to have access to non-identifying information about birth relatives, generally on written request. These laws usually require that the adopted person be an adult, usually at least 18 years of age. More than half of the states allow birth parents to access non-identifying information, and a number of states give such access to adult birth siblings. How non-identifying information is collected, maintained, and disclosed varies from state to state.

Identifying information is any data that may lead to the positive identification of an adopted person, birth parents, or other birth relatives. Identifying information includes the current name of the person and an address or other contact information that would allow adopted persons or birth relatives to make personal contact. Almost all states permit the release of identifying information when the person whose information is sought has consented to the release of the information. In many states, birth parents are asked to specify at the time of consent or relinquishment whether they are willing to have their identity disclosed to the adopted person when he or she reaches age 18 or 21. If there is no consent, state laws vary as to whether identifying information may be released. In some states, information may not be released without a court order documenting good cause to release the information. A person seeking a court order must be able to demonstrate a compelling reason for disclosure that outweighs the need to maintain the confidentiality of a party to an adoption. Some states have imposed limitations on the release of identifying information. In Connecticut, release of identifying information is allowed only when a court determines that the requested information will not be detrimental to the public interest or the welfare of the adoptee or birth or adoptive parents.[47]

In some states, the law provides for confidential intermediaries who act on behalf of a member of the adoption triad (birth parent, adoptive parent, adopted person) to make contact with the other members of the triad. Acting as a go-between for the parties involved, the confidential intermediary determines the willingness of each member to allow confidential information to be shared. Finally, there are several states that have open aspects of the adoption records for adult adopted persons. In these states, an adult adoptee can obtain an original birth certificate and, in some instances, additional adoption record information. States with laws that broadly provide adopted persons access to their birth certificates and other information in their adoption records are described in Table 3-2.

Table 3-2. State Laws Providing Adult Adopted Persons With Direct Access to Birth/Adoption Information

Alabama	Original birth certificate is made available to adopted persons, aged 18 years or older, on request. Birth parents may file a nonbinding contact preference form requesting direct contact with the adopted adult, contact through an intermediary, or no contact at all.
Alaska	Provides access to adopted persons aged 18 years and older and birth parents of adopted persons aged 18 years and older, if the adopted person gives written permission for release of the information.
Delaware	Adult adopted persons may request their original birth certificates. Birth parents have the option of filing a veto against disclosure. If a disclosure veto is filed, the original birth certificate is not released to the adopted person.
Kansas	Grants access to the adoption file and the original birth certificate to adopted persons, aged 18 years and older; birth parents; and adoptive parents of a minor child. Birth parents may contact the adopted adult if he or she agrees to contact.
Maine	As of January 1, 2009, adult adopted persons who were born in Maine will have the right to obtain copies of their original birth certificates. Birth parents may file a nonbinding preference form.
New Hampshire	The original birth certificate is made available to the adopted person, aged 18 years or older, on request. Birth parents may file a nonbinding contact preference form.
Oregon	The original birth certificate is made available to the adopted adult, aged 21 years or older, on request. Birth parents may file a nonbinding contact preference form.
Tennessee	Adopted persons, aged 21 years or older, may access their original birth certificates and adoption records unless the record indicates that birth was the result of rape or incest and the birth parent victim does not consent to disclosure. Birth parents also may veto contact.

Post-adoption Contact Agreements Between Birth and Adoptive Families

Post-adoption contact agreements, sometimes referred to as *cooperative adoption* or *open adoption* agreements, are arrangements that provide for some degree of contact between a child's adoptive family and members of the child's birth family after the child's adoption has been finalized. These arrangements may range from informal, mutual understandings between the birth and adoptive families to written, formal contracts. In general, state law does not prohibit post-adoption contact or communication given the right of adoptive parents to decide who may have contact with their adopted child. These contacts often are arranged by mutual understanding without any formal agreement and are not legally enforceable. As of 2012, 34 states and the District of Columbia have statutes in place that provide for legally enforceable written agreements for post-adoption contact or communication. The written agreements specify the type and frequency of contact and are signed by the parties to an adoption prior to finalization. The modes of contact can range from an exchange of information about the child between adoptive and birth parents; to the exchange of cards, letters, and photos; to personal visits with the child by birth family members.[48] These statutes provide mechanisms for parties to return to court to enforce these agreements if necessary. Many require that the parties first seek mediation before resorting to judicial enforcement.[49]

Conclusion

Adoption is governed by state, federal, and international law. These laws address a range of issues that are vital to the success of adoption placement and finalization. This chapter has identified a number of the legal issues, but it is not intended to be a comprehensive listing of all relevant adoption law issues, nor does it provide an in-depth description of the issues that are discussed. Hopefully, it provides professionals and families with an enhanced understanding of the legal considerations in domestic infant, foster care, and international adoption.

References

1. Huard LA. The law of adoption: ancient and modern. *Vanderbilt Law Rev.* 1956;9(23):743–758
2. Hollinger JH. Introduction to adoption law and practice. In: Hollinger JH, ed. *Adoption Law and Practice, Volume 1.* New York, NY: Matthew Bender & Co; 2002:1–84
3. Kempin FG. *Legal History: Law and Social Change.* Englewood Cliffs, NJ: Prentice-Hall; 1963
4. Presser SB. The historical background of the American law of adoption. *J Fam Law.* 1971; 11:446–461
5. Leiby L. *A History of Social Welfare and Social Work in the United States.* New York, NY: Columbia University Press; 1978
6. Grossberg M. *Governing the Hearth: Law and Family in Nineteenth Century America.* Chapel Hill, NC: University of North Carolina Press; 1985
7. Peck EF. *Adoption Laws in the United States, Publication #148.* Washington, DC: US Department of Labor, Children's Bureau, US Government Printing Office; 1925
8. Cahn NR. Perfect substitutes or the real thing? *Duke Law J.* 2003;61:39–47

9. Ross CJ. Society's children: the care of indigent youngsters in New York City, 1875–1903. In: Cahn NR, Hollinger JH, eds. *Families by Law: An Adoption Reader.* New York, NY: New York University Press; 2004:11–18

10. Parker IR. *Fit and Proper? A Study of Legal Adoption in Massachusetts.* Boston, MA: Church Home Society; 1927

11. Folks H. *The Care of Destitute, Neglected and Delinquent Children.* New York, NY: Macmillan; 1902

12. Samuels EJ. The idea of adoption: an inquiry into the history of adult adoptee access to birth records. *Rutgers Law Rev.* 2001;53:367–392

13. Samuels EJ. The idea of adoption: an inquiry into the history of adult adoptee access to birth records. In: Cahn NR, Hollinger JH, eds. *Families by Law: An Adoption Reader.* New York, NY: New York University Press; 2004:136–141

14. Zainaldin J. The emergence of a modern family law: child custody, adoption, and the courts, 1796–1851. *Northwestern Univ Law Rev.* 1979;72:1038–1089

15. Zelizer V. *Pricing the Priceless Child.* Princeton, NJ: Princeton University Press; 1985

16. Hollinger JH. Adoption law. *Future Child.* 1995;3(1):43–61

17. Official California Legislative Information. California Family Code §§8600; 9300; 9302; 9320; 9326. http://www.leginfo.ca.gov/.html/fam_table_of_contents.html. Accessed February 11, 2014

18. Child Welfare Information Gateway. *Who May Adopt, Be Adopted, or Place a Child for Adoption?* Washington, DC: US Department of Health and Human Services, Children's Bureau; 2006

19. Cornell University Law School. Adoption: an overview. http://topics.law.cornell.edu/wex/Adoption. Accessed February 11, 2014

20. American Academy of Pediatrics Committee on Psychosocial Aspects of Child and Family Health. Promoting the well-being of children whose parents are gay or lesbian. *Pediatrics.* 2013;131(4):827–830

21. American Academy of Pediatrics Committee on Psychosocial Aspects of Child and Family Health. Coparent or second-parent adoption by same-sex parents. *Pediatrics.* 2002;109(2):339–340

22. Perrin EC, American Academy of Pediatrics Committee on Psychosocial Aspects of Child and Family Health. Technical report: coparent or second-parent adoption by same-sex parents. *Pediatrics.* 2002;109(2):341–344

23. Mabry CR, Kelly L. *Adoption Law: Theory, Policy and Practice.* Buffalo, NY: William S. Hein Publishing; 2006

24. Child Welfare Information Gateway. *Consent to Adoption.* Washington, DC: US Department of Health and Human Services, Children's Bureau; 2012

25. Adoption.com. Adoption facilitators. http://adopting.adoption.com/child/adoption-facilitators.html. Accessed February 11, 2014

26. Child Welfare Information Gateway. *Use of Advertising and Facilitators in Adoptive Placements.* Washington, DC: US Department of Health and Human Services, Children's Bureau; 2008

27. Adamec C, Miller LC. *The Encyclopedia of Adoption.* Washington, DC: Infobase Publishing; 2007

28. Child Welfare Information Gateway. *Regulation of Private Domestic Adoption Expenses.* Washington, DC: US Department of Health and Human Services, Children's Bureau; 2008

29. US Department of Health and Human Services Administration for Children & Families. Trends in foster care and adoption FY2002–FY2007. http://www.acf.hhs.gov/programs/cb/resource/trends-in-foster-care-and-adoption. Accessed February 11, 2014

30. Child Welfare Information Gateway. *Grounds for Involuntary Termination of Parental Rights.* Washington, DC: US Department of Health and Human Services, Children's Bureau; 2007

31. Child Welfare Information Gateway. *Adoption Assistance for Children Adopted From Foster Care.* Washington, DC: US Department of Health and Human Services, Children's Bureau; 2004

32. US Department of Health and Human Services Administration for Children & Families. The AFCARS report: preliminary FY2011 estimates as of July 2012 (#19). http://www.acf.hhs.gov/programs/cb/resource/afcars-report-19. Accessed February 11, 2014

33. Child Welfare Information Gateway. Adoption assistance by state. http://www.childwelfare.gov/adoption/adopt_assistance. Accessed February 11, 2014

34. Official California Legislative Information. Welfare and Institutions Code Section 16135–16135.30. http://www.leginfo.ca.gov/cgi-bin/displaycode?section=wic&group=16001-17000&file=16135-16135.30. Accessed February 11, 2014

35. State of Connecticut cga General Assembly. Chapter 319a: Child Welfare Sec. 17a-121a . http://www.cga.ct.gov/current/pub/chap_319a.htm#sec_17a-121a. Accessed February 11, 2014

36. Office of the Revisor of Statutes. 2013 Minnesota Statutes. 259.85 Postadoption Service Grants Program. http://www.revisor.mn.gov/statutes/?id=259.85. Accessed February 11, 2014

37. Oklahoma State Legislature. Oklahoma Statutes. Title 10. Children §10-22.2. http://webserver1.lsb.state.ok.us/OK_Statutes/CompleteTitles/os10.rtf. Accessed February 11, 2014

38. Texas Constitution and Statutes. Family Code Title 5. The Parent-Child Relationship and the Suit Affecting the Parent-Child Relationship. Subtitle B. Suits Affecting the Parent-Child Relationship. Chapter 162. Adoption Sec. 162.306. http://www.statutes.legis.state.tx.us/Docs/FA/htm/FA.162.htm#162.306. Accessed February 11, 2014

39. US Department of State Bureau of Consular Affairs. Intercountry adoption. http://adoption.state.gov/index.php. Accessed February 11, 2014

40. US Citizenship and Immigration Services. Before your child immigrates to the United States. http://www.uscis.gov/adoption/your-child-immigrates-united-states. Accessed February 11, 2014

41. Child Welfare Information Gateway. *State Recognition of Intercountry Adoptions Finalized Abroad.* Washington, DC: US Department of Health and Human Services, Children's Bureau; 2006

42. Joint Commission on International Children's Services. Readopting your child from overseas. http://www.rainbowkids.com/ArticleDetails.aspx?id=185. Accessed February 11, 2014

43. Lyford CJ. "Readoption"—what is it? Do you need to do it? Should you do it? What does it involve? Some things to consider regarding readoption. http://www.fwcc.org/index.php?option=com_content&view=article&id=181. Accessed February 11, 2014

44. US Department of Health and Human Services Office of Inspector General. Interstate Compact on the Placement of Children: implementation. http://oig.hhs.gov/oei/reports/oei-02-95-00044.pdf. Accessed February 11, 2014

45. Association of Administrators of the Interstate Compact on Medical Assistance. ICAMA the compact. http://aaicama.org/cms/index.php/icama-aaicama/the-icama. Accessed February 11, 2014

46. ChildAdoptionLaws.com. Child adoption laws: Idaho. http://www.childadoptionlaws.com/child_adoption_laws/adoption_laws_idaho.htm. Accessed February 11, 2014

47. Connecticut Ann. Stat. Section 7-53. http://www.cga.ct.gov/asp/menu/statutes.asp. Accessed February 11, 2014

48. Child Welfare Information Gateway. *Postadoption Contact Agreements Between Birth and Adoptive Families.* Washington, DC: US Department of Health and Human Services, Children's Bureau; 2012

49. Child Welfare Information Gateway. *Postadoption Contact Agreements Between Birth and Adoptive Families.* Washington, DC: US Department of Health and Human Services, Children's Bureau; 2005

CHAPTER 4

Pre-adoption Considerations for Pediatricians

Paul J. Lee, MD, FAAP, and Linda D. Sagor, MD, MPH, FAAP

A basic understanding of domestic and international adoption issues is important for all pediatricians. Within the US foster care system, more than 100,000 children are eligible for adoption, with approximately 50,000 children adopted each year.[1] There are more than a quarter million international adoptees in the United States, and more than 10,000 international adoptions occur annually, although this number continues to fall.[2]

Prospective adoptive parents routinely consult health care professionals to help them navigate the process leading to a successful adoption. These parents want to utilize a practitioner's medical knowledge and experience to prepare them and will likely continue to seek advice and guidance from these health care professionals before, during, and after the adoption process.

Health care professionals are often asked to review medical information but may also be asked other questions about the basics of adoption and how to begin the journey. Although pediatricians may be comfortable discussing pre-adoption medical issues involving children who are in foster care or being adopted, they receive minimal exposure to adoption issues during their training. As a result, they typically have little or no knowledge of the procedures involved in adoption or the specific social and medical issues of children who have been in the foster care system or an international orphanage. There is even less familiarity and comfort with the complex questions and topics asked by prospective parents of international adoptees (eg, "Which country do you think we should adopt from?"; "Can we realistically expect his or her growth and development to catch up to his or her chronologic age?"). Pediatricians in the United States may not understand the medical terminology and health care procedures of other countries and rarely see common global health issues in their practices. This chapter will review important aspects of domestic and international adoption and discuss specific concerns that families bring to their pediatricians prior to the actual adoption.

Types of Adoptions

Families who are considering adopting a child born within the United States have 2 main options: an agency adoption (through the public foster care system or a private licensed agency) or an independent adoption. A third option is adopting a child born outside the United States, referred to as intercountry or international adoption.

There are approximately half a million children in the US foster care system at any given time. Each state has specific child welfare agencies to supervise the care of children in state custody. While the goal for most of these children is reunification with their birth families, there are many children, from infancy through adolescence, who are free to be adopted because their parents have had their rights terminated. In 2011, there were more than 104,000 children in the United States waiting for adoption from the foster care system.[1]

Children enter foster care for many reasons, most because of physical abuse and neglect related to parental mental illness, substance abuse, and family violence and dissolution. The majority come from backgrounds of poverty. A smaller percentage of children come into state custody because of cognitive and physical disabilities of parents, their own intensive medical issues, and sexual abuse. Because these children often have risk factors for physical or mental health problems, they are sometimes considered to be children with special needs. However, it is also important to note that, despite a history of difficult circumstances, many children are healthy and resilient and will flourish in a nurturing environment. Emphasizing the importance of health, safety, and permanence, the Adoption and Safe Families Act of 1997 increased adoption incentives, especially for children with chronic medical problems, and laid out strict guidelines to terminate parental rights in a timely fashion.[3]

There are 3 types of private adoptions: domestic through a licensed agency, independent domestic, and international. The first approach for a domestic adoption would include birth and prospective parents working with a licensed private agency to explore their options, which include

- *Agency-identified adoption:* Birth and prospective adoptive parents request services within the same agency.
- *Agency-assisted adoption:* Prospective adoptive parents use services of one agency for home study (see The Adoption Process on page 76) while using another to locate the birth parents.
- *Parent-identified adoption:* Prospective adoptive parents are aware, through the Internet, friends, or other informal channels, of birth mother/parents considering adoption; they then work with an agency to develop a plan.

The second type of domestic adoption is an independent adoption, handled by attorneys or adoption facilitators, with no agency involvement. While attorneys are licensed and regulated by state laws (and often belong to the American Academy of Adoption Attorneys), facilitators are not. About 65% of states allow facilitators to work with prospective adoptive parents to find an expectant birth mother, but very few states allow them to charge a fee for this service.[4] And although most facilitators are professionals who adhere to ethical business practices, it is still important that parents check the references and credentials of the agency, attorney, or facilitator they choose to use to avoid any possibility of inexperience, misrepresentation, or fraud.

Lastly, in international adoption, most prospective parents choose and work with an agency, usually based on its reputation, recommendations from others, or the countries in which it works. These adoptions are, of course, agency identified or agency assisted. Occasionally, there are independent international adoptions using attorneys or adoption facilitators. Some countries permit parents to do the adoption themselves with in-country assistance. A common example of an independent international adoption is an intercountry adoption of a relative by a US citizen.

While it might seem less costly and more desirable to "do it yourself," this option certainly entails more emotional and financial risk, hard work, and a steep learning curve. There is little supervision or oversight to protect prospective parents' rights or costs and to ensure regulations and laws of both countries are followed correctly. An adoption attorney with experience in international adoptions will still be necessary to finalize an independent international adoption.

Openness of Adoption

Prior to 1950, most states had legislation that kept adoption records sealed and unavailable to birth or adoptive parents as well as the adopted child. In the following years, however, many adult adoptees requested their records from agencies and, finding them sealed, began to advocate for change. Many states then developed policies so that people involved in adoptions could get easier access to medical and other important information.[5]

In confidential adoptions, no identifying information is given to any of the parties involved. Semi-open or mediated adoptions allow information to be relayed through a mediator, usually a caseworker or an attorney, but do not involve direct communication. Open or fully disclosed adoptions allow adoptive parents and child to interact directly with birth parents. This process may help to decrease the child's, as well as the birth parents', sense of grief and loss and allow the child to maintain connections grounded in reality rather than imagination and fantasy. Though open adoptions are not recommended in some situations (eg, history of extreme violence with birth parent, mental illness that would preclude appropriate boundary setting), research from the Minnesota/Texas Adoption Research Project indicates some benefits in the right setting.[6] Almost all international adoptions would be considered semi-open, as information is obtained through an agency, attorney, or facilitator, and communication with birth parents is often impossible (eg, birth parents are unknown, deceased, lost to follow-up, not interested) or not allowed (ie, parental rights have been terminated). Although not typical, in some cases, information may be available, and for some, a meeting with the parents might be possible.

The Adoption Process
(See also Chapter 2, The Process of Adoption in the United States, on page 25.)

Obviously, after much thought and research, the first step in the adoption process is for prospective parents to decide whether they wish to adopt domestically or internationally and then whether they will use an agency or proceed independently. If parents chose to use an agency, they should be advised to find one that will provide support and assistance throughout the application process, during the adoption, and as for many years post-adoption as needed.

Regardless of the type of adoption chosen, a home study must be completed by the prospective parents before the process can continue. A home study is a formal review of the parents and home environment by a social worker and is used to determine whether the parents and their home are suitable to nurture and support a child. While requirements vary by state and country, the typical home study will include

- A personal interview with each adult in the household and a home visit with prospective parents to learn more about them, their reasons for adoption, and their background. Some agencies will also obtain input from children already in the household through a personal interview, written statement, or even drawings (for very young children).
- An evaluation of the physical, mental, and emotional capacity of the parents and any other adults in the household. A physical examination and screening tests may be necessary.
- A full report of the prospective parents' home and living conditions, including the neighborhood, community, and school system, to ensure the child will have a safe and nurturing environment.
- A detailed financial analysis, including financial statements and records, of the prospective parents.
- A description of pre-adoption counseling provided to the prospective parents or a post-adoption counseling plan.
- A background check of the parents and any other adults in the household, including criminal record, history of child abuse, substance abuse, sexual abuse, and domestic violence.
- An appraisal of the prospective parents' ability to provide an appropriate level of care, if they are considering a child with special needs.
- A complete explanation for any adult in the household who ever had an unfavorable home study or was rejected for adoption.
- Several personal references.

- A specific assessment of how all of these factors affect the prospective parents' ability to care for an adopted child, how many children can be adopted, and any restrictions on children who could be placed with the family.

The home study can take anywhere from 3 to more than 9 months to complete. Once the home study has been submitted, the actual placement process can begin. The agency, attorney, or facilitator now starts identifying prospective adoptable children for the parents. It can take weeks, months, and sometimes years for a suitable match to be made, based on the home study recommendations and the parents' preferences. Once a specific child is identified, the parents will receive a written referral, which contains medical and other information about the child. They then have an opportunity to review the referral information to decide whether they should proceed with adoption or decline and wait for another referral.[7]

International Adoption

International adoption follows the same domestic adoption procedures described previously; however, there are many additional steps and considerations. There are many exclusion criteria set by placement countries that may limit options, such as parental age, parental health issues, length of marriage, ethnic background, and being a single or same-sex parent. Not all countries participate in international adoption with the United States, and a separate application must be submitted to US Citizenship and Immigration Services (USCIS). There are 3 separate forms— the I-800A, I-600A, and I-600—depending on whether the foreign country is a party to the Hague Convention (I-800A) or not (most commonly the I-600A, unless the child is already known).[8-10]

The Hague Convention on Protection of Children and Co-operation in Respect of Intercountry Adoption is an international agreement between 80 countries, including the United States. It is intended to safeguard intercountry adoptions by preventing the abduction, exploitation, sale, or trafficking of children and by considering what is in the best interest of children who are being adopted from another country. The United States signed the Hague Convention in 1994; it became effective in April 2008. Convention countries from which US parents commonly adopt children include China, Colombia, India, Mexico, and the Philippines.[11,12] The current list of convention countries is available at http://adoption.state.gov/hague_convention/countries.php.[13]

Although international adoption from a non-convention country (ie, Russia, Ethiopia, South Korea, Ukraine, Haiti, and Kazakhstan) is very similar to the Hague process, there are theoretically more transparency and protection for parents who adopt from convention countries. Convention countries are required to have a central authority to be the source of adoption information and point of contact for that country. Agencies who work with convention countries must be accredited at the federal level by one of the US Department of State accrediting entities. All fees must be itemized and disclosed to prospective parents. A US consular official in the birth country must certify that the adoptee has met the requirements of the convention and the Intercountry Adoption Act of 2000. The official also determines whether the child meets visa eligibility criteria for entering the United States before the adoption is finalized (or custody is granted) in the birth country.

Convention country adoptions also carry additional stipulations. The home study must meet state and federal requirements and be prepared by an accredited or approved adoption service provider, supervised provider, or exempted provider (ie, a social worker who only does the home study and does not provide any other adoption services for the case). An exempted provider home study must still be approved by the accredited/approved adoption service provider. Parents must choose the convention country before completion of the home study and submit it to the USCIS with the I-800A form. Lastly, at the time of this writing, parents must receive 10 hours of adoption education.[14] For more information, see http:// adoption.state.gov.

Convention and non-convention countries usually require a dossier as well. This is a collection of documents required by the foreign country central authority. While many of the documents are the same as required for the home study and USCIS, countries may request additional paperwork including birth and marriage certificates, verification of employment, the adoption agency license, and personal and passport photographs. These documents must be notarized and apostilled (governmental authentication of the notary public's notarization), often with strict criteria that reject the notarization if the notary's commission expires within 6 to 12 months.

If the USCIS approves the I-800A, I-600A, or I-600 application, parents will be issued the I-797 Notice of Action or the I-171H Notice of Favorable Determination Concerning Application for Advanced Processing of an Orphan Petition. Although parents have now been cleared by the United States for an international adoption, many months can elapse before parents receive a referral from the foreign country. The USCIS documents expire after 15 to 18 months, and parents must sometimes file for extensions and resubmit updated paperwork if the adoption is unlikely to be finalized prior to the USCIS expiration dates.[15]

Finally, parents must apply for the appropriate type of immigrant visa for the prospective adoptee to enter the United States, issued by the US Department of State at the embassy or consulate in the foreign country where the child resides.[16]

Financial Considerations

Costs of adoption can vary from free to minimal in foster care adoptions to many thousands of dollars in agency and independent adoptions. Expenses common to all types of adoption include home study and legal fees. While the cost of the home study is usually the responsibility of prospective parents, there may be no fee associated with adoption from foster care.

Adoption-specific expenses include

- *Domestic adoption: foster care.* Fees are generally low and may include some attorney, medical, and travel fees. Children with special health care needs may be eligible for adoption assistance payments or Supplemental Security Income. Adoption assistance from the federal government is administered under the Title IV-E adoption assistance program. Payments to parents of an eligible child with special needs can take the form of one-time (nonrecurring) or ongoing (recurring) adoption assistance. These funds are paid through the state agency or another public or nonprofit private agency. Parents can determine if they will qualify for federal or state adoption subsidies to help with the expenses incurred in adopting a child with special health care needs at www.childwelfare.gov/pubs/f_subsid.cfm.[17]

- *Domestic adoption: licensed private agency.* Unlike adoption of a child from foster care, which involves fairly minimal fees, in a private or independent adoption the adoptive family is expected to pay many of the expenses. Fees generally include home study, birth parent counseling, and adoptive parent preparation and training. Some agencies may have a sliding scale, depending on the number of children adopted and whether the child has special needs.[18]

- *Domestic adoption: independent.* This is the same as domestic adoption through a licensed private agency but may also include additional fees for the birth mother's medical costs, advertising, and legal representation.

- *Intercountry adoption.* The same as domestic private agency adoption but will include an adoption program fee for the country, which varies by country. If not already included in the agency fee, an optional dossier fee to expedite the application through the government and country's authentication process can save months of time. There are governmental fees for filing and processing the I-800A, I-600A, and I-600 applications and fingerprinting for a US Federal Bureau of Investigations criminal background check. Parents must also factor in the cost of travel (often without the benefit of advance prices because most countries give little advance notice when parents must travel), prolonged hotel stays, and meals. For those who choose to do an independent international adoption, there will be legal fees and additional fees for the child's foster and medical care, plus the same governmental and travel costs. In most cases, children with special health care needs who are adopted internationally do not meet the eligibility requirements of the federal Title IV-E adoption assistance program.[19]

Health Care Considerations of Adopted Children

Foster Care/Domestic Adoption

As noted previously, children in foster care have higher rates of chronic disabilities, serious emotional and behavioral problems, significant developmental delays, and poor school performance than other children from similarly impoverished backgrounds. Studies over the past 15 years have noted that between 50% and 80% of children in foster care have mental health and developmental issues.[20-24] It is not surprising that many of these children have considerable mental health needs, given that the life of a child in foster care is often filled with separation, loss, powerlessness, and discontinuity.[25] Children with frequently changing placements have a greater likelihood of mental health problems resulting from sudden and distressing interruptions in their relationships as well as insecure attachments to caregivers with multiple problems.[26] In 2010, the average amount of time spent in foster care was 26.74 months, with an average of 3 different placements during that time.[27] This may lead to further placement disruptions if foster parents become overwhelmed with the emotional needs of their child.[28]

Disruptive behavior disorders such as conduct disorder, attention-deficit/hyperactivity disorder (ADHD), and oppositional defiant disorder are the most prevalent diagnoses. Other common diagnoses include post-traumatic stress disorder, mood disorders and depression, adjustment reaction, and reactive attachment disorder. Developmental delays are found in 30% to 60% of children in foster care but only in 4% to 10% of the general population.[29-31] While speech and language delays are most common, cognitive problems and gross motor delays are also noted. Children in foster care are also more likely (30%–40%) to have a special education classification related to an emotional or behavioral disturbance.[32] Despite the prevalence of mental health and developmental issues, only one quarter of those needing services receive them.[21,33]

Children in foster care are at increased risk for physical health issues as well. The health care they received prior to placement (indeed, sometimes during placement) is often fragmented, inconsistent, and incomplete. Newborns of mothers who have been abusing alcohol or drugs may have immediate problems after birth as well as long-term issues (see Chapter 5, Prenatal Substance Exposure: Alcohol and Other Substances—Implications for Adoption, on page 97).

The most common medical concerns include obesity, dental caries, respiratory disease (especially asthma), and incomplete immunizations. While growth delay, short stature, and failure to thrive have been reported in previous studies, recent research has indicated that being significantly overweight or obese (body mass index >85%) is a more prevalent and more common diagnosis in this population. In a study done in 2001 to 2004 in Utah, 35% of all children older than 3 years entering foster care were overweight or obese, compared with 15% to 20% in the general population.[24] Results from research in Massachusetts[34] indicated that 25% of children aged 2 to 12 years evaluated at a foster care clinic shortly after placement were overweight or obese.

International Adoption

Internationally adopted children face the same emotional, behavioral, and developmental issues and concerns as children in foster care. However, the resulting disorders may be more severe and exacerbated by their placement in orphanages or other institutions. One of the best known and documented examples of the adverse effects of institutionalization is the devastating impact found on the physical, emotional, behavioral, and developmental health of children in Romanian orphanages in the 1980s.[35]

Behavioral problems are common in internationally adopted children and stem from psychosocially depriving institutionalization prior to adoption and emotional neglect.[36] In addition to disruptive behavior disorders reported in children adopted from domestic foster care, sensory integration disorders and institutional autism occur as well. Previous studies have shown that early institutional care is a risk factor for mental health problems years after adoption, such as increased rates of ADHD and social problems.[37,38] Unfortunately, there is little evidence that the likelihood of these behavioral problems wanes with time post-adoption.[39]

Despite all of these caveats, foster care has been shown to have a positive influence on the social development of institutionalized children who have experienced deprivation, as long as placement in foster care occurs early enough in life. The Bucharest Early Intervention Project is an ongoing longitudinal study examining the effects of early institutionalization on the brain and behavior development by monitoring areas such as physical growth, cognitive function, social-emotional development, attachment, and brain development. This project has also been examining and documenting the significant effect of high-quality foster care as an intervention for institutionalized children.[40]

Children in orphanages also experience emotional neglect from inadequate numbers of orphanage caregivers and low caregiver-to-child ratios, lack of primary caregivers, frequent changes in caregivers, and inadequately trained caregivers who simply cannot provide the level of attention a child requires. Without enough caregiver contact, orphans experience physical and emotional neglect in a non-stimulating environment. Lack of a consistent and constant model to learn from leads to developmental delays, especially cognitive and language skills.[41] The absence of appropriate supervision puts these children at risk for physical and sexual abuse.[42] Information about possible sexual or physical abuse, especially for children who are older at the time of adoption, can unfortunately be common and is typically not revealed in pre-adoption paperwork. Families need to be prepared to address these issues as they arise.

Poverty, weak economies, and lower standards of living compared with the United States mean that orphans in many countries do not have access to the health care and behavioral services they may need, let alone basic necessities like adequate nutrition, particularly protein, and micronutrients like iron. Malnutrition inhibits growth and has deleterious effects on a child's health, immune system, and brain development. Poverty also increases the likelihood that the birth mother had little to no prenatal care and poor nutrition and health herself, further decreasing the chances of a healthy, normal baby. Children living in other countries are at risk of acquiring global infections not commonly seen in the United States, such as intestinal parasites, malaria, and Chagas disease, while living in a crowded institutionalized setting increases their exposure to respiratory and gastrointestinal infections, such as tuberculosis and hepatitis A. The net result is that their location and circumstances exacerbate the negative effect of being an orphan while precluding any preventive or palliative measures.

Special Needs

Some children have been placed in the foster care system because of significant medical issues that the birth parent(s) may not be emotionally or financially prepared to handle. There have also been a growing number of international children, especially from China, identified with a known disability. These adoptees are often classified as having special needs, including preexisting medical conditions such as cleft palate, congenital heart disease, orthopedic issues such as clubfoot and amniotic bands, and infections such as HIV and chronic hepatitis B. Adoptees with special needs also include children with cognitive, behavioral, developmental, and psychiatric disorders. Box 4-1 lists some of the medical and developmental concerns that can cause a child to be labeled as having special needs.

Technically, almost all domestic adoptions from foster care could be considered special needs because this is terminology used by state laws to indicate eligibility for federal financial assistance. It is a phrase commonly heard and used but disliked by adoption professionals and youth in foster care because of its negative connotations. Each state has its own specific definition of special needs, based on some or all of the following criteria: ethnic or racial background; age; membership in a sibling group; medical, physical, or emotional disabilities; risk of physical, mental, or emotional disabilities based on birth family history; and any condition that makes it more difficult to find an adoptive family. Specific state definitions are found at https://www.childwelfare.gov/adoption/adopt_assistance/questions.cfm?quest_id=1.[43] According to Title IV-E of the Social Security Act, a child or youth with special needs must also meet the following 2 requirements to be eligible for federal adoption assistance: the child or youth cannot or should not be returned home to his or her parent(s), and an unsuccessful attempt was made to place the child or youth without adoption (financial) assistance, except in cases in which

Box 4-1. Conditions Classified as Special Needs

This is not intended to be a comprehensive list but to give health care professionals an idea of what medical conditions might result in a child being identified as having special needs.

General
- Failure to thrive
- Prematurity
- Maternal alcohol use during pregnancy
- Maternal smoking during pregnancy
- Maternal drug use during pregnancy
- Age/older child

Genetic
- Down syndrome
- Turner syndrome
- Inborn errors of metabolism (eg, phenylketonuria)
- Dwarfism
- Neurofibromatosis

Infectious Diseases
- Tuberculosis
- Hepatitis B (chronic, carrier, exposed)
- Hepatitis C (chronic, carrier, exposed)
- Syphilis
- HIV
- Cytomegalovirus

Hematologic
- Hemophilia
- Thalassemia
- Sickle cell disease

Facial
- Cleft lip or palate
- Microsomia

Vision
- Partial/total vision loss, unilateral/bilateral
- Strabismus
- Amblyopia
- Malformed eye
- Eye trauma/missing eye
- Ptosis
- Nystagmus

Hearing
- Partial/total hearing loss
- Ear deformity (eg, microtia, atresia)

Respiratory
- Asthma
- Cystic fibrosis
- Pectus excavatum/carinatum

Cardiovascular
- Heart murmur
- Congenital heart disease (eg, atrial septal defect, ventricular septal defect, patent foramen ovale, patent ductus arteriosus, tetralogy of Fallot, pulmonary hypertension)

Gastrointestinal
- Malabsorption
- Gastroesophageal reflux
- Pyloric stenosis
- Feeding/swallowing issues
- Umbilical/inguinal hernia
- Imperforate anus/anal atresia

Genitourinary
- Kidney disease/malformations
- Urinary tract malformations
- Vesicoureteral reflux
- Genital malformations (eg, hypospadias)
- Intersex conditions/ambiguous genitalia
- Cryptorchidism
- Rectovaginal/vesicovaginal/rectovesical fistula

Neurologic
- Brain atrophy
- Cerebral hemorrhage
- Cerebral palsy
- Epilepsy/seizure disorder
- Spina bifida/meningocele/myelomeningocele
- Paraplegia/hemiplegia
- Spinal fusion
- Hypotonia/hypertonia
- Hydrocephalus
- Microcephaly

Box 4-1. Conditions Classified as Special Needs, continued

Orthopedic
- Arthrogryposis
- Bow legs
- Rickets
- Syndactyly
- Missing digits/limbs (congenital [amniotic band sequence] or traumatic)
- Partially formed digits/limbs (congenital or traumatic)
- Talipes equinovarus (clubfoot)
- Talipes varus
- Hip dysplasia/congenital hip dislocation
- Scoliosis

Dermatologic
- Albinism
- Burns/scars
- Disfiguring birthmark(s) (eg, hemangioma, nevus)

Neurodevelopmental
- Significant developmental delay
- Language delays
- Fetal alcohol syndrome

---

such a placement would not have been in the best interests of the child or youth.[44] As discussed previously, a child or youth with special needs from another country does not qualify for federal adoption assistance.

The appeal of a child with special needs to parents is that the adoption process is usually expedited, considerably shortening the lengthy waiting time. Unfortunately, many of these parents choose speed of adoption at the expense of a complete understanding of the medical, developmental, and emotional needs of the child. These parents may then be poorly equipped to deal with all of the concerns of the child following adoption. Some parents, on the other hand, have carefully researched or already have experience with a child with a particular medical issue and are comfortable or even eager to adopt such a child. Although the reason for classifying the child as special needs is usually quite clear, in some referrals it may not be as evident, especially with international referrals, in which details are lacking or, to a lesser extent, the specific reason(s) for the concern would not be considered a significant issue in the United States.

Obtaining Information on a Prospective Adopted Child

Though obtaining information may be a challenging process, it is well worth the time and energy. The information parents obtain will help their health care professional identify specific or potential problems, discuss treatment, and hopefully prevent unnecessary repetition of certain tests, evaluations, and immunizations. As parents understand the unique needs of the child, they will be able to consider what resources will be necessary and whether they will be able to care for this child, enabling them to make the best informed and appropriate decision about the prospective adoption. Finally, if parents have decided to proceed with adoption, it will ultimately be helpful for them to know as much as possible about the child's medical, educational, and family background.

In domestic adoptions from foster care, the first resource for information is the child's caseworker, whether at a public child welfare or private agency. This may then lead to other sources of information, such as previous primary care physicians, subspecialty consultations, hospitalizations, child care and school records, early intervention, and behavioral and mental health evaluations. Box 4-2 lists important data that will help pediatricians guide parents in their quest for information about the child and his or her potential medical and developmental issues and status. When prospective parents have difficulty obtaining information, medical professionals may be able to access health records (with parental permission) for them.

In international adoptions, information on the child can come from one or more sources, such as the orphanage, caregivers, in-country adoption or governmental agency, physicians, and social workers. Typically it will include photos; some basic and background information; and medical, social, and development history, although the amount provided and usefulness varies widely. Some countries, such as Russia and the Ukraine, may do "blind" referrals in which parents are given an invitation to visit but receive no information about a particular child prior to their travels. Once there, parents are shown a child and given some information. During this visit, parents must then decide whether or not to accept the referral and begin the actual adoption process. Box 4-2 lists useful referral information for children adopted internationally.

The Medical Review

Overview

For domestic and international adoptions, the first encounter between a health care professional and prospective parents may be to discuss medical information, also known as the *medical review*. The purpose of the medical review is 4-fold— to identify and discuss pertinent medical and developmental issues in the information provided, to provide an overall risk assessment of the short- and long-term implications of these issues, to address and clarify any additional parental concerns or questions, and to identify critical missing information that the family needs to go back and try to obtain.

Reviewing an adoption referral puts pediatricians in the uncomfortable position of giving medical advice about a child whom neither they nor the parents have actually seen. Pediatricians may be reluctant to offer advice based on such limited data or fear of medicolegal risk. However, parents are usually aware of the limitations in the medical information and are seeking an opinion on any potential health or medical issues by having a professional with medical knowledge and experience review the data to identify risks that a nonmedical person might not recognize.

Box 4-2. Useful and Relevant Referral Information to Assess a Prospective Adoptee's Medical Condition

It is important to understand that this is an idealized list and that most referrals will be missing much of this information. Further details may not be forthcoming or available.

1. *Health history of parents, siblings, and extended family:* ages, current medical issues, developmental or cognitive delays, mental health problems, history of smoking, alcohol or drug abuse, genetic conditions, medications.

2. *Social history of parents, siblings, and extended family:* educational attainment, history of incarcerations and other legal issues, domestic violence, previous foster care placement, history of abuse or neglect, current and past relationships with family and friends, cultural and religious background. Are sibling(s) with the birth parent(s), in foster care, adopted, or in an orphanage*?

3. *Why child is available for adoption:* If voluntarily, why? If not voluntarily, why not?

4. *Child's birth history:* pregnancy history (including number of pregnancies, births/outcomes, health issues during pregnancy[s], and any problems); prenatal care; gestational age; labor and delivery; Apgar scores (if hospital birth); type of delivery (vaginal, cesarean); birth measurements including weight, length, and head circumference; health at delivery and in the perinatal period; problems in nursery (eg, hyperbilirubinemia, opiate withdrawal, sepsis, poor feeding).

   Also: date or estimated date of birth, current or estimated age, place of birth (country/region/city), date of admission to infant hospital (if applicable; eg, Russia, where baby may be transferred to another hospital after birth), date(s) of admission, age when placed in orphanage or foster care (can be multiple).*

5. *Child's past medical history:* previous health issues, chronic illness, hospitalizations, operations, developmental milestones, physical examinations, behavioral/mental health evaluations and interventions, presence of well-child/preventive and dental care, immunizations (which ones and dates given). Weight, height, head circumferences (eg, at 3 months, 6 months, 9 months, 1 year, as appropriate for age of child)—a pattern of growth determines reliability of the measurements; head circumference is a surrogate marker for brain size and growth. Is there any evidence of fetal alcohol syndrome/fetal alcohol spectrum disorders? Laboratory tests (tests, dates, and results) including a complete blood cell count and HIV, hepatitis B, and syphilis test results. The American Academy of Pediatrics *Red Book* lists appropriate laboratory testing for international adoptions,[45] but these recommendations are applicable to domestic adoptions as well.

6. *Child's past social history:* previous placements (number, length); reason for disruptions in placement; school performance; special educational needs; history of abuse, neglect, or early childhood trauma.

7. *Child's current medical and social issues:* acute illnesses, chronic illness, medications, allergies, physical examination, developmental/behavioral/mental health problems, temperament, language skills, school placement and needs, most recent health care, dental, mental health professionals, ongoing relationships with family, laboratory test results and immunizations (also see item 5).

8. Child's strengths, special interests and abilities, talents, and hobbies. For older children, does the child want to be adopted, and is the child prepared for it?

---

*Information particular to international adoption.

When discussing limitations of the information with parents, it is important to realize that they have typically pored over the review repeatedly, focusing on anything that they don't understand or seems abnormal. Many have already discussed their concerns with family, friends, and online support groups and used Internet search engines and resources to obtain information and opinions that run the gamut from accurate to misleading.

If a pediatrician agrees to do a medical review of a prospective adoptee, the first step is to identify relevant medical information (see boxes 4-1 and 4-2) and assess and evaluate its importance and usefulness. A formal consultation discussion can then be arranged, which should include an explanation of medical terms (plus foreign medical diagnoses for international adoptions) and assessment of their significance, if any; laboratory test results; somatic growth trends; and a developmental assessment of degree and signs of developmental delays or other issues such as alcohol-related neurodevelopmental disorders. Finally, there should be an overall risk assessment of the need for any medical or developmental intervention after arrival.

The purpose of the risk assessment is to give parents a realistic appraisal of the likely types and degree of interventions that may be required for the prospective adoptee. It is up to the parents to decide whether the level of risk is within their personal level of comfort to proceed with the referral. It is important for parents to understand that adoption is a "leap of faith" and that there are no guarantees or promises that "everything will be fine." Parents will have to be the ones who make the decision whether or not to adopt; a health care professional cannot and should not be making it for them. Care should be taken not to give a personal opinion if asked, "Should we take this child?" or "Would you take this child?" When concluding the review, it should be emphasized that any advice provided is a professional opinion based on limited data and selective information and not a recommendation and that accurate diagnoses or outcome predictions cannot be made without being able to examine or interact with the child in person and perform necessary and appropriate tests.

The mnemonic HOUR can be a helpful guideline for the medical review discussion.

- **H**onest
- **O**bjective
- **U**ncomplicated
- **R**ealistic
- *Be honest—know your limitations and be open about them.* No one knows the answer to every question, and there isn't always a definitive answer for every question. Health care professionals shouldn't be afraid to admit that they don't know the answer to a question. Incorrect advice is always worse than no advice. There's nothing wrong with saying that an answer needs to be researched further

or discussed with another colleague or specialist before addressing a parental concern. Parents cannot develop a relationship of trust if they realize a pediatrician is giving incorrect information. Many prospective parents have immersed themselves in adoption and foster care information and know more than many medical professionals about certain topics. However, parents are still gathering information and opinions from those they trust and respect. If a pediatrician doesn't feel qualified to address a topic, parents can be referred to an appropriate specialist or resource.

- *Be objective, professional, and nonjudgmental.* The medical review is an opinion based on a health care professional's medical experience and interpretation of the facts. Although it may sound like an oxymoron to give an objective opinion, a professional opinion is one based on facts and verified knowledge and information, not hearsay or emotion. Avoid the urge to editorialize or insert any personal bias. Again, it's up to the parents, not the pediatrician, to decide whether to proceed with the adoption based on their assessment of the potential risks and ability to provide care for a child with those risks.

- *Be uncomplicated, clear, and straightforward.* Avoid the use of medical jargon and try to discuss issues in terms that a non–medically trained person would understand. Even the most intelligent parents can be emotionally overwhelmed during the referral process and have difficulty following all the nuances of a discussion. It is OK to repeat and reinforce important issues and ask questions to make sure that parents have really understood what they have heard. Encourage and give them ample opportunities to ask questions. Conversely, there is no need to be patronizing or oversimplify the discussion.

- *Be realistic.* Advice should be based on the information provided. Nothing should be assumed that cannot be verified from the provided information or personal experience. Ultimately, it does not help prospective parents to underplay negative information or be overly optimistic. It's also important that a pediatrician find balance between being cautious with the advice given and completely pessimistic because the desired level of information and detail is not available. The goal is to keep parental expectations grounded in facts and likely evidence-based outcomes, not hopes and fantasies. Parental satisfaction with an adoption depends on how closely their expectations for the child correlate with the child's actual status and abilities. If parental expectations are set unrealistically high or overly optimistic compared with reality, parents will be unhappy and resentful of their situation. The closer a child matches or exceeds the parents' preconceptions, the more positive the overall experience will be for the child and parents. This is why it is so critical to be honest and realistic when discussing a prospective adoptee's medical issues and risks.

The mnemonic HOUR is also important because it emphasizes taking enough time to speak with parents. This is a potential life-altering decision for parents and should not be based on a hurried chat between patients or some thoughts based on a quick perusal of the information. It is appropriate to set up an appointment or block out time to speak with parents and be able to discuss matters fully. It is also appropriate to discuss payment for providing a professional opinion and for the time spent with parents, depending on the amount of time and effort expended by the health care professional. As a practical point, medical insurance typically will not cover a pre-adoption referral because the child is not actually part of the family at the time of service. Parents should be aware that any fees charged will be out of pocket.

If parents decide not to proceed with the referral, it is important to remain professional and nonjudgmental, as many feel guilty about making such a decision. If necessary, parents can be reminded that the adoption is supposed to be a positive addition to the family, and if dealing with a potential medical or developmental issue will result in stress and unhappiness, it is probably better not to proceed. It is also important to assess the level of stress and depression the parents may feel following a declined referral. Many families may have overwhelming feelings of guilt or become depressed. They may have feelings of being alone and not know how to ask for help. It is important to discuss this with them and refer them to appropriate psychological resources if needed.

Medical Review for an Adoption of a Child With Special Needs

In doing a medical review for an adoption of a child with special needs, it is important to go over some basic authoritative references (eg, American Academy of Pediatrics *Red Book* [www.aapredbook.org], standard pediatrics textbook, online resources such as *Pediatric Care Online* [www.pediatriccareonline.org]) as well as appropriate references regarding the type of adoptee (eg, foster care, international) because a full discussion of special medical and developmental concerns is well beyond the scope of this chapter. Many parents may have already searched the Internet for any potential medical or developmental issue and spoken with other families online through adoption electronic mailing lists and user groups or through their agency. However, it is still important to discuss special needs with parents at length, as some have misconceptions about the severity of a condition and may underestimate or overestimate the level of care and services required. For example, some parents may not realize that a cleft palate may require multiple surgeries and ongoing consultations with orthodontists, feeding specialists, geneticists, plastic surgeons, and otolaryngologists. Conversely, some parents may not realize the benign nature of many common congenital heart abnormalities like small ventricular septal defect or patent foramen ovale.

International Adoption Medical Review

It is important to recognize that a medical review for an international adoption is quite different from the usual US health care record. Useful information is often missing, translation mistakes and transcription errors frequently occur, medical terminology may not be familiar to US practitioners, and reliability of source materials can be questionable. As mentioned previously, some countries like Russia only offer blind referrals—no official information is provided prior to travel to the country, although adoption agencies may obtain some information through other sources. If parents wish to discuss pretravel information from a blind referral country, such information should be considered of uncertain reliability, and that fact should be conveyed to parents as part of the referral assessment. Some health care professionals and international adoption practices will meet with parents who are doing a blind international adoption to coach and help prepare them to identify children with significant medical, behavioral, and developmental issues while they are overseas. Some practitioners will also make themselves available by e-mail or phone to parents who are traveling to help them with their decision. Parents or the agency will occasionally provide a video of the child being considered. This is usually helpful, although to a limited degree because the videos are usually short (a few minutes), are not translated, and can capture the child at an exceptionally good (or bad) moment, based on the setting, time of day, child's mood, and persons present.

International Travel for International Adoption

Most countries require parents to travel to the birth country to complete the adoption and take custody of the child. Some, like Russia and Ethiopia, require multiple visits. Parents should be advised to prepare themselves for international travel. This involves seeing their own physician to discuss their travel plans and address their health, medications, making sure their immunizations are up to date, and possibly seeing a travel physician for travel immunizations. Proper preparation is important because parents will be the primary caregiver for the new adoptee and must be in good health to be able to take care of the child and optimize bonding. Obviously, the initial interaction and bonding with the child will be negatively affected if a parent is too ill to interact with the child in a meaningful way, especially when the child has just started his or her new life with the family. Boxes 4-3 and 4-4 include a sample questionnaire and checklist for prospective parents to help organize and optimize their travel health issues.

Similar guidelines should be followed for children and young adults who may be accompanying the travelers. Again, a referral to a travel clinic for specific travel recommendations and immunizations may be necessary depending on the primary care physician's comfort, experience with international travel to underdeveloped countries, and access to travel vaccines.[47]

Box 4-3. Sample Health Questionnaire for International Travel

1. When are you traveling? How long will you be at each location?
2. Where are you traveling (eg, countries, regions, towns/cities, urban vs rural)?
3. What kinds of accommodations exist where you will be staying (eg, hotel with air-conditioning, outdoor camping)?
4. What's the purpose of the trip (business, vacation, both)?
5. How will you be traveling—airplane, ship, train, motor vehicle?
6. Have you traveled internationally in the past? Where did you go and when?
7. How old are you?
8. What is your current health status?
9. Do you have any significant medical history (eg, past major illnesses, surgery, chronic health problems, immune disorder, underlying medical conditions)?
10. Do you have any food or environmental allergies? To what (eg, eggs, latex, yeast)?
11. What medications (prescription, nonprescription) are you currently taking or have you taken in the past 3 months?
12. What vaccinations have you had previously, how many doses did you receive, and when (as precisely as possible) were the doses given?
13. Did you have any reaction to any previous vaccinations? Which vaccines and what happened?
14. If you are female, are you pregnant now? Are you trying to become pregnant or planning on becoming pregnant in the next 3 months? Are you breastfeeding?

Box 4-4. Checklist to Prepare for International Travel

1. Learn about the destination(s)—eg, accommodations, food, water, medical services, infectious risks—from reputable, up-to-date sources such as the Centers for Disease Control and Prevention Travelers' Health Web site (wwwnc.cdc.gov/travel/default.aspx) or the World Health Organization International Travel and Health Web site (www.who.int/ith/en).
2. Schedule an appointment with your physician or a travel medicine clinic well in advance of the trip—at least 2 weeks, preferably more.
3. Discuss the answers to the pretravel health questionnaire (Box 4-3).
4. Have a complete medical examination if not done recently or if a trip longer than a month is planned.
5. Obtain a letter from your physician about your health history, medications, allergies, and immunization records.
6. Obtain extra prescriptions for your medications, as well as a letter from your physician explaining your need for the drug, as some countries have strict laws on narcotics. Know the generic names of your medications because pharmaceutical companies overseas may use different brand names from those in the United States.
7. Discuss with your physician how you will take medication as you cross time zones.

Box 4-4. Checklist to Prepare for International Travel, continued

8. Get the appropriate immunizations for your travel.

   Routine: includes tetanus, diphtheria, pertussis (whooping cough), varicella (chickenpox), measles, mumps, rubella (German measles), influenza (see www.cdc.gov/vaccines/schedules/easy-to-read/adult.html)[46]

   Recommended: depends on the destination—includes hepatitis A, hepatitis B, typhoid, polio, Japanese encephalitis

   Required: yellow fever for most sub-Saharan African and tropical South American countries; meningococcal for Saudi Arabia during the hajj

9. Make sure you have an ample supply of medication in original, labeled containers. Do not use pill cases or other unlabeled containers.

10. Consider a dental checkup, especially if not done recently, or if a trip longer than one month is planned.

11. Check insurance coverage for travel abroad.

12. Have insurance information cards and claim forms with you.

13. Have an emergency release form.

14. Complete the inside page of your passport with important identification and emergency contact information.

15. Keep a photocopy of your passport at home or separate from your passport in case of loss or theft.

16. If you wear eyeglasses, bring an extra pair with you.

17. As an extra precaution, pack extra eyeglasses and medication in carry-on luggage in case checked baggage is lost.

18. Consider wearing a medical alert bracelet if you have allergies or reactions to medications, insect bites, certain foods, or other unique medical problems.

19. If traveling with children, preteens, or teens, complete all of these steps, including steps 2 through 10 with the child's pediatrician or travel medicine clinic.

Many families will make a medical kit to take with them, often containing basic over-the-counter medications for fever, pain, rashes, diarrhea, and first aid supplies. Box 4-5 is a sample traveler's emergency medical kit. Although there may be some disagreement within the adoption community, it is generally advised that the family not bring antibiotics to administer to their new child while traveling. The family is ill equipped to make a diagnosis of a bacterial infection that would be responsive to antibiotics. In addition, antibiotics for diarrhea may make the diarrhea worse and delay obtaining an accurate stool culture when the child comes to his or her new country. Lastly, there are concerns related to possible allergic reactions to antibiotics given, especially when treating a viral infection, which will not be responsive to the antibiotic.

The pre-adoption experience can be exciting and terrifying for the new adoptive family. By understanding the multiple processes associated with adoptions and the information that may be provided, pediatricians can help significantly reduce

---

Box 4-5. Sample Traveler's Emergency Medical Kit

Prescription Medications for Parents
- Parents should pack all of their prescription medications in their carry-on bag. Bringing extra is also recommended in case originals are lost or broken while traveling.
- Include a list of all parental medications and any medical conditions, including a list of known allergies.

Over-the-counter Medicines and Supplies
- Analgesics/antipyretics for pain/fever (eg, acetaminophen, ibuprofen).
- Antihistamine (for allergic reactions).
- Topical antibiotic/antifungal preparations, topical hydrocortisone.
- Bismuth subsalicylate (available as tablets, caplets, liquid), antacid.
- Bandages, gauze, tape, elastic bandage wraps.
- Insect repellent, sunscreen, lip balm.
- Tweezers, scissors, thermometer.
- Obtain a directory of English-speaking physicians at your destination(s); the International Association for Medical Assistance to Travelers is a good starting point (www.iamat.org/index.cfm). Parents may also ask their adoption agency for a list of health care professionals whom other families have used.
- If traveling with infants or children, schedule an appointment with the child's pediatrician or travel medicine clinic and complete all steps.

---

parents' anxiety and fear, obtain and interpret information for families adopting domestically, and better prepare families for their new arrival. With international adoption, pediatricians can evaluate and interpret any information that may be provided. If the pediatrician is unfamiliar with the specifics of international adoptions, a referral can be made to a number of international adoption specialty clinics (see www2.aap.org/sections/adoption/directory/map-adoption.cfm).[48] The ultimate goal is to help prepare families for the successful integration of an adopted child into their new family.

References

1. US Department of Health and Human Services Administration for Children and Families. Trends in foster care and adoption FY2002–FY2011. http://www.acf.hhs.gov/programs/cb/resource/trends-in-foster-care-and-adoption. Accessed February 11, 2014
2. US Department of State Bureau of Consular Affairs. Intercountry adoption: statistics. http://adoption.state.gov/about_us/statistics.php. Accessed February 11, 2014
3. US Government Printing Office. HR 867: Adoption and Safe Families Act of 1997. http://www.gpo.gov/fdsys/pkg/BILLS-105hr867enr/pdf/BILLS-105hr867enr.pdf. Accessed February 11, 2014
4. Child Welfare Information Gateway. *Use of Advertising and Facilitators in Adoptive Placements.* Washington, DC: US Department of Health and Human Services, Children's Bureau; 2012
5. Child Welfare Information Gateway. *Openness in Adoption.* Washington, DC: US Department of Health and Human Services, Children's Bureau; 2003

6. University of Massachusetts Amherst Department of Psychology. Minnesota/Texas Adoption Project. http://www.psych.umass.edu/adoption. Accessed February 11, 2014

7. Child Welfare Information Gateway. The adoption home study process. https://www.childwelfare. gov/pubs/f_homstu.cfm. Accessed February 11, 2014

8. US Citizenship and Immigration Services. Hague process. http://www.uscis.gov/adoption/ immigration-through-adoption/hague-process. Accessed February 11, 2014

9. US Citizenship and Immigration Services. Orphan process. http://www.uscis.gov/adoption/ immigration-through-adoption/orphan-process. Accessed February 11, 2014

10. US Citizenship and Immigration Services. Adoptions based forms. http://www.uscis.gov/forms/ adoptions-based-forms. Accessed February 11, 2014

11. Hague Conference on Private International Law. Welcome to the intercountry adoption section. http://www.hcch.net/index_en.php?act=text.display&tid=45. Accessed February 11, 2014

12. Convention of 29 May 1993 on Protection of Children and Co-operation in Respect of Intercountry Adoption. http://www.hcch.net/index_en.php?act=conventions.text&cid=69. Accessed February 11, 2014

13. US Department of State Bureau of Consular Affairs. Convention countries. http://adoption.state. gov/hague_convention/countries.php. Accessed February 11, 2014

14. US Department of State Bureau of Consular Affairs. Hague adoption process. http://adoption.state. gov/adoption_process/how_to_adopt/hague.php. Accessed February 11, 2014

15. US Citizenship and Immigration Services. After approval of orphan and Hague application. http:// www.uscis.gov/adoption/after-approval/after-approval-orphan-and-hague-application. Accessed February 11, 2014

16. US Citizenship and Immigration Services. Before your child immigrates to the United States. http://www.uscis.gov/adoption/your-child-immigrates-united-states. Accessed February 11, 2014

17. Child Welfare Information Gateway. *Adoption Assistance for Children Adopted From Foster Care.* Washington, DC: US Department of Health and Human Services, Children's Bureau; 2011

18. Child Welfare Information Gateway. *Regulation of Private Domestic Adoption Expenses.* Washington, DC: US Department of Health and Human Services, Children's Bureau; 2010

19. US Department of Health and Human Services Administration for Children and Families. Child welfare policy manual: title IV-E, adoption assistance program, international adoptions. http:// www.acf.hhs.gov/cwpm/programs/cb/laws_policies/laws/cwpm/policy_dsp.jsp?citID=175. Accessed February 11, 2014

20. Takayama JI, Wolfe E, Coulter KP. Relationship between reason for placement and medical findings among children in foster care. *Pediatrics.* 1998;101:201–207

21. Landsverk JA, Burns BJ, Stambaugh LF, Rolls Reutz JA. *Mental Health Care for Children and Adolescents in Foster Care: Review of Research Literature.* Report prepared for Casey Family Programs, 2006. http://www.casey.org/Resources/Publications/pdf/MentalHealthCareChildren.pdf. Accessed February 11, 2014

22. Simms MD, Dubowitz H, Szilagyi MA. Health care needs of children in the foster care system. *Pediatrics.* 2000;106:909–917

23. Harman J, Childs G, Kelleher K. Mental health care utilization and expenditures by children in foster care. *Arch Pediatr Adolesc Med.* 2000;154:1114–1117

24. Steele J, Buchi K. Medical and mental health of children entering the Utah foster care system. *Pediatrics.* 2008;122:e703–e709

25. Szilagyi M. The pediatrician and the child in foster care. *Pediatr Rev.* 1998;19:39–50

26. Rubin D, O'Reilly A, Luan X, Localio R. The impact of placement stability on behavioral well-being for children in foster care. *Pediatrics.* 2007;119:336–344

27. Children's Rights. Facts about foster care. http://childrensrights.org/issues-resources/foster-care/ facts-about-foster-care. Accessed February 11, 2014

28. Austin L. Mental health needs of youth in foster care: challenges and strategies. *The Connection: Quarterly Magazine of the National Court Appointed Special Advocate Association.* 2004;20:6–13

29. Leslie LK, Gordon JN, Ganger W, Gist K. Prevalence of developmental delay in young children in child welfare by placement type. *Infant Ment Health J.* 2002;23:496–516

30. Leslie LK, Hurlburt MS, Landsverk J, Barth R, Slymen DJ. Outpatient mental health services for children in foster care: a national perspective. *Child Abuse Negl.* 2004;28:697–712

31. Stahmer AC, Leslie LK, Hurlburt M, et al. Developmental and behavioral need and service use for young children in child welfare. *Pediatrics.* 2005;116:891–900

32. Smithgall C, Gladden RM, Howard E, George R, Courtney M. *Educational Experiences of Children in Out-of-home Care.* Chicago, IL: Chapin Hall Center for Children at the University of Chicago; 2004

33. Burns BJ, Phillips SD, Wagner HR, et al. Mental health need and access to mental health services by youth involved with child welfare: a national survey. *J Am Acad Child Adolesc Psychiatry.* 2004;43:960–970

34. Colman E, Forkey H, Sagor L. Unexpected anthropometric findings in children entering foster care: experience of the UMass FaCES Clinic. Platform presentation, Pediatric Academic Society Annual Meeting, Honolulu, Hawaii, 2008

35. Johnson DE. Medical and developmental sequelae of early childhood institutionalization in international adoptees from Romania and the Russian Federation. In: Nelson CA, ed. *The Effects of Early Adversity on Neurobehavioral Development.* Mahwah, NJ: Lawrence Erlbaum Associates; 2000:113–162

36. Merz EC, McCall RB. Behavior problems in children adopted from psychosocially depriving institutions. *J Abnorm Child Psychol.* 2010;38:459–470

37. Juffer F, van IJzendoorn MH. Behavior problems and mental health referrals of international adoptees: a meta-analysis. *JAMA.* 2005;293:2501–2515

38. Hawk B, McCall RB. CBCL problems of post-institutionalized international adoptees. *Clin Child Fam Psychol Rev.* 2010;13:199–211

39. Gunnar MR, Van Dulmen MHM. Behavior problems in post-institutionalized international adoptees. *Dev Psychopathol.* 2007;19:129–148

40. Zeanah CH, Egger HL, Smyke AT, et al. Institutional rearing and psychiatric disorders in Romanian preschool children. *Am J Psychiatry.* 2009;166:777–785

41. Fox NA, Almas AN, Degnan KA, Nelson CA, Zeanah CH. The effects of severe psychosocial deprivation and foster care intervention on cognitive development at 8 years of age: findings from the Bucharest Early Intervention Project. *J Child Psychol Psychiatry.* 2011;52:919–928

42. Miller LC. *The Handbook of International Adoption Medicine.* New York, NY: Oxford University Press; 2005

43. Child Welfare Information Gateway. "Special needs" adoption: what does it mean? http://www.childwelfare.gov/pubs/factsheets/specialneeds. Accessed February 11, 2014

44. Child Welfare Information Gateway. Adoption assistance by state. http://www.childwelfare.gov/adoption/adopt_assistance. Accessed February 11, 2014

45. American Academy of Pediatrics. Medical evaluation of internationally adopted children for infectious diseases. In: Pickering LK, Baker CJ, Kimberlin DW, Long SS, eds. *Red Book: 2012 Report of the Committee on Infectious Diseases.* Elk Grove Village, IL: American Academy of Pediatrics; 2012:191–199

46. Centers for Disease Control and Prevention. Immunization schedules for adults in easy-to-read formats. http://www.cdc.gov/vaccines/schedules/easy-to-read/adult.html. Accessed February 11, 2014

47. American Academy of Pediatrics. International travel. In: Pickering LK, Baker CJ, Kimberlin DW, Long SS, eds. *Red Book: 2012 Report of the Committee on Infectious Diseases*. Elk Grove Village, IL: American Academy of Pediatrics; 2012:103–109

48. American Academy of Pediatrics Council on Foster Care, Adoption, and Kinship Care. Adoption search. http://www2.aap.org/sections/adoption/directory/map-adoption.cfm. Accessed February 11, 2014

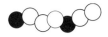

CHAPTER 5

Prenatal Substance Exposure: Alcohol and Other Substances— Implications for Adoption

Claire D. Coles, PhD

The phone call. "Should we adopt this child?"

When it is a newborn, the parents call directly or through a friend to ask about the effects of substance abuse on the child's development. Often, they are referred by an adoption agency. The stories are very similar—the child is about to be born or has just been born and is about to become available for adoption. The prospective parents have a day or two to decide if they will accept this baby. They have been waiting a long time for a baby, and if they turn down this chance, they are not sure when the next one will come. Drug testing at the hospital reveals that the mother has been using cocaine, methamphetamines, opiates, or, most commonly, marijuana. The specter of drug exposure turns a potentially joyous moment into an anxious one. There are several reactions to this dilemma; one is to seek expert information about the child's prognosis.

This scenario highlights the dilemma that many parents will go through as they think about an adoption. Regardless of how the child may join the family—adopted as a newborn, through foster care, from an international orphanage—concerns of drug abuse or alcohol exposure may be present. These issues are also a problem for the "expert" on the other end of the phone call or in the primary care office. Although the pediatrician's role is vital in supporting families during the pre-placement period and later providing a medical home that will support the family by monitoring the developing child and offering appropriate care, health care professionals can sometimes find it difficult to answer parents' underlying questions, including, "Will this child be healthy?" "Will there be long-term developmental problems?" and "Should we adopt this child?"

For a newborn, these answers cannot be provided for several reasons. First, there is often only minimal information about the mother and baby, and in the case of the newborn, the "expert" may not have any opportunity to evaluate the actual people who are the focus of the discussion. Thus, the discussion has to be in general terms, referring to the research on the effects of these substances on a child's development. Because there is considerable heterogeneity in outcomes seen in exposed newborns and older children, it is impossible to predict whether a given child will be affected simply on the basis of knowledge of exposure. Drug screens may have revealed marijuana or cocaine use, but the potential parent often has not thought to ask about alcohol, cigarettes, or prescription drugs, which are more common than illicit drugs. There is no reliable screening test for prenatal alcohol exposure, and hospitals or agencies may not have this information. Information about alcohol and cigarettes is usually based solely on the birth parent's report and thus may be absent or unreliable. Prospective or adoptive parents who are warned about cocaine, methamphetamines, or heroin may not be as concerned about exposure to alcohol and cigarettes, but because it is highly likely there was polysubstance exposure, it seems responsible to ask whether they have considered these further issues. In addition, there are a number of social and medical problems associated with maternal substance use that will likely affect the successful integration of the child into the new family.

One important role for the pediatrician is helping prospective parents understand what questions should be asked as they consider adoption. These questions may concern the birth mother's substance use and lifestyle but may also focus on prospective parents' tolerance for dealing with developmental problems in an adopted child. In raising these issues, medical professionals may increase the concerns parents are feeling, which can affect their decision about adoption or reactions to their child's behavior later in development. There is also a potential ethical dilemma for the expert in talking with parents. What are the effects of the information provided on prospective parents and vulnerable neonates? If prospective parents decide to reject a child based on their concerns about substance exposure, the child may not be placed in a supportive caregiving environment and may, therefore, have a less positive outcome. If parents decide to accept the child, the outcomes cannot be predicted—they may be positive or negative.

When a child has been adopted, different questions are asked, such as, "What should parents expect?" "How should they interpret behavior?" "What are appropriate services?" "Where can they find resources?" In working with children and families, it is important for the pediatrician to understand the nature and extent of the risks as well as how prenatal exposure and parental substance abuse affect the developing child and to have the tools available to support positive outcomes.

Substance Abuse and Adoption: How Great Is the Risk?

Children from substance-abusing families make up a significant percentage of those available for adoption in the United States. In 2009, 57,466 children with public child welfare agency involvement were adopted in the United States,[1] with 107,011 children in these systems waiting for adoption. It is estimated that among those families whose children entered foster care at birth or later, 70% to 80% had some involvement with substance abuse.[2] In addition, in comparison with other

---

Case Study: Domestic Adoption Through Protective Services System

Estivan is an 11-year-old Hispanic male. His adoptive mother, a college graduate, is 40 years old, unmarried, and employed as a restaurant manager. Estivan is the fourth of 11 known pregnancies to his birth mother. He was born at 28 weeks' gestational age and had a number of medical problems associated with prematurity, including respiratory distress syndrome, hypoglycemia, and a long term on a respirator. He remained in the nursery for 4 months postnatally. Currently, he is described as in good health.

The adoptive mother is a relative of the birth mother. The birth father is unknown. The child's mother, 30 years old at his birth, abandoned him in the hospital. The birth mother was observed to use drugs—crack cocaine and marijuana—and alcohol during the pregnancy. The child had positive urine toxicology at birth. Estivan's adoptive mother describes their relationship as "very close," although he was taken into custody earlier this year when bruises were noted at school and he was found to have been beaten with a belt. His adoptive mother described Estivan as moody and oppositional and reports that he does things "just to get his own way" and "fake cries" at times. In discussion with the pediatrician, his adoptive mother reported that Estivan is negative and oppositional and tries to have his own way all the time.

Estivan is in the fifth grade in a regular classroom setting. He is reported to have difficulty in school in academics and socially and does not do his homework. He is also reported to have problems getting along with other children. His adoptive mother has raised questions about learning disabilities, attention-deficit/hyperactivity disorder, and effects of prenatal drug exposure. The family has received a number of services through county agencies this year and also in the previous year through a nonprofit faith-based agency. Currently, Estivan and his adoptive mother are in family counseling with a psychologist. When given psychologic and academic testing, he was found to be of average ability and have appropriate achievement scores. He was also noted to show restlessness, inattentiveness, and anxiety that could interfere with learning. On questionnaires completed by his adoptive mother, Estivan was rated as demonstrating relative delays in adaptive performance and a moderate level of behavior problems. Problems in the parent/child relationship were noted. A multidisciplinary team led by a pediatrician made the following diagnoses:

- Prenatal exposure to noxious substance (cocaine)
- Disorders related to preterm infants unspecified weight
- Abuse of a child
- Parent/child relational problem

The team recommended that Estivan and his mother participate in Parent-Child Interaction Therapy to address the parent/child problems identified during the assessment and that his pediatrician monitor Estivan's subsequent adjustment with a yearly assessment of his emotional and educational status. It was also recommended that his mother have supportive counseling and that she be provided with information about family support groups.

groups, a higher percentage of children of substance abusers are eventually placed for adoption rather than reunited with their families.[3] If these statistics are applied to the number adopted, it can be assumed that more than 40,000 children with a history of parental substance abuse are adopted each year domestically. Thus, more than 7 million children younger than 18 years born in the United States may have experienced parental substance abuse that was severe enough to have led to loss of custody. The number of these children with prenatal exposure is unknown, but it is likely that the number is significant.

The number of internationally adopted children who have been prenatally exposed is difficult to establish and probably varies depending on the country of origin. The total number of intercountry adoptions between 1999 and 2010 is reported to be 224,615 by the US Department of State (2010),[4] with 2002 through 2007 the period during which the greatest number of children were adopted. The countries from which the most children were adopted in these years were China, Guatemala, and Russia.[5] The number of children exposed to alcohol and other drugs probably varies by country of origin, with Eastern European countries believed to have the highest percentage, with perhaps as many as 20% of children adopted from countries making up the former Soviet Union affected by alcohol and other drugs.[6]

Effects of Prenatal Exposure to Various Substances of Abuse

At the present time, many of the children who become available for adoption have a history of exposure to potentially teratogenic substances due to maternal use during pregnancy. The most common exposures include alcohol, tobacco, marijuana, and a variety of prescription medications that may have been used with or without medical supervision (Figure 5-1).[7] Less likely but still relatively common are so-called "hard drugs"—cocaine, methamphetamines, heroin, and other opiates.

One of the reasons for concern about children born to women who use and abuse substances during pregnancy is the potential for a teratogenic effect of these substances on the embryo and fetus. The areas that are generally considered to be of concern are prenatal and postnatal growth, physical malformations of various kinds, and neurodevelopment as a result of effects of the substances on the central nervous system (CNS). Many of the substances of abuse (alcohol, cigarettes, prescription drugs including narcotics and depressants, and illicit drugs such as cocaine, heroin, marijuana, and methamphetamines) have been the subject of study. Although not all of these have been comprehensively researched (particularly prescription medications), it is known that some are teratogens that will affect development of the child. This information can be of use in managing the care of adopted children with such exposures.

It can be difficult, however, to determine whether any developmental issues are related to substances of abuse or other factors. Variables such as socioeconomic

Case Study: Internationally Adopted Child

Tatiana is a 6-year-old white female adopted from an Eastern European orphanage at 15 months. The older adoptive parents are well educated, upper-middle-class professionals who have no other children. Records from the country of origin note that her birth mother, age 37, was a "registered alcoholic" and used "drugs." (In the birth country, this description generally refers to injected heroin.) The child was born at 32 weeks' gestational age (8 weeks preterm) and was noted to have a number of medical problems at birth including positive tests for hepatitis C, cytomegalovirus, and toxoplasmosis. Test results for hepatitis B, HIV, and syphilis were negative. The child was abandoned in the hospital following birth and when stable was transferred to a "baby home," where she remained until adopted. It appeared that the orphanage did not provide adequate stimulation and that there was no opportunity to form an attachment with a caregiver while in this facility. By report, she was severely delayed at 15 months; she couldn't sit up and she had very low muscle tone when her parents first brought her home. There is a history of bilateral strabismus and she is followed by pediatric ophthalmology. Previous chromosome studies, microarray analysis, and fragile X (autism panel) are normal.

In the United States, Tatiana received services from her county's early intervention programs until 3 years of age and then was entered into a preschool for children with special needs with a diagnosis of autism. The preschool referred her for further evaluation to rule out fetal alcohol syndrome (FAS).

Medical examination for physical signs associated with prenatal exposure revealed the following signs: weight less than the fifth percentile, hirsutism of the skin, posterior rotation of the ears, short palpebral fissures, epicanthal folds, bilateral strabismus, upturned nares, small philtrum, and thin vermillion border of upper lip. Toxoplasmosis and herpes simplex were no longer noted, and hepatitis C was not active. Developmental evaluation performed by a psychologist resulted in an overall IQ score of 50, with all other measures of language and adaptive functioning consistent with intellectual disabilities in the mild to moderate range. Language and communication abilities (scores in the 60s) were higher than nonverbal and motor skills, consistent with patterns often observed in FAS disorders. The child was noted to have problems with motor tone and graphomotor planning and hand grasp. No behavioral characteristics consistent with a diagnosis of autism spectrum disorder were noted. The psychologist noted that behaviors associated with institutionalization are often mistaken for autism. Fetal alcohol syndrome, mild intellectual disabilities, and motor coordination disorder were diagnosed in addition to the previously noted medical problems.

Recommendations for future care were made in several domains.

1. *Medical:* follow-up care with developmental pediatrics, with attention to effects of prenatal infections; ophthalmology, with regard to persistent strabismus.
2. *Physical and occupational therapy:* to address delays in motor and graphomotor skills.
3. *Educational:* special educational services. Based on her level of intellectual functioning, Tatiana will require special educational services for the foreseeable future and is eligible for these based on federal law and state regulation.
4. *Social and family support:* There are a number of support groups and agencies that provide information and support for families with children with FAS and intellectual disabilities and who have adopted internationally.
5. *Monitor development and provided anticipatory guidance:* Tatiana will require specialized care over her lifetime. She should be followed closely by her pediatrician, and developmental assessments should be carried out by appropriate professionals during childhood and adolescence to monitor development and behavior. Her parents may need support in adjusting to her diagnosis and providing care.

Figure 5-1.
Percentage of Pregnant Women in Each Age Group Reporting Type of Drug Use

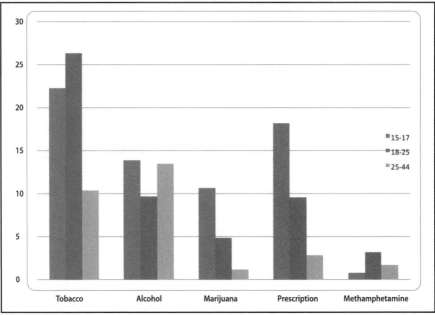

Based on Substance Abuse and Mental Health Services Administration. *Results from the 2003 National Survey on Drug Use and Health: National Findings.* Rockville, MD: Substance Abuse and Mental Health Services Administration; 2004

status, access to medical and social services, and the presence or absence of a male figure in the household have a significant influence on child development. Maternal mental health, social support networks, and stressful life events such as exposure to violence or domestic abuse are also important variables that affect long-term developmental outcomes. Many of these environmental risk factors are directly associated with maternal use of substances of abuse, making it difficult to identify the effect of prenatal exposure in isolation.

Polysubstance Use

In reviewing the effects of various substances, it is important to keep in mind that women who use drugs during pregnancy, which is currently considered to be socially unacceptable, generally use more than one such substance.[8] Cigarettes and alcohol are the most common, with prescription drugs and marijuana being almost equally frequent.[7] Illicit substances, like cocaine, methamphetamines, and narcotics, are used relatively less frequently, probably by fewer than 5%.[9] Some of these substances are readily identifiable through urine toxicology, while alcohol, probably the exposure of greatest concern, does not have a reliable biomarker in pregnancy. Research on the effects of individual substances follows but should be considered in the likely context of polysubstance abuse.

Tobacco

Although increasing pressure is being placed on women who smoke to stop during pregnancy, the majority of smoking mothers fail to do so, with 15% to 25% of all expectant mothers continuing tobacco use during gestation.[10] Nicotine and its by-product, cotinine, are found in fetal serum and amniotic fluid at 15% higher concentrations than in maternal blood. These substances can last for 15 to 20 hours[11] and can be further ingested postnatally by nursing newborns.[12] There is no consistent evidence that smoking during pregnancy is associated with major structural anomalies; however, physical and medical outcomes that have been linked to tobacco exposure, after controlling for pertinent demographic and confounding variables, include decreased growth[13] as well as increased risk for spontaneous abortion[14,15] and sudden infant death syndrome.[16] In reviews of effects of maternal smoking during pregnancy, evidence for the association with lower birth weight is overwhelming, even when demographic and other potentially confounding variables are controlled.[17,18] Interestingly, this growth retardation does not persist, and older children who were exposed prenatally to tobacco smoke may show excessive weight gain as they age.[19,20]

In early childhood, tobacco exposure is associated with decreased lung function, increased airway responsivity,[21] and higher risk for obstructive sleep apnea.[22] An increased incidence of asthma, although not allergic-based asthma, is also reported.[23] Multiple reviews of the relationship between tobacco exposure and otitis media conclude that there is an increased risk in this area,[24,25] with prenatal exposure associated with a greater risk than postnatal exposure.[26]

Finally, there have been concerns about the effects of tobacco exposure on cognition and behavior. Evidence for a general cognitive deficit during infancy and early childhood is mixed,[27–30] as is evidence for effects on academic achievement,[29,31,32] leading many to suggest that social factors account for observed differences. There is more support for a specific deficit in auditory processing and early language development. Fried and Watkinson[27] found evidence of an effect on language development in the preschool period and later in the middle-class Ottawa Prenatal Prospective Study cohort,[33] as well as on phonology and articulation[29] and later verbal memory skills.[33,34] In other samples that provide converging evidence, pre-linguistic skills in 6-month-olds[35,36] and vocalization of vowel-consonant combinations were delayed in smokers' children at 8 months.[37] In older children, vocabulary expression and receptive language was impaired,[38–40] and problems in reading have been found.[28,41,42]

Auditory processing deficits may be the basis for problems in language and reading. In children of smokers, poorer auditory habituation on standardized infant assessment has been found repeatedly.[43–45] Franco and colleagues[46] reported that newborns and 12-week-olds of smokers showed decreased arousal to auditory stimuli compared with newborns and infants of nonsmokers. Evidence in older infants and children is more limited but consistent,[47] suggesting that there may be an underlying auditory processing deficit associated with prenatal exposure to tobacco smoke that manifests in delays in early language development and specific aspects of reading development.

There is a great deal of evidence that tobacco exposure is associated with arousal dysregulation and behavior problems of various severities, including attention-deficit/hyperactivity disorder (ADHD), antisocial behavior, and criminality in adulthood.[48] Alterations in responsiveness have been observed over the whole of childhood beginning in the fetal period[49] as well as later infancy[50–52] and in older children in the areas of poorer attentional control[53,54] and behavioral and conduct problems.[55–63] In summary, although the effects of tobacco exposure on development have been somewhat overlooked, accumulating evidence suggests that there may be grounds for concern in certain areas, particularly in language, auditory processing, and behavior.

Alcohol

Despite 40 years of prevention efforts, almost 2% of pregnant women report drinking heavily (7 or more drinks/week) and 10% to 12% report drinking at lower levels.[64,65] There are a range of negative outcomes associated with such exposure that have been labeled fetal alcohol spectrum disorders (FASDs). The most severe is fetal alcohol syndrome (FAS), which is diagnosed based on knowledge of maternal alcohol use during gestation and the presence of growth retardation (<10th percentile) in weight, length, or height; dysmorphology, including certain sentinel features (Figure 5-2); and evidence of damage to the CNS, which may include a reduced head circumference, neurologic signs (eg, seizures, cerebral palsy), or neurodevelopmental deficits.[66] Neurodevelopmental deficits range from developmental delays that can be observed in infancy and global deficits in learning and adaptive functioning in older individuals to milder expressions that manifest as learning disabilities and behavioral problems.[67] In addition, alcohol-related neurodevelopmental disorder has been described, which does not involve facial dysmorphology or growth retardation but instead affects only cognition and behavior.[68]

The *facial dysmorphia* associated with heavy exposure is 1 of the 3 aspects of teratogenic exposure used to define FAS. These features include midface hypoplasia; short palpebral fissures; flattened or indistinct philtrum, usually associated with a thin or flattened upper vermillion; and anteverted nares. Other minor anomalies are also commonly found in affected children, including epicanthal folds, low

Figure 5-2.
Facial Features Associated With Prenatal Alcohol Exposure

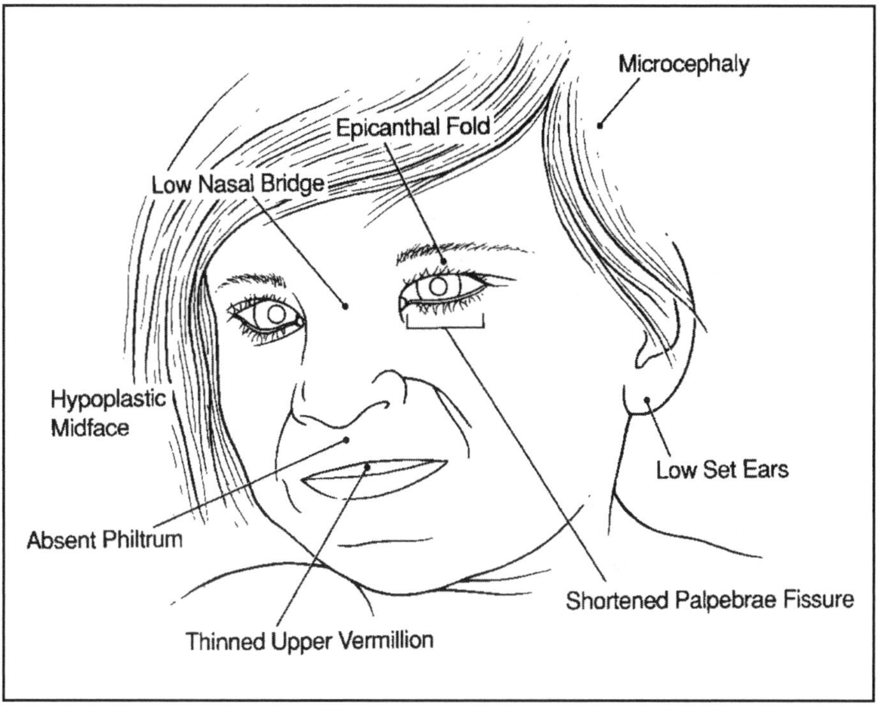

Facial features associated with prenatal alcohol exposure, including those that are considered sentinel features of fetal alcohol syndrome—microcephaly, shortened palpebral fissures, absent philtrum, and thin upper vermillion. Other features that are frequently observed include ptosis, strabismus, epicanthal folds, low nasal bridge, high arched palate, low-set ears, and hypoplastic mandible.

Illustration Credit: Claire D. Coles, PhD

nasal bridge, ear anomalies (low set and rotated), and micrognathia.[66,68] In practice, assessment of these anomalies is complicated by variance associated with age and ethnicity. When affected individuals are followed over childhood into early adulthood, some of the individual features that are salient during infancy and early childhood become harder to identify, particularly after puberty.[69]

Growth retardation, the second of the criteria features of FAS during infancy and the preschool period, is found less consistently in older children and youth.[70,71] In addition, in clinical samples, it can be difficult to establish that growth is affected by alcohol exposure and not by environmental neglect or institutionalization in the case of the internationally adopted child (see Chapter 12, Long-term Growth and Puberty Concerns for Adopted Children, on page 239). Research studies of children with prenatal exposure provide more reliable evidence for the persistence of growth effects. Generally, in exposure samples,[71,72] children exposed to alcohol appear to be smaller than controls or national norms. However, mean heights are often within normal ranges, so while this characteristic is statistically "real," it may or may not be of clinical significance and not necessarily helpful in identification of specific at-risk individuals if maternal alcohol use is unknown. Whether the lower birth weight, height, and head circumference associated with prenatal alcohol exposure (and perhaps associated polysubstance use) will be a risk factor for other conditions that occur later in life (eg, obesity, metabolic disorders) has not yet been established.

Neurodevelopmental effects of prenatal alcohol exposure is the third criteria. Effects of alcohol teratogenesis on the brain and, by extension, behavior have been investigated in a variety of ways. Neuroimaging studies indicate that there are substantial and specific effects of alcohol on brain volume and structure that can be measured over the life span.[73,74] More specifically, effects on white matter integrity have been documented,[75] arguing that this is one of the mechanisms for the observed behavioral deficits. Functional neuroimaging (ie, electroencephalogram, functional magnetic resonance imaging) is limited in this population, but results indicate that functional differences exist in alcohol-affected individuals.[76]

Using behavioral measures, neurodevelopmental effects of alcohol exposure have been extensively documented.[67,77] Global intellectual deficits are often observed as a result of alcohol exposure, and deficits in general intellectual functioning (ie, scores on intelligence or other ability tests) are observed in children diagnosed with FAS and FASD. However, children meeting diagnostic criteria for FAS may show a relatively broad range of intellectual outcomes ranging from severe intellectual deficiency to above average-levels of functioning,[78,79] with the mean level of performance typically in the borderline to mildly intellectually deficient range (IQ 65 to 75).[68] There has also been discussion of the effect of prenatal exposure to low or moderate levels of alcohol, and most research studies have reported that in such cohorts, there is a decrement of several IQ points (4 to 6) attributable to the exposure.[80]

In some individuals, global deficits are not noted, but there may be specific decrements in certain cognitive and functional areas.[81] Motor problems or delays are often noted in infancy,[82,83] and deficits in visual-motor integration[67,84] and fine-motor strength and coordination are often found in older children.[85,86] Other areas of concern include balance,[87] increased clumsiness,[86] abnormal gait,[86] and tremors.[88,89] In addition, a number of neurocognitive functions have been examined and appear to be affected by prenatal alcohol exposure. These include specific deficits in visual-spatial processing[67,70,78,89]; arousal and regulation of attention[90,91]; aspects of executive functioning, including memory, working memory, and planning and organizational skills[84,92–94]; academic achievement, particularly in mathematics[95,96]; as well as behavior and emotional regulation.[97,98]

In summary, alcohol is a teratogen that when used in pregnancy has been found to be associated with a number of negative developmental outcomes. However, not all exposed children are affected, and there is substantial evidence that appropriate care postnatally can improve outcomes even in those who are affected.

Marijuana

In the 1996 National Institute on Drug Abuse survey of the prevalence and patterns of substance use among pregnant women, 2.8% reported marijuana use during their first trimester of pregnancy.[99] This is probably a low estimate, as other studies using urine toxicology measures report much higher rates (20%–27%).[100] If these studies are accurate, marijuana, which is the most commonly used illicit drug, is also, after alcohol and tobacco, the most commonly used substance during pregnancy.[101] Dysmorphology associated with marijuana exposure has not been found, and there is similarly little evidence for an effect on growth.[102] There have only been a few epidemiologic studies of the effects on child development. Most of the existing information concerning the behavioral effects of prenatal exposure to marijuana comes from reports of the Ottawa Prenatal Prospective Study[103] and the work of Nancy Day and her colleagues. According to Goldschmidt, Day, and Richardson,[101] it is difficult to isolate the effects of marijuana exposure from its correlates and environmental risk factors.

In the examination of outcomes, the Ottawa study found that prenatal exposure to marijuana was associated with less optimal responses on learning paradigms at birth and over the first month,[43] but when the same children were examined at 12 months, no adverse effects of exposure were noted.[27] Later, an effect on verbal ability and memory was observed in 4-year-olds but not at ages 2, 3, 5, or 6 years after statistically adjusting for other important variables such as ratings of the home environment.[34] Effects on child behavior problems at preschool and school age and on child behavior problems at age 10 were reported with prenatal marijuana exposure in the first and third trimesters, predicting significantly increased hyperactivity, inattention, and impulsivity symptoms.[34,104] O'Connell and Fried[104] also found that mothers who used marijuana heavily during pregnancy rated their children as being more impulsive or hyperactive. After statistically controlling for maternal personality and home environment conditions, many of the neurobehavioral consequences of prenatal exposure to marijuana do not remain significant. According to Fried,[103] the only definitive statement about prenatal exposure to marijuana would be that if there are long-term consequences, such effects are very subtle. At this point, human studies are relatively sparse, and no precise mechanism of action has been substantiated.[105]

Cocaine and Other Stimulants

Although the epidemic of cocaine and crack use that began in the 1980s has waned to some extent (perhaps replaced by methamphetamine), the problem of prenatal exposure to cocaine and other stimulants persists. Women reporting cocaine use also reported use of tobacco and alcohol, and some combine the use of cocaine or crack with heroin.[106] According to the Substance Abuse and Mental Health Services Administration,[7] 4.3% of pregnant women report using an illicit drug within the past month, although the number using cocaine and amphetamines is likely to be 1% to 2% based on previous studies.[107] Because of concerns raised during the "crack baby" period,[108] there has been extensive examination of the teratogenic potential in animal models and clinical studies.[109-112] Cocaine does not seem to be associated with any physical dysmorphology, but exposure has been associated with lower gestational age and reduced birth weight and length (see Gouin et al for a meta-analysis).[113] However, most cocaine-exposed children do not have "clinically significant" growth failure and appear to have a postnatal catch-up in growth. For instance, in comparing preterm and full-term cocaine-exposed infants to socioeconomic status–matched contrast groups, Coles et al[114] found that growth differences could no longer be observed by 8 weeks of age and that over 24 months, there were no differences in growth rate for weight, length, or ponderal index. In the same sample, at 8 years postpartum, there were no effects of prenatal exposure on growth, including height, weight, and head circumference.[115]

Studies of neurodevelopmental effects of cocaine have found few direct effects on intellectual development that cannot be accounted for by caregiving environment.[116,117] Kilbride et al[118] reported that at 36 months, no effects on cognition, psychomotor skills, or language were observed in exposed children who had received case management services compared with those who did not and a nonexposed contrast group. They did find that those exposed children who remained with their mothers and did not receive services had lower verbal scores on intelligence tests and measures of language development than those in contrast groups. Similarly, in a follow-up study examining outcomes at 4 to 6 years, Chasnoff et al[119] reported that differences in developmental functioning in their clinical samples can be accounted for by environmental factors, principally caregiver behavior. In contrast, Mayes et al[120] reported that cocaine-exposed children show "delayed developmental indices" relative to controls and children exposed to other illicit drugs but that their developmental trajectories from 3 to 36 months are parallel to those of other groups. Examination of mean scores suggests that none of the groups tested can be defined as delayed, although by 36 months, all groups are scoring about one standard deviation below the mean on standardized tests, a phenomenon commonly associated with environmental deprivation. Similarly, Richardson and colleagues[121,122] found that 3-year-old cocaine-exposed children followed in 2 different longitudinal samples had different cognitive outcomes, demonstrating the extent to which these outcomes are dependent on sampling and other methodologic considerations.

An effect of cocaine on cognition is suggested by its reported effects on attention. Mayes et al[123] reported that cocaine exposure affected 3-month-olds' ability to complete a procedure measuring attention. Brown et al[116] found differences in attentional response associated with prenatal cocaine but not other illicit drug exposure at 8 weeks. However, as these authors note, the caregiving instability associated with maternal drug use independently accounted for more variance in attentional response than did the direct effect of cocaine. In a sample of older children, Savage and colleagues[124] report "subtle" effects on errors of commission and task efficiency on a vigilance task in prenatally exposed 10-year-olds who were otherwise not different from controls on a number of behavioral measures. These findings raise concerns about the vulnerability of exposed children who, in addition to physiological dysregulation associated with prenatal exposure to cocaine and other drugs, are clearly also at environmental risk for an increased incidence of developmental psychopathology.

The most persuasive evidence for a behavioral effect of cocaine concerns the effect on regulation of physiological arousal that has been observed from early infancy through adolescence and may be associated with an effect on dopamine regulation.[125] Physiological arousal is associated with temperament and social-emotional development. Several investigators have identified increased irritability in newborns and young infants[126–129] and alterations in psychophysiology, including heart rate and respiration.[130] These effects persist beyond the neonatal period and appear to be associated with the ability to modulate stress responses using executive functioning skills.[131–133]

Prenatal stimulant exposure is a marker for a constellation of risk factors that appear to have negative consequences for the infant and developing child. An increased incidence of behavior problems has been reported in children of illicit drug-using mothers, in particular with prenatal cocaine exposure.[115,134,135] Accornero et al[136] argued that such behavior was more related to maternal psychologic functioning than to cocaine exposure. No specific "cocaine syndrome" has yet emerged, and many of the problems previously anticipated have not manifested. However, the weight of the evidence suggests that cocaine exposure may produce an increased vulnerability to certain environmental stressors. The interactions of these factors may have long-term negative consequences for children.

Methamphetamine presents a similar problem, but there is as yet a limited body of research on the effects of this drug. Recently published studies focus on maternal characteristics and infancy status.[137–139] These studies note that maternal characteristics are similar to those found in women using heroin and cocaine[137,138] and that neonates present with behavior responses characteristic of exposure to other stimulants, including decreased arousal postnatally and greater vulnerability to stress.[139] These results suggest that methamphetamine may have effects similar to those associated with cocaine; however, it is important to reserve judgment until further research is available.

Opiates

Studies report prevalence for opiate use during pregnancy to range from fewer than 1% to 2% to as high as 21%.[140,141] Opiates include illegal drugs (eg, heroin) as well as certain prescription medications, like oxycodone, which may be misused by addicts. Methadone maintenance has become accepted as the standard of care for opiate addiction during pregnancy[142] but has similar effects on the fetus. The literature on developmental outcomes for infants prenatally exposed to opiates is relatively sparse and was primarily generated in the 1970s and early 1980s. The literature is also made more problematic because of the issue of polysubstance abuse, as research investigating prenatal opiate exposure includes exposure to heroin, methadone, or both and may also include exposure to amphetamines, barbiturates, benzodiazepines, cocaine, alcohol, and nicotine.[143] There is no evidence of a dysmorphic syndrome associated with opiates, and according to Kandall et al,[142] no study has identified malformations or an increase in any specific dysmorphic syndrome that could be related to maternal methadone maintenance. The most consistently reported effects of prenatal opiate exposure are fetal growth retardation and neonatal abstinence syndrome.[106] Neonatal abstinence is described by Kaltenbach and Finnegan[144] as a generalized disorder characterized by signs and symptoms of CNS hyperirritability, gastrointestinal dysfunction, respiratory distress, and vague autonomic symptoms that include yawning, sneezing, mottling, and fever. These signs are observed in the neonatal period and do not persist.[145]

Studies of the early development of heroin- and methadone-exposed offspring indicate relatively normal intellectual development, at least during infancy.[146] In studies by Hans and Marcus, no differences in mental development were found at 4, 12, and 24 months of age when comparing opiate-exposed and nonexposed children.[147,148] Kaltenbach and Finnegan[144] found no differences in mental development scores at 6, 12, and 24 months when the 2 groups were compared. Between 3 and 6 years of age, heroin-exposed children performed more poorly than their peers on a cognitive index in one study but the same on behavior and skills in another study.[148] Kaltenbach[143] concludes her review of the effects of prenatal opiate exposure by stating that opiate-exposed children through 2 years of age function well within the normal range of development and that children between 2 and 5 years of age do not differ in cognitive function from other high-risk populations.

Illicit drug use is associated with late and inadequate prenatal care, poverty, poor nutrition, domestic and stranger violence, and other severe threats to maternal and infant health.[149] It is especially difficult to identify the effect of a specific illicit substance such as heroin because of the issue of polysubstance abuse. As with cocaine exposure, outcomes of heroin and methadone exposure are more strongly related to home and parenting environment variables than direct drug effects.[143] Thus, early caregiving history should be taken into account in working with the child prenatally exposed to opiates.

In summary, substance use and abuse during pregnancy is common, and children of mothers who abuse drugs during pregnancy are affected by a range of biological and environmental factors. At the present time, it is clear that there are negative effects of substance abuse on fetal development and family function and that these consequences must be taken into consideration in working with exposed children, including those who have been adopted. The physical and behavioral problems seen in children with prenatal exposure to drugs and other substances are the result of many related factors such as poverty, exposure to violence, and lack of access to medical and social services. These factors likely interact with the initial prenatal substance exposure to negatively affect long-term developmental outcomes for the child.

Supporting the Child and Family

To treat adopted children with prenatal substance exposure and provide support to their families, health care professionals must address a series of issues. First, when acting as a pre-placement resource, the goal is to best provide appropriate guidance to families who are considering adopting an exposed child. The Evan B. Donaldson Adoption Institute, in discussing adoptive parent preparation, notes that the more informed and realistic the pre-adoptive parents, the more positive the outcomes for parents and child.[150] As discussed in the initial example, the problem of polysubstance exposure and the variability in outcomes would make definitive recommendations difficult even if such recommendations were appropriate. Although the risk of developmental and behavioral problems is elevated, many children with prenatal exposure escape serious problems, and in addition to the direct effects of the exposure, there are a variety of associated factors that may affect outcomes. These include the child's genetic background, effects of the birth mother's medical history, extent to which the child has had a nonoptimal early caregiving experience, and availability of resources to support positive developmental outcomes. During pre-adoption planning, pediatricians can discuss the risks of exposure to various substances with prospective parents and counsel them on other lifestyle factors that often co-occur with maternal substance abuse. This information can support the family in asking the right questions during the process and also help them to have appropriate expectations as the child grows. Information about maternal substance abuse and health is usually available to social service agencies and in medical records and should be obtained in the pre-adoption period if possible as part of the process of finalizing the adoption.

The circumstances are different when a child enters the practice and is identified as adopted. Then, pediatricians must be cognizant of the possibility of prenatal exposure and the recommendations of the American Academy of Pediatrics (AAP) in caring for such children.[151,152] The first step will be to take a good history that includes information about the birth parent. When there is suspicion of prenatal exposure, pediatricians may be able to confirm by requesting birth records and social service reports. When the child is in a family placement, relatives of the birth mother may be available to provide information about the pregnancy. While it may feel awkward to ask a grandmother about her daughter's substance abuse, this is often an excellent source of information, and family members are usually open to such discussion when the well-being of the child is a concern. Because family members are aware of the birth mother's problems, they will not be offended if the physician asks focused and direct questions about prenatal exposure. Such questions should be open-ended (eg, "How many days a week did [birth mother] drink alcohol during her pregnancy with [child]? And how many drinks did she have on the days she was drinking?"). Further questions about cigarette smoking (eg, "Was she a cigarette smoker? Did she use a pack a day or more? Less?") and other drug use ("How frequently did she smoke marijuana?") flow directly from this conversation. For the child adopted internationally, information may be more fragmentary, although in some cases, medical records are available from the country of origin and can be translated.

After the child is adopted, the goal is to anticipate any difficulties that may present as a result of the prenatal exposure or postnatal environment, without inducing excessive anxiety or labeling the child in a way that may have negative effects. The ongoing medical home provided by pediatricians is the best way to provide such care. As recommended in 2012 by the AAP,[151] pediatricians can support the child and family by monitoring the child during the developmental process, guided by an understanding of the problem of prenatal exposure, teratogenic effects of various substances on child development immediately and in the long term, and their manifestation at different points during development. In 2000,[152] the AAP made the following specific recommendations for working with families in which alcohol exposure is a factor:

- First, pediatricians should familiarize themselves with the effect of various substances of abuse on child and family outcomes.
- Second, children suspected of such exposure should be evaluated by a pediatrician knowledgeable in the diagnosis of FASD and neurodevelopmental problems that accompany these conditions as early as possible. When necessary, referrals to other specialists are encouraged.
- Finally, parents and other caregivers should be provided with support and anticipatory guidance.

One frequent dilemma for pediatricians is that of differential diagnosis. It may be difficult to decide whether to attribute developmental and behavioral problems to the teratogenic effects of exposure or to co-occurring factors like family genetics or postnatal environmental problems. When the basis for the problem is not obvious (eg, FAS), further evaluation may help to identify contributing factors. Differential diagnosis is important because while the effects of alcohol and other substance use in pregnancy may present as similar to other behavioral disorders (eg, ADHD, conduct disorder), the underlying pathology is different and there is evidence that different treatment modalities are required.[81]

In supporting families, it is helpful to have guidelines that can be used when a prenatally exposed child has been adopted. In some cases, such guidelines have been suggested by public health agencies[66] and professional organizations, such as those on the treatment of alcohol-affected children provided by the AAP.[152] Information about other exposures is less comprehensive, although there are well-evaluated protocols for the treatment of neonates who are experiencing neonatal abstinence syndrome due to opiate exposure.[153] In other cases, such as the appropriate follow-up care for children with cocaine and methamphetamine exposure, there are no standard recommendations available at this time.

Intervention for Children Affected by Alcohol and Substance Use

One concern for many families is how to provide the best care to support optimal learning and development in children who have experienced prenatal substance exposure. Until recently, there was no literature on this topic, and pediatricians did not have access to evidence-based treatment recommendations. However, recent research in this area suggests that children affected by alcohol and other substances of abuse can benefit from standard behavioral and educational interventions[154] as well as from more focused approaches that take into account the specific characteristics of affected children.[155,156] In their summary of 5 innovative studies that worked with alcohol-affected children, Bertrand et al[155] recommend that interventionists adapt existing treatments, such as behavioral management, to accommodate the neurodevelopmental deficits characteristic of FASD. The reviewed studies all used empirically validated methods that were modified to work with children who had difficulties with speed of processing of information, working memory deficits, and executive functioning problems as well as difficulties with self-regulation.

Another important element was explicit instruction. While the typical child is able to acquire most knowledge through observation and a process of abstracting rules, skills, and knowledge from an ongoing situation, children affected by alcohol require explicit instruction to master the same skills. When such modifications are in place, affected children can be served within community settings. Central to the success of such interventions were caregiver involvement and investment in the treatment process. Other authors have emphasized the importance of early identification and anticipatory guidance to avoid the development of secondary disabilities.[154,156] Given that there is a great deal of heterogeneity in the effects of exposure to alcohol and other substances, it is important to plan interventions that target the individual needs of the affected child.

Because of the complexity of presentation as well as the multiple problems that can present, pediatricians may need to act as the leader of a team of knowledgeable professionals who can each contribute their expertise to support more positive outcomes. Developmental problems in young children may require the involvement of occupational, physical, or speech therapists to achieve optimal outcomes. If behavioral or educational problems are noted in the older child, referral for psychological and educational evaluation can be very useful in designing individualized treatment plans and implementing appropriate interventions. In all cases, parental involvement in treatment is highly recommended, as sometimes specialized techniques are helpful in supporting behavioral change.[157]

In summary, many adopted children have experienced prenatal exposure to alcohol and other substances. Fortunately, not all children will be negatively affected by such exposure; however, some are significantly impaired and will require careful monitoring during development to ensure optimal outcomes. Understanding the potential teratogenic effects as well as other familial and environmental factors that may influence a child's development will allow early recognition and addressing of problems to hopefully minimize the development of secondary disabilities and ensure the most positive outcomes.

References

1. US Department of Health and Human Services Administration for Children and Families. Children's Bureau. http://www.acf.hhs.gov/programs/cb. Accessed February 12, 2014
2. National Center on Substance Abuse and Child Welfare. Fact sheet 3—research studies on the prevalence of substance use disorders in the child welfare population. http://ncsacw.samhsa.gov/files/Research_Studies_Prevalence_Factsheets.pdf. Accessed February 12, 2014
3. Wulczyn F. Epidemiological perspectives on maltreatment prevention. *Future Child.* 2009;19(2):39–66
4. US Department of State Bureau of Consular Affairs. Intercountry adoption: statistics. http://adoption.state.gov/about_us/statistics.php. Accessed February 12, 2014
5. US Department of State Bureau of Consular Affairs. FY 2010 annual report on intercountry adoptions, December 2010. http://adoption.state.gov/content/pdf/fy2010_annual_report.pdf. Accessed February 12, 2014
6. Robert M, Carceller A, Domken V, et al. Physical and neurodevelopmental evaluation of children adopted from Eastern Europe. *Can J Clin Pharmacol.* 2009;16(3):e432–e440
7. Substance Abuse and Mental Health Services Administration. *Results from the 2003 National Survey on Drug Use and Health: National Findings.* Rockville, MD: Substance Abuse and Mental Health Services Administration; 2004

8. Howell KH, Coles CD, Kable JA. The medical and developmental consequences of prenatal drug exposure. In: Brick J, ed. *Handbook of the Medical Consequence of Alcohol and Drug Abuse*. New York, NY: The Haworth Press, Taylor & Francis Group; 2008:219–249

9. Substance Abuse and Mental Health Services Administration. *Results from the 2009 National Survey on Drug Use and Health: Volume I. Summary of National Findings*. Rockville, MD: Substance Abuse and Mental Health Services Administration; 2010

10. Ebrahim SH, Floyd RL, Merritt RK, Decoufle P, Holtzman D. Trends in pregnancy-related smoking rates in the United States, 1987–1996. *JAMA*. 2000;283(3):361–366

11. Slotkin T. Fetal nicotine or cocaine exposure: which one is worse? *J Pharm Exp Therapeutics*. 1998;285:931–945

12. Polifka JE. Drugs and chemicals in breast milk. In: Slikker W, Chang LW, eds. *Handbook of Developmental Neurotoxicology*. San Diego, CA: Academic Press; 1998:383–400

13. Landesman-Dwyer S, Emanuel I. Smoking during pregnancy. *Teratology*. 1979;19:119–126

14. Himmelberger DU, Brown BW, Cohen EN. Cigarette smoking during pregnancy and the occurrence of spontaneous abortion and congenital abnormality. *Amer J Epi*. 1978;108:470–479

15. Kline J, Levin B, Shrout P, Stein Z, Susser M, Warburton D. Maternal smoking and trisomy among spontaneously aborted conceptions. *Amer J Hum Gen*. 1983;35:421–431

16. Haglund B, Cnattinghus S. Cigarette smoking as a risk factor for sudden infancy death syndrome: a population-based study. *Am J Health*. 1990;80:29–32

17. Abel EL. Smoking and pregnancy. *J Psychoactive Drugs*. 1984;16:327–338

18. Werler MM, Pober BR, Holmes LB. Smoking and pregnancy. *Teratology*. 1985;32:473–481

19. Cornelius M, Goldschmidt L, Day N, Larkby C. Prenatal substance use among pregnant teenagers: a six-year follow-up of effects on offspring growth. *Neurotox Teratol*. 2002;24:703–710

20. Huang JS, Lee TA, Lu MC. Prenatal programming of childhood overweigh and obesity. *Matern Child Health J*. 2007;11:461–473

21. Moshammer H, Hoek G, Luttmann-Gibson H, et al. Parental smoking and lung function in children: an international study. *Am J Resp Crit Care Med*. 2006;173(11):1255–1263

22. Sawnani H, Jackson T, Murphy T, Beckerman R, Simakajornboon N. The effect of maternal smoking on respiratory and arousal patterns in preterm infants during sleep. *Am J Resp Crit Care Med*. 2004;169:733–738

23. Jaakkolla JJK, Gissler M. Maternal smoking in pregnancy, fetal development, and childhood asthma. *Am J Public Health*. 2004;94(1):136–140

24. Adair-Bischoff CD, Sauve RS. Environmental tobacco smoke and middle ear disease in preschool-age children. *Arch Pediatr Adolesc Med*. 1998;152:127–133

25. Ilicali OC, Keles N, Deier K, Saiun OF, Guldiken Y. Evaluation of the effect of passive smoking on otitis media in children by an objective method: urinary cotinine analysis. *Laryngoscope*. 1998;111:163–167

26. Stathis SL, O'Callaghan M, Williams GM, Najman JM, Anderson MJ, Bor W. Maternal cigarette smoking during pregnancy is an independent predictor for symptoms of middle ear disease at five years' postdelivery. *Pediatrics*. 1999;104:1–6

27. Fried PA, Watkinson B. Thirty-six- and forty-eight-month neurobehavioral follow-up of children prenatally exposed to marijuana, cigarettes, and alcohol. *J Dev Behav Pediatr*. 1990;11:49–58

28. Sexton M, Fox NL, Hebel JR. Prenatal exposure to tobacco: II. Effects on cognitive functioning at age three. *Int J Epi*. 1990;19:72–77

29. Makin J, Fried PA, Watkinson B. A comparison of active and passive smoking during pregnancy: long-term effects. *Neurotox Teratol*. 1991;13:5–12

30. Streissguth AP, Barr HM, Sampson PD, Darby BL, Martin DC. IQ at age 4 in relation to maternal alcohol use and smoking during pregnancy. *Dev Psych*. 1989;25:3–11

31. Fergusson DM, Lloyd M. Smoking during pregnancy and its effects on child cognitive ability from the ages of 8 to 12 years. *Paediatr Perinatal Epidemiol.* 1991;5:189–200

32. Hardy JB, Mellits ED. Does maternal smoking during pregnancy have a long-term effect on the child? *Lancet.* 1972;2:1332–1336

33. Fried PA, O'Connell CM, Watkinson B. 60- and 72-month follow-up of children prenatally exposed to marijuana, cigarettes, and alcohol: cognitive and language assessment. *J Dev Behav Pediatr.* 1992;13:383–391

34. Fried PA, Watkinson B, Gray R. A follow-up study of attentional behavior in 6-year-old children exposed prenatally to marijuana, cigarettes, and alcohol. *Neurotox Teratol.* 1992;14:299–311

35. Kable JA. Auditory vs. general information processing deficits in infants of mothers who smokes during their pregnancy. Unpublished doctoral dissertation, Purdue University, West Lafayette, IN, 1995

36. Coles CD, Kable JA, Lynch MA, Johnson KC. Language development at 6 and 15 months in children of smokers. Unpublished manuscript. 2008

37. Obel C, Henriksen TB, Hedegaard M, Secher NJ, Ostergaard J. Smoking during pregnancy and babbling abilities of the 8-month-old infant. *Paediatr Perinat Epidemiol.* 1998;12(1):37–48

38. Kukla L, Hruba D, Tyrlik M. Smoking of mothers during pregnancy in relation to mental and motoric development disorders in 4- and 5-year-old children. The ELSPAC study results. *Psychologia a Patopsychologia Dietata.* 2006;41:39–49

39. Lewis BA, Kirchner HL, Short EJ, et al. Prenatal cocaine and tobacco effects on children's language trajectories. *Pediatrics.* 2007;120:78–85

40. Bauman KE, Flewelling RL, LaPrelle J. Parental cigarette smoking and cognitive performance of children. *Health Psychol.* 1991;10(4):282–288

41. Fogelman K. Smoking in pregnancy and subsequent development of the child. *Child Care Health Dev.* 1980;6:233–249

42. Fried PA, Watkinson B, Siegel LS. Reading and language in 9- to 12-year olds prenatally exposed to cigarettes and marijuana. *Neurotoxic Teratol.* 1997;19:171–183

43. Fried PA, Makin JE. Neonatal behavioral correlates of prenatal exposure to marihuana, cigarettes and alcohol in a low risk population. *Neurotoxic Teratol.* 1987;9:1–7

44. Jacobson SW, Fein GG, Jacobson JL, Schwartz PM, Dowler JK. Neonatal correlates of prenatal exposure to smoking, caffeine, and alcohol. *Inf Ment Health J.* 1984;7:253–265

45. Picone TA, Allen LH, Olsen PN, Ferris ME. Pregnancy outcome in North American women. II. Effects of diet, cigarette smoking, stress, and weight gain on placentas, and on neonatal physical and behavioral characteristics. *Am J Clin Nutrit.* 1982;36:1214–1224

46. Franco P, Groswasser J, Hassid S, Lanquart JP, Scaillet S, Kahn A. Prenatal exposure to cigarette smoking is associated with a decrease in arousal in infants. *J Pediatr.* 1999;135:34–38

47. Kristjansson EA, Fried PA, Watkinson B. Maternal smoking during pregnancy affects children's vigilance performance. *Drug Alcohol Dep.* 1989;24:11–19

48. Brennen P, Grekin E, Mednick S. Maternal smoking during pregnancy and adult male criminal outcomes. *Arch Gen Psychiatry.* 1999;56:215–219

49. Zeskind PS, Gingras JL. Maternal cigarette-smoking during pregnancy disrupts rhythms in fetal heart rate. *J Pediatr Psychol.* 2006;31:5–14

50. Horne RS, Franco P, Adamson T, Groswasser J, Kahn A. Influences of maternal cigarette smoking on infant arousability. *Early Human Dev.* 2004;79:49–58

51. Leech S, Richardson GA, Goldschmidt L, Day N. Prenatal substance exposure: effects on attention and impulsivity of 6-year-olds. *Neurotoxic Teratol.* 1999;21:109–118

52. Schuetze P, Eiden RD. The association between maternal smoking and secondhand exposure and autonomic functioning at 2-4 weeks of age. *Inf Behav Dev.* 2006;29:32–43

53. Noland JS, Singer LT, Short EJ, et al. Prenatal drug exposure and selective attention in preschoolers. *Neurotox Teratol.* 2005;27:429–438

54. Streissguth AP, Martin DC, Barr HM, Sandman BM. Intrauterine alcohol and nicotine exposure: attention and reaction time in 4-year-old children. *Dev Psychol.* 1984;20:533–541

55. Brook DW, Zhang C, Rosenberg G, Brook JS. Maternal cigarette smoking during pregnancy and child aggressive behavior. *Amer J Addict.* 2006;15(6):450–456

56. Cornelius M, Leech S, Larkby C. Prenatal substance exposure: growth outcomes among 10-year-old offspring of teenage mothers. *Neurotox Teratol.* 2007;29:409

57. Day NL, Richardson GA, Goldschmidt L, Cornelius MD. Effects of prenatal tobacco exposure on preschoolers' behavior. *J Dev Behav Pediatr.* 2000;21:180–188

58. Fergusson DM, Woodward LJ, Horwood LJ. Maternal smoking during pregnancy and psychiatric adjustment in late adolescence. *Arch Gen Psychiatry.* 1998;55(8):721–727

59. Linnet KM, Dalsgaard S, Obel C, et al. Maternal lifestyle factors in pregnancy risk of attention deficit hyperactivity disorder and associated behaviors: review of the current evidence. *Am J Psychiatry.* 2003;160:1028–1040

60. Monuteaux MC, Blacker D, Biederman J, Fitzmaurice G, Buka SL. Maternal smoking during pregnancy and offspring overt and covert conduct problems: a longitudinal study. *J Child Psych Psychiatry.* 2006;47:883–890

61. Orlebeke JF, Knol DL, Verhulst FC. Child behavior problems increased by maternal smoking during pregnancy. *Arch Environ Health.* 1999;54:15–19

62. Thapar A, Fowler T, Rice F, et al. Maternal smoking during pregnancy and attention deficit hyperactivity disorder symptoms in offspring. *Am J Psychiatry.* 2003;160:1985–1989

63. Wakschlag LS, Pickett KE, Cook E, Benowitz NL, Leventhal BL. Maternal smoking during pregnancy and severe antisocial behavior in offspring: a review. *Am J Public Health.* 2002;92:966–974

64. Centers for Disease Control and Prevention. Alcohol use among pregnant and nonpregnant women of child bearing age—United States, 1991–2005. *MMWR.* 2009;58(19):529–532

65. Substance Abuse and Mental Health Services Administration. *Results from the 2007 National Survey on Drug Use and Health: National Findings.* Rockville, MD: Substance Abuse and Mental Health Services Administration; 2008

66. National Center on Birth Defects and Developmental Disabilities, Centers for Disease Control and Prevention. *Fetal Alcohol Syndrome: Guidelines for Referral and Diagnosis.* Atlanta, GA: US Department of Health and Human Services; 2004

67. Mattson SN, Crocker N, Nguyen TT. Fetal alcohol spectrum disorders: neuropsychological and behavioral features. *Neuropsychol Rev.* 2011;21(2):81–101

68. Stratton K, Howe C, Battaglia F; Committee to Study Fetal Alcohol Syndrome. *Fetal Alcohol Syndrome: Diagnosis, Epidemiology, Prevention, and Treatment.* Washington, DC: National Academy Press; 1996

69. Streissguth AP. *Fetal Alcohol Syndrome: A Guide for Families and Communities.* Baltimore, MD: Paul Brooks Publishing Company; 1997

70. Coles CD, Platzman KA, Lynch MA, Freides D. Auditory and visual sustained attention in adolescents prenatally exposed to alcohol. *Alcohol Clin Exp Res.* 2002;26:263–271

71. Day NL, Zuo YU, Richardson GA, Goldschmidt L, Larkby CA, Cornelius MD. Prenatal alcohol use and off spring size at 10 years of age. *Alcohol Clin Exp Res.* 1999;23:863–869

72. Day NL, Leech SL, Richardson GA, Cornelius MD, Robles N, Larkby C. Prenatal alcohol exposure predicted continued deficits in offspring size at 14 years of age. *Alcohol Clin Exp Res.* 2002;26:1584–1591

73. Lebel C, Roussotte F, Sowell ER. Imaging the impact of prenatal alcohol exposure on the structure of the developing human brain. *Neuropsychol Rev.* 2011;21(2):102

74. Chen X, Coles CD, Lynch ME, Hu X. Understanding specific effects of prenatal alcohol exposure on brain structure in young adults. *Hum Brain Mapp.* 2012;33(7):1663–1676

75. Wozniak JR, Muetzel RL. What does diffusion tensor imaging reveal about the brain and cognition in fetal alcohol spectrum disorders? *Neuropsychol Rev.* 2011;21(2):133–147

76. Coles CD, Li Z. Functional neuroimaging in the examination of effects of prenatal alcohol exposure. *Neuropsychol Rev.* 2011;21(2):119–132

77. Jacobson JL, Jacobson SW. Effects of prenatal alcohol exposure on child development. *Alcohol Res Health.* 2002;26(4):282–286

78. Mattson SN, Riley EP. A review of the neurobehavioral deficits in children with fetal alcohol syndrome or prenatal exposure to alcohol. *Alcohol Clin Exp Res.* 1998;24:226–231

79. Streissguth AP, Herman CS, Smith DW. Intelligence, behavior and dysmorphogenesis in the fetal alcohol syndrome: a report on 20 patients. *J Pediatr.* 1978;92:363–367

80. Streissguth AP, Bookstein FL, Sampson PD, Barr HM. Attention: prenatal alcohol and continuities of vigilance and attentional problems from 4 through 14 years. *Dev Psychopathol.* 1995;7:419–446

81. Coles CD. Discriminating effects of prenatal alcohol exposure from other behavioral and learning disorders. *Alcohol Res Health.* 2011;34(1):42–50

82. Coles CD, Smith IE, Fernhoff PM, Falek A. Neonatal neurobehavioral characteristics as correlates of maternal alcohol use during gestation. *Alcohol Clin Exp Res.* 1985;9(5):454–460

83. Jacobson SW, Jacobson JL, Sokol RJ, Martier SS, Ager JW. Prenatal alcohol exposure and infant information processing ability. *Child Dev.* 1993;64:1706–1721

84. Coles CD, Brown RT, Smith IE, Platzman KA, Erickson S, Falek A. Effects of prenatal alcohol exposure at school age: I. Physical and cognitive development. *Neurotox Teratol.* 1991;13(4):357–367

85. Conry J. Neuropsychological deficits in fetal alcohol syndrome and fetal alcohol effects. *Alcohol Clin Exp Res.* 1990;14:650–655

86. Marcus JC. Neurological findings in the fetal alcohol syndrome. *Neuropediatrics.* 1987;18:158–160

87. Roebuck TM, Simmons RW, Mattson SN, Riley EP. Prenatal exposure to alcohol affects the ability to maintain postural balance. *Alcohol Clin Exp Res.* 1998;22:1992–1997

88. Steinhausen HC, Willms, J, Spohr HL. Long-term psychopathology and cognitive outcome of children with fetal alcohol syndrome. *J Am Acad Child Adol Psychiatry.* 1993;32:990–994

89. Aronson M, Kyllerman M, Sabel KG, Sandin B, Olegard R. Children of alcoholic mothers. Developmental, perceptual and behavioral characteristics as compared to matched controls. *Acta Paediatr Scand.* 1985;74:27–35

90. Coles CD, Kable JA, Drew-Botsch C, Falek A. Early identification of risk for effects of prenatal alcohol exposure. *J Stud Alcohol.* 2000;61(4):607–616

91. Coles CD, Platzman KA, Raskind-Hood CL, Brown RT, Falek A, Smith IE. A comparison of children affected by prenatal alcohol exposure and attention deficit, hyperactivity disorder. *Alcohol Clin Exp Res.* 1997;21(1):150–161

92. Coles CD, Lynch ME, Kable JA, Johnson KC, Goldstein FC. Verbal and nonverbal memory in adults prenatally exposed to alcohol. *Alcohol Clin Exp Res.* 2010;34(5):897–906

93. Mattson SN, Riley EP. Implicit and explicit memory functioning in children with heavy prenatal alcohol exposure. *J Int Neuropsychol Soc.* 1999;5:462–471

94. Kodituwakku PW, Handmaker NS, Cutler SK, Weathersby EK, Handmaker SD. Specific impairments in self-regulation in children exposed to alcohol prenatally. *Alcohol Clin Exp Res.* 1995;19:1558–1564

95. Howell KK, Lynch MA, Platzman KA, Smith GH, Coles CD. Prenatal alcohol exposure and academic functioning in adolescence: a longitudinal follow-up. *J Pediatr Psychol.* 2006;31(1):116–126

96. Streissguth AP, Barr HM, Carmichael-Olson H, Sampson PD, Bookstein FL, Burgess DM. Drinking during pregnancy decreases word attack and arithmetic scores on standardized tests: adolescent data from population-based prospective study. *Alcohol Clin Exp Res*. 1994;18:248–254

97. Streissguth AP, Barr HM, Kogan J, Bookstein FL. *Understanding the Occurrence of Secondary Disabilities in Clients with Fetal Alcohol Syndrome (FAS) and Fetal Alcohol Effects (FAE). Final Report to the Centers for Disease Control and Prevention (CDC)*. Seattle, WA: University of Washington, Fetal Alcohol and Drug Unit; 1996

98. Kelly SJ, Day N, Streissguth AP. Effects of prenatal alcohol exposure on social behavior in humans and other species. *Neurotox Teratol*. 2001;22:143–149

99. National Institute on Drug Abuse. *National Pregnancy and Health Survey*. Rockville, MD: National Institute on Drug Abuse; 1996

100. Ebrahim SH, Gfroerer J. Pregnancy-related substance use in the United States during 1996–1998. *Obstet Gynecol*. 2003;101(2):374–379

101. Goldschmidt L, Day NL, Richardson, GA. Effects of prenatal marijuana exposure on child behavior problems at age 10. *Neurotox Teratol*. 2000;22:325–336

102. Day N, Sambamoorthi U, Taylor P, et al. Prenatal marijuana use and neonatal outcome. *Neurotox Teratol*. 1991;13:329–334

103. Fried PA. Behavioral outcomes in preschool and school-age children exposed prenatally to marijuana: a review and speculative interpretation. In: Wetherington CL, Smeriglio VL, Finnegan LP, eds. *Behavioral Studies of Drug-Exposed Offspring: Methodological Issues in Human and Animal Research*. Rockville, MD: National Institute on Drug Abuse; 1996:242–260

104. O'Connell CM, Fried PA. Prenatal exposure to cannabis: a preliminary report of postnatal consequences in school-age children. *Neurotox Teratol*. 1991;13:631–639

105. Behnke M, Eyler FD. The consequences of prenatal substance use for the developing fetus, newborn, and young child. *Int J Addict*. 1993;28(13):1341–1391

106. Day NL, Cottreau CM, Richardson GA. The epidemiology of alcohol, marijuana, and cocaine use among women of child-bearing age and pregnant women. *Clin Obstet Gynecol*. 1993;36:232–245

107. Brantley M, Rochat R, Floyd V, et al. Population-based prevalence of perinatal exposure to cocaine—Georgia, 1994. *MMWR*. 1996;41:887–891

108. Coles CD. Saying "goodbye" to the "crack baby." *Neurotox Teratol*. 1993;5:290–292

109. Eyler FD, Behnke M. Early development of infants exposed to drugs prenatally. *Clin Perinatol*. 1999;26(1):107–150

110. Frank DA, Augustyn M, Knight WG, Pell T, Zuckerman B. Growth, development, and behavior in early childhood following prenatal cocaine exposure: a systematic review. *JAMA*. 2001;285:1613–1625

111. Lester BM, Lagasse LL. Children of addicted women. *J Addict Dis*. 2010;29(2):259–276

112. Tronick EZ, Beeghly M. Prenatal cocaine exposure, child development, and the compromising effects of cumulative risk. *Clin Perinatol*. 1999;26:151–171

113. Gouin K, Murphy K, Shah PS. Knowledge synthesis on determinants of low birth weight and preterm births. Effects of cocaine use during pregnancy on low birthweight and preterm birth: systematic review and metaanalysis. *Am J Obstet Gynecol*. 2011;204(4):340.e1–e12

114. Coles CD, Bard KA, Platzman KA, Lynch ME. Attentional response at 8 weeks in prenatally drug-exposed and preterm infants. *Neurotox Teratol*. 1999;21(5):527–537

115. Kable JA, Coles CD, Lynch ME, Platzman KA. Physiological responses to social and cognitive challenges in 8-year-olds with a history of prenatal cocaine exposure. *Dev Psychobiol*. 2008;50:251–265

116. Brown JV, Bakeman R, Coles CD, Platzman KA, Lynch ME. Prenatal cocaine exposure: a comparison of two-year-old children in parental and non-parental care. *Child Dev*. 2004;75(4):1282–1295

117. Frank DA, Jacobs RR, Beeghly M, et al. Level of prenatal cocaine exposure and scores on the Bayley Scales of Infant Development: modifying effects of caregiver, early intervention, and birth weight. *Pediatrics.* 2002;110:1143–1152

118. Kilbride H, Castor C, Hoffman E, Fuger KL. Thirty-six-month outcome of prenatal cocaine exposure for term or near-term infants: impact of early case management. *J Dev Behav Pediatr.* 2000;21:19–26

119. Chasnoff IJ, Anson A, Hatcher R, Stenson H, Iaukea K, Randolph LA. Prenatal exposure to cocaine and other drugs: outcome at four to six years. *Ann NY Acad Sci.* 1998;846:314–328

120. Mayes LC, Cicchetti D, Acharyya S, Zhang H. Developmental trajectories of cocaine-and-other-drug-exposed and non-cocaine-exposed children. *J Dev Behav Peds.* 2003;24:323–335

121. Richardson GA. Prenatal cocaine exposure: a longitudinal study of development. *Ann NY Acad Sci.* 1998;846:144–152

122. Richardson GA, Conroy ML, Day NL. Prenatal cocaine exposure: effects on the development of school-age children. *Neurotox Teratol.* 1996;18:627–634

123. Mayes LC, Bornstein MH, Chawarska K, Granger RH. Information processing and developmental assessments in three-month-olds exposed prenatally to cocaine. *Pediatrics.* 1995;95:539–545

124. Savage J, Brodsky NL, Malmud E, Giannetta JM, Hurt H. Attentional functioning and impulse control in cocaine-exposed and control children at age ten years. *J Dev Behav Pediatr.* 2005;26:42–47

125. Mayes LC. Developing brain and in utero cocaine exposure: effects on neural ontogeny. *Dev Psychopathol.* 1999;11:685–714

126. Brown JV, Bakeman R, Coles CD, Sexson WR, Demi A. Maternal drug use, fetal growth and newborn behavior: are preterms and fullterms affected differently? *Dev Psychol.* 1998;34(3):540–554

127. Bada HS, Bauer CR, Shankaran S, et al. Central and autonomic system signs with in utero drug exposure. *Arch Dis Child.* 2002;87:F106–F112

128. Mehta SK, Super DM, Connuck D, et al. Autonomic alterations in cocaine-exposed infants. *Amer Heart J.* 2002;144:1109–1115

129. Bard KA, Coles CD, Platzman KA, Lynch MA. The effects of prenatal drug exposure, term status and caregiving on arousal and arousal modulation in 8-week-old infants. *Dev Psychobiol.* 2000;36:194–212

130. Bendersky M, Lewis M. Arousal modulation in cocaine-exposed infants. *Dev Psychol.* 1998;34:555–564

131. Karmel BZ, Gardner JM, Freedland RL. Arousal-modulated attention at four months as a function of intrauterine cocaine exposure and central nervous system injury. *J Pediatr Psychol.* 1996;21:821–832

132. Bendersky M, Gambini G, Lastella A, Bennett DS, Lewis M. Inhibitory motor control at five years as a function of prenatal cocaine exposure. *J Dev Behav Pediatr.* 2003;24(5):345–351

133. Li Z, Coles CD, Lynch ME, et al. Prenatal cocaine exposure alters emotional arousal regulation and its effects on working memory. *Neurotoxicol Teratol.* 2009;31(6):342–348

134. Bendersky M, Bennett D, Lewis M. Aggression at age 5 as a function of prenatal exposure to cocaine, gender, and environmental risk. *J Pediatr Psychol.* 2006;31(1):71–84

135. Delany-Black V, Covington C, Templin T, Ager JW, Martier SS, Sokol RJ. Prenatal cocaine exposure and child behavior. *Pediatrics.* 1998;102:945–950

136. Accornero VH, Morrow CE, Bandstra ES, Johnson AL, Anthony JC. Behavioral outcome of preschoolers exposed prenatally to cocaine: role of maternal behavioral health. *J Pediatr Psychol.* 2002;27(3):259–269

137. Derauf C, LaGasse LL, Smith LM, et al. Demographic and psychosocial characteristics of mothers using methamphetamine during pregnancy: preliminary results of the infant development, environment, and lifestyle study (IDEAL). *Am J Drug Alcohol Abuse.* 2007;33(2):281–289

138. Good MM, Solt I, Acuna JG, Rotmensch S, Kim MJ. Methamphetamine use during pregnancy: maternal and neonatal implications. *Obstet Gynecol.* 2010;116(2 Pt 1):330–334

139. Smith LM, LaGasse LL, Derauf C, et al. Prenatal methamphetamine use and neonatal neurobehavioral outcome. *Neurotoxicol Teratol.* 2008;30(1):20–28

140. McCalla S, Minkoff HL, Feldman J, et al. The biologic and social consequences of perinatal cocaine use in an inner-city population: results of an anonymous cross-sectional study. *Am J Obstet Gynecol.* 1991;164:625–630

141. Ostrea EM, Brady M, Gause S, Raymondo AL, Stevens M. Drug screening of newborns by meconium analysis: a large-scale, prospective, epidemiologic study. *Pediatrics.* 1992;89:107–113

142. Kandall SR, Doberczak TM, Jantunen M, Stein J. The methadone-maintained pregnancy. *Clin Perinatol.* 1999;26(1):173–183

143. Kaltenbach KA. Exposure to opiates: behavioral outcomes in preschool and school-age children. In: Wetherington CL, Smeriglio VL, Finnegan LP, eds. *Behavioral Studies of Drug-Exposed Offspring: Methodological Issues in Human and Animal Research.* Rockville, MD: National Institute on Drug Abuse; 1996:230–241

144. Kaltenbach KA, Finnegan LP. Neonatal abstinence syndrome: pharmacotherapy and developmental outcome. *Neurobehav Toxicol Teratol.* 1986;8:353–355

145. Finnegan LP. Pathophysiological and behavioral effects of the transplacental transfer of narcotic drugs to the fetuses and neonates of narcotic-dependent mothers. *Bull Narc.* 1979;31(3):1–58

146. de Cubas MM, Field T. Children of methadone-dependent women: developmental outcomes. *Amer J Orthopsychiatry.* 1993;63(2):266–276

147. Hans SL. Developmental consequences of prenatal exposure to methadone. *Ann N Y Acad Sci.* 1986;562:195–207

148. Hans SL, Marcus J. Motor and attentional behavior in infants of methadone maintained women. In: Harris L, ed. *Problems of Drug Dependence.* Rockville, MD: National Institute on Drug Abuse; 1983

149. Frohna JG, Lantz PM, Pollack H. Maternal substance abuse and infant health: policy options across the life course. *Milbank Q.* 1999;77(4):531–570

150. Brodzinsky DM. *Adoptive Parent Preparation Project, Phase I: Meeting the Mental Health and Developmental Needs of Adopted Children.* New York, NY: Evan B. Donaldson Adoption Institute; 2008

151. American Academy of Pediatrics. AAP endorses statement of alcohol-related neurodevelopmental disabilities. *AAP News.* 2012;33(9):18

152. American Academy of Pediatrics Committee on Substance Abuse and Committee on Children with Disabilities. Fetal alcohol syndrome and alcohol related neurodevelopmental disorders. *Pediatrics.* 2000;106(2):358–361

153. Finnegan LP, Connaughton JF Jr, Kron RE, Emich JP. Neonatal abstinence syndrome: assessment and management. *Addict Dis.* 1975;2:141–158

154. Coles CD, Taddeo E, Millians M. Innovative educational interventions with school-aged children affected by fetal alcohol spectrum disorders (FASD). In: Adubato SA, Cohen DE, eds. *Prenatal Alcohol Use and FASD: Historical and Future Perspectives.* United Arab Emirates: Bentham eBooks; 2011

155. Bertrand J; Interventions for Children with Fetal Alcohol Spectrum Disorders Research Consortium. Interventions for children with fetal alcohol spectrum disorders (FASDs): overview of findings for five innovative randomized control research projects. *Res Dev Disabil.* 2009;30:986–1006

156. Peadon E, Rhys-Jones B, Bower C, Elliott EJ. Systematic review of interventions for children with fetal alcohol spectrum disorders. *BMC Pediatr.* 2009;9:35

157. Olson HC, Gelo J, Beck S. "Family matters": fetal alcohol spectrum disorders and the family. *Dev Disabil Res Rev.* 2009;15(3):235–249

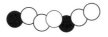

CHAPTER 6

Relating Genetics to Psychiatric Issues for Children With a History of Adoption

Jonathan Picker, MBChB, PhD

Families enter the adoption process with a range of expectations for their child and family. Extended birth family history, which may be shared with prospective adoptive families, or information that is later learned about mental health concerns of birth family members often raise questions for families and pediatricians about what this information means for the adopted child. As with children entering families by birth, future concerns are not always predictable, but legal frameworks exist to support appropriate disclosure of information during the adoption process to prospective parents.[1] This chapter will review the current state of understanding of the implications of genetic and environmental risk factors with respect to later mental health concerns.

Potential Post-adoption Concerns

Though most children appear to adjust well after adoption into families, even when there have been psychologic issues present prior to adoption,[2–4] psychiatric issues are more common for children with a history of adoption than in the general pediatric population. This is the case particularly in older adoptees.[5] While the majority of children who are adopted as infants do very well, there is an approximately 2-fold increase in behavioral issues relative to the general pediatric population.[4] In the highest risk group, including those adopted later in childhood and adolescence or who entered care because of abuse and neglect, about half have behavioral or emotional problems, but about half still appear to adjust well psychologically, despite the adversity.[6]

Potential Reasons for Psychopathology

The reason for the overall increased risk in psychiatric concerns for children with a history of adoption is not completely clear. Evidence supports a role for genetic, teratogenic, and social risk factors as well as issues specific to adoption itself, including the pathogenesis of the adoption process, long-term effects of pre-adoption rearing, referral bias in adopting parents, and impaired adopter/adoptee relationships.[7-9] In addition to considering pre-adoptive factors, it is also important to bear in mind that environmental risk factors include post-adoption risk factors, eg, issues from the adopting family's side such as psychopathology within the parents or other siblings already in the family.[10,11] Depression in adolescents, for example, has been shown to be increased in adopted as well as the biological offspring of depressed (nonbiological) rearing mothers.[12]

The Role of Genetics

In recent years, as the human genome project began to have clinical implications, there has been an increasing possibility of understanding the role genes play in predisposing an adopted (or any other) child to later behavioral and emotional challenges. Genetics is very rarely, if ever, the only factor contributing to psychiatric disease, although risk or resilience genes may be essential to determining whether an individual will or will not develop psychopathology within his or her given environment. As a result, genetics offer the opportunity to provide prognostic information, as well as potentially guide therapy.[13-15] While genetic knowledge offers a real opportunity for proactive interventions, much misinformation is available online and elsewhere. In addition, even if data are reliable, it can be challenging for professionals in the field to correctly interpret the often very complex and incomplete information currently available.[16] The state of knowledge with respect to genetics and their role in later behaviors is extremely dynamic, and as a result, our determinations of whether a particular genetic variant is or is not pathogenic is evolving as our understanding of genetic markers and susceptibility genes becomes more comprehensive and sophisticated. As a result of decades of research, we are only now beginning to appreciate that reliable interpretation of psychiatric-risk genes must take into account the role of other genetic polymorphisms present in the individual.

Given the very rapid ongoing revolution in our knowledge of the genetic underpinnings of psychopathology, it is clearly not possible to provide definitive information about psychopathology predispositions for any person. However, guidelines with respect to risk factors and interpretation of family histories of particular psychiatric illnesses, as well as genetic disorders predisposing to psychiatric illness, are helpful as an aid to assist families pre- and post-adoption.

As consumer-direct personalized medicine becomes increasingly available, knowledge of the potential pitfalls of interpretation of genetic results is particularly important when considering risk or resilience prediction for any individual.

Personalized Medicine

The increasing availability of personalized medicine as a concept and practice raises the possibility that children who are being adopted will be genotyped prior to or as part of their adoption process. This may occur as result of institutional, local, or national directives or because potentially adoptive parents may request genotyping as part of a background prerequisite. Furthermore, companies offering genotyping appear to support the notion of genotyping children, although it is unclear how this information will or could be used. Proponents of broad-screen genotyping argue that the information will allow caregivers to screen for and proactively anticipate and act on identified risk factors. Proponents of screening also suggest that proactive genotyping will ensure that when needed, prescriptions can be provided that are more closely tailored to the individual's "pharmacogenetic background," thereby increasing likely efficacy and decreasing side effects. One example would be knowledge of an individual's cytochrome oxidase P450 polymorphisms.[14] However, with few exceptions, our understanding of identified polymorphisms is still very limited, though slowly improving, as demonstrated by recent findings of polymorphisms involved in metabolism of antipsychotic drugs.[17]

Clearly the potential to over-interpret or misinterpret results to the detriment of the tested individual remains high and may have specific additional social consequences for the psychiatric population.[18] It is unclear when this situation will change, as our understanding of genetic variability continues to expand rather than becoming more defined. As whole genome sequencing, with the exponentially increased amount of raw data that comes with it, becomes a feasible reality for individuals, it is likely that the difficulties interpreting available data will become significantly greater for the foreseeable future. The research community is working

What are genetic polymorphisms (or polymorphic alleles)?

Polymorphisms are natural variations in a gene, DNA sequence, or chromosome that are thought to have no adverse effects on the individual and occur with fairly high frequency in the general population. Polymorphisms may involve 1 of 2 or more variants of a particular DNA sequence. The most common type of polymorphism involves variation at a single base pair. Polymorphisms can also be much larger in size and involve long stretches of DNA. Single nucleotide polymorphisms, or SNP (pronounced "snip"), are being studied by scientists to determine how SNPs in the human genome correlate with disease, drug response, and other phenotypes.

hard to change this, and more than 100 genome-wide association studies (GWAS) targeting psychiatric disorders have been conducted using microarray platforms to assay for polymorphisms, which are predicted to cover greater than 80% of the genome.[19,20]

Unfortunately, though the single nucleotide polymorphism markers are well covered by this testing, they appear to account for only a small proportion of genetic variability for most diseases. Therefore, the gene variants implicated by current testing, while relevant and important in their own right,[21] do not play a sufficient role in disease prediction. There is also concern that the statistical methods used to predict disease risk, which are based on odds ratios or association studies, are not appropriate for individual counseling.[22] In addition, because the clinical value of a genetic test depends on its sensitivity, specificity, and positive and negative predictive values, as we discover more "risk" polymorphisms, most people will be at similar risk. Therefore, for less-common diseases (with a prevalence of ≤1%), the positive predictive value of a genetic test will almost always be low. Thus, despite extensive studies, it appears that GWAS have not provided predictive value for psychiatric diseases in individuals.[23] To some degree, this challenge may reflect the attempt to amalgamate traditional psychiatric phenotypic measurements, which are expressed symptoms and signs rather than biologically based measures, with genetic variations that are, at most, indirectly related to these measures.

Genetics and International Adoption

Most data available with respect to genetic polymorphisms in the literature are specific to white people of European descent. The amount known about polymorphic variability in other populations is significantly more limited. It is clear that international adoption has a multitude of trans-ethnic possibilities, as there is an ever-evolving geographic arena in which adoption takes place.

With respect to behavior problems, there are a number of potential issues involving children with a history of international adoption. The risk for suicidal behavior is increased in adoptees generally, but it is unclear if this risk is increased in international versus domestic adoptees, as studies have presented conflicting results. In Sweden, a country with a relatively high rate of international adoption, the adjusted odds ratio increased 3.6-fold for attempted and completed suicidal acts, as well as having a 3.2-fold increase for psychiatric admissions in international adoptees relative to the general population.[24–26]

However, no increase in behavioral problems reported by adoptees themselves or parents was found in studies.[27,28] A recent meta-analysis of international adoption across the globe found that though international adoptees were referred to mental health services more frequently than non-adopted children and extreme deprivation and adversity increased risk for mental health problems in the international group, the rate of referral was less than for domestic adoptees who appeared to have greater internalizing and externalizing symptoms.[29]

Within the United States, children adopted in infancy domestically appeared to have approximately twice the risk of having an externalizing disorder (eg, attention-deficit/hyperactivity disorder) relative to international infant adoptees.[4] It also appears that girls may be at increased risk for internalizing disorders (eg, anxiety disorder) relative to boys.[30] A meta-analysis of adolescent international adoptees rather encouragingly found that though the level of externalizing psychiatric symptoms is elevated in the population, this likely reflected pre-adoption adversity rather than the nature of the adoption itself.[31] Not surprisingly, increasing age at adoption, degree of institutionalization, and pre-adoption stresses increase the risk of psychologic problems in international adoptees.[32]

In summary, practice is evolving with respect to evaluation of genetic risk factors for all individuals, and one might expect that genotyping may continue to be considered with respect to a pre-adoption assessment, not just for psychopathology but for health issues generally. When this will be able to be carried out reliably and predictively is not really clear.[33]

Genetics of Psychiatric Disorders

Although broader genotyping may not be helpful with respect to predicting long-term behavioral and emotional concerns, some more focused questions based on extended family can be answered from a genetic perspective with respect to long-term risk. The implication of family histories of schizophrenia, mood disorders (including bipolar disorder and depression), suicide, and anxiety disorders will be reviewed herein.

Schizophrenia

Schizophrenia is a common disorder with significant morbidity. Affecting approximately 1% of the world population, it appears to affect most global populations to the same degree. This appears to be the case whether it is considered a single entity with varying expressivity or an umbrella disorder encompassing various different subtypes (eg, paranoid, catatonic). Heritability estimates from twin studies range from 0.6 to 0.85, suggesting a strong genetic component,[34,35] possibly the highest of any psychiatric disorder. First-degree relatives of an individual with schizophrenia are reported to have an 8% to 15% chance of having the disorder.

Though significant overlap has been proposed between risk genes for schizophrenia and bipolar disorder, the heritability is much higher in schizophrenia (Table 6-1). This may be reflected in changes in copy number variants in the genome (regions that are deleted or duplicated) that appear to be more common in schizophrenia as opposed to bipolar disorder, in which background copy number

Table 6-1. Genetic Risk for Common Psychiatric Disorders

Disorder	Incidence	Heritability	Risk to First-degree Relatives[a]	MZ/DZ Twin Concordance Rates
Anxiety Disorders	15%/25%[b]	40%	20%	
Phobias or Panic	5%/12%[b]	40%	8%/31%[b]	
Major Depression	4%/8%[b]	30%/42%[b]	9%/18%[b]	40%/11%
Bipolar	1%	60%	9%/27%[b]	
Schizophrenia	1%	80%	5%/15%[b]	50%/13%
OCD	3%		10%/35%[b]	
ADHD	5%	70%/80%[b]	15%/60%[b]	
Alcohol Dependence	14%/3%[b]		27%/5%[b]	

Abbreviations: ADHD, attention-deficit/hyperactivity disorder; MZ/DZ, monozygotic/dizygotic; OCD, obsessive-compulsive disorder.

Counseling data from National Coalition for Health Professional Education in Genetics.

[a]With one affected relative.

[b]Male percentage/female percentage.

Adapted from Tsuang D, Faraone SV, Tsuang MT. Psychiatric genetic counseling. In: Bloom FE, Kupfer DJ, eds. Back to Psychopharmacology—the Fourth Generation of Progress. 4th ed. Baltimore, MD: Lippincott Williams & Wilkins; 1995

variations in the chromosomal makeup are similar to those found in the general population.[36] Numerous candidate genes have been proposed as predisposing individuals to schizophrenia and are under active investigation. Linkage studies and GWAS have identified potential risk loci, some of which include candidate genes. However, for the vast majority of cases, evidence is leaning toward a multifactorial model of multiple genes of small risk aggregating toward risk for the disorder, rather than a few genes putting an individual at increased risk irrespective of whether schizophrenia is viewed as a single disorder with variable phenotypic expression or a number of different disorders that fall under the umbrella term of schizophrenia.[37] At this time, definitive evidence for specific risk genes remains insufficient to offer genetic testing, although as noted in Table 6-1, risk counseling can be provided on the basis of family history.[38–40]

Bipolar Disorder

Like schizophrenia, bipolar disease has a high heritability of approximately 60%, with first-degree relatives having approximately a 9% to 27% chance of presenting with bipolar disorder themselves. Candidate genes have been proposed for bipolar disorder, but the evidence has been less compelling than for schizophrenia and likely reflects a greater polygenic and environmental basis for this disorder.[40] Furthermore, with respect to pediatric epidemiology, the degree to which children are affected by bipolar disorder is currently unclear, with wide-ranging disparate views. A European consensus meeting in 2007 generally determined that in prepubertal children, bipolar disease is a rare disorder, with onset typically occurring only in adolescence or adulthood.[41] Importantly, there is substantial evidence for overlap between bipolar disease and depression. It is unclear if this overlap is because of a shared risk from a genetic predisposition to mood disorders (which may lead to solely depression or bipolar disorder) or possibly because of difficulties classifying these disorders correctly.[42]

Major Depression

Major depression has a heritability of approximately 37%, with an odds-ratio risk of 2.84 for first-degree relatives for major depression.[43] It appears that for a diagnosis of depression, there is an additive genetic effect.[44] With respect to childhood depression, while twin studies appear to support genetic influences, adoption studies did not show sufficient evidence for the same degree of genetic loading.[45,46] Interestingly, a genetic component becomes clearer in a stressful environment such as a high level of family conflict,[47,48] indicating that genetics may act primarily as a susceptibility factor rather than as a primary etiology for major depression in children.

Suicide

Suicidality appears to be more common among adoptees than for non-adopted children growing up with their birth parents.[47,48] Suicide is closely associated with depression in Western and Eastern cultures,[49] but only a proportion of individuals with depression will attempt or complete suicide. A mixture of psychiatric and environmental factors appears to increase one's risk for suicidal behavior, including social and familial issues along with genetic predisposition.[50] A seminal study among Danish adoptees who committed suicide found a 6-fold increase in the rate of suicidality among birth relatives compared with non-related family members, suggesting a genetic link or predisposition for completion of suicide.[51] This has been supported by twin studies demonstrating an increased risk among monozygotic over dizygotic twins. More than one-third of individuals attempting suicide have a first-degree relative with a history of suicidality, particularly completed episodes.[52–54]

A genetic link to aggression has been reported and shared 30% to 55% heritability, suggesting that transmission of suicidality and aggression was interlinked.[55] Interestingly, although shared environmental factors appear to explain 18% of the variance for suicide attempts, there did not appear to be any shared environmental factors for suicidal ideation (which is known to be associated with depression). One could hypothesize that the unique genetic factors predisposing toward suicidal behavior represent the impulse to act on thoughts, rather than the thoughts themselves being responsible for the suicidal behavior, and that the same impulsivity may also explain the link between aggression and suicidality. Familial transmission of suicide and major depression, while partially overlapping, is distinct. Importantly, consistent emotional warmth and discipline with close parental monitoring appear to mitigate suicide risk even among predisposed youth.[55,56]

Anxiety Disorders

On a population level, females have an approximately 2-fold increase in risk of meeting criteria for anxiety-related disorders including generalized anxiety disorder (GAD), panic disorders and phobias, and depression.[57–59] Overall there appears to be a heritability of 0.43 for panic disorder and 0.32 for GAD. For panic disorder, the remaining variance in liability appears to be attributed primarily to environment. For GAD, this was true for men, but for women, a potentially significant role of familial environment was also seen. Modeling has suggested that anxiety-related disorders (ie, GAD, panic disorders, and phobias) share common genetic and environmental risk factors, although agoraphobia appears to also have a unique genetic component not shared by the other disorders.[59,60] Genetic risk for personality disorders may also underlie the genetic component of anxiety-related disorders. A shared genetic risk correlates with increased risk of neurotic symptoms but correlates negatively with extravert traits.[61]

Substance Abuse

The role of genetic predisposition to alcohol and substance abuse is a complex one because individuals who abuse substances may have a genetically based predisposition for alcohol and substance abuse or may have an increased risk for abuse related to a behavioral component of another disorder, such as an attentional, anxiety, or conduct disorder or antisocial personality traits.[62–64] Interestingly, adoptive parental smoking appears to increase the risk for substance abuse in adopted children but to a much smaller degree than for biological offspring.[4]

Heritability for abuse of various substances ranges from several percent up to approximately 50%.[65] Candidate risk genes are under investigation and appear to have some overlap. Twin studies have suggested that there is a greater than 60% genetic overlap between dependency to alcohol and tobacco.[66] Candidate genetic susceptibility loci and genes for alcohol and tobacco dependency appear to segregate within specific ethnic groups. Candidate genes for other substances are also under investigation.[65]

It is important to note that alcohol use itself may have an epigenetic effect on expression of susceptibility genes, leading to increased risk of substance abuse.[67] Overall, risk for substance abuse is clearly a complex issue, with societal factors clearly compounding other environmental and genetic risk factors.

Gender Identity Disorder

Gender identity disorder is the display of a strong and persistent desire to be of the opposite sex, including persistent discomfort with one's phenotypic sex, which is not concurrent with a sexual dysmorphism syndrome. Transsexualism, on the other hand, is the desire to live publicly as a member of the opposite sex and may or may not have any morbidity attached to it.[68] The incidence of gender identity disorder is approximately 1 of 3,000 to 1 of 30,000 of the population, and the male-to-female ratio is 3:1.[69] It should be noted that cross-gender behavior in children is common (2%–12%).[70]

Gender identity disorder appears to have a 62% heritability,[71] although the literature is very limited and has some variance.[72–74] In monozygotic twin studies, there is a 30% to 50% concordance for desire by males to become female (MTF) and to a lesser degree female MZ twin concordant desire to become male (FTM).[75–79] With respect to etiology, hormonal levels may differ in utero, with increased androgens found in twice as many FTM as in the control population. Prenatal stress hormones have also been suggested as playing a role in transgenderism.[80,81] Candidate genes have been proposed for MTF and FTM populations.[82,83]

Sex chromosome aneuploidy (SCA) has also been reported, though this likely reflects coincidence, as SCAs are relatively common in the general population. There have only been a few reports, which is not really consistent with an increased risk.[84–87] However, while SCAs do not appear to have a primary role in gender identity disorders, they are associated with psychopathology, as are other genetic syndromes.

Inherited Genetic Syndromes With Associated Psychopathology

While the majority of individuals with psychopathology do not have other problems, many genetic syndromes are associated with psychopathology. While individually rare, genetic syndromes collectively affect 3% to 6% of the pediatric population. Cognitive and physical disorders increase the risk for behavioral problems, although many individuals with the same syndromes are well adjusted. Awareness of the potential that children may have a syndrome predisposing them to a psychiatric problem is essential for making an appropriate diagnosis, which may have additional physical consequences.

Table 6-2. Syndromic Disorders With a Significant Behavioral Component[88-104]

Syndrome	Typical Psychiatric Problems	Gene Mutation or Chromosomal Deletion
Velocardiofacial	Psychosis, autism, mood disorders	del22q11.2
Angelman	Autism	*UBE3A* or del15q11-13
Prader-Willi	OCD, mood disorders	del15q11-13
Smith-Magenis	Multiple, sleep disorder	*RAI1* or del17p11.2
Williams	ADHD, disinhibition, depression (as adult)	*ELN* or del7q11.23
Rubinstein-Taybi	Mood disorder, aggression	*CREBBP* or del16p13
Homocystinuria	Psychosis, depression, aggression	*MTHFR*
PKU	Anxiety, depression	*PH*
Metachromatic leukodystrophy	Psychosis, depression	*ASA*
Lesch-Nyhan	Self-injurious behavior	*HGPRT*
Smith-Lemli-Opitz	Bipolar, sad, aggressive	*DHCR7*
CHARGE	OCD, immaturity	*CHD7*
Fragile X	ADHD, anxiety, hyperarousal, autism	*FMRP*
Rett	Autism	*MeCP2*
FG	ADHD, anxiety, aggression	*MED12*
Turner	ADHD, immaturity	Loss of all or part of X
XXY, XYY	ADHD	Additional X or Y

Abbreviations: ADHD, attention-deficit/hyperactivity disorder; OCD, obsessive-compulsive disorder; PKU, phenylketonuria.

Note: These are typical problems but do not represent the complete spectrum of psychopathology reported in the disorders; in addition, all of these problems are not present in all cases of the specific disorders.

Many genetic disorders predispose individuals to psychopathology, but it is critical to realize that this is an increased risk and not inevitable. Examples of specific genetic syndromes with often-seen psychiatric problems and associated genetic findings are outlined in Table 6-2. It is noteworthy that teratogenic disorders such as fetal alcohol syndrome are a significant cause of psychopathology in affected individuals and may or may not exist with an underlying genetic disorder in the birth mother or father.

Conclusion

Our understanding of how genetics affects the likelihood of developing a psychiatric disorder is only in its infancy. Although our understanding of the role of genetic factors is evolving, awareness of a potential role of genetic contributors plays an important role for those working with families hoping to adopt or trying to manage behavioral problems in an adopted child.[105] Although there is good reason to believe that the information from the human genome project will have enormous benefit for many people in the future, currently available data are typically inadequate for prospective counseling purposes. As a result, the typically generic genetic screening currently available should only be undertaken or interpreted with extreme caution.

References

1. Myers ED. The English adoption law. *Soc Serv Rev.* 1930;4:53–63
2. Sharma AR, McGue MK, Benson PL. The psychological adjustment of United States adopted adolescents and their nonadopted siblings. *Child Dev.* 1998;69:791–802
3. Brand AE, Brinich PM. Behavior problems and mental health contacts in adopted, foster, and nonadopted children. *J Child Psychol Psychiatry.* 1999;40:1221–1229
4. Keyes MA, Sharma A, Elkins IJ, Iacono WG, McGue M. The mental health of US adolescents adopted in infancy. *Arch Pediatr Adolesc Med.* 2008;162:419–425
5. Rees CA, Selwyn J. Non-infant adoption form care: lessons for safeguarding children. *Child Care Health Dev.* 2009;35:561–567
6. Rushton A, Dance C. The adoption of children from public care: a prospective study of outcome in adolescence. *J Am Acad Child Adolesc Psychiatry.* 2006;45:877–883
7. Peters BR, Atkins MS, McKay MM. Adopted children's behavior problems: a review of five explanatory models. *Clin Psychol Rev.* 1999;19:297–328
8. Colvert E, Rutter M, Beckett C, et al. Emotional difficulties in early adolescence following severe early deprivation: findings from the English and Romanian adoptees study. *Dev Psychopathol.* 2008;20(2):547–567
9. Robert M, Carceller A, Domken V, et al. Physical and neurodevelopmental evaluation of children adopted from Eastern Europe. *Can J Clin Pharmacol.* 2009;16:e432–e440
10. Rueter MA, Keyes MA, Iacono WG, McGue M. Family interactions in adoptive compared to nonadoptive families. *J Fam Psychol.* 2009;23:58–66
11. Gottesman II, Laursen TM, Bertelsen A, Mortensen PB. Severe mental disorders in offspring with 2 psychiatrically ill parents. *Arch Gen Psychiatry.* 2010;67:252–257
12. Tully EC, Iacono WG, McGue M. An adoption study of parental depression as an environmental liability for adolescent depression and childhood disruptive disorders. *Am J Psychiatry.* 2008;165:1148–1154
13. Faraone SV, Tsuang MT, Tsuang DW. *Genetics of Mental Disorders.* New York, NY: The Guilford Press; 1999
14. de Leon J. Pharmacogenomics: the promise of personalized medicine for CNS disorders. *Neuropsychopharmacology.* 2009;34:159–172
15. Moldin SO. Psychiatric genetic counseling. In: Guze SB, ed. *Washington University Adult Psychiatry.* St. Louis, MO: Mosby; 1997
16. Finn CT, Smoller JW. Genetic counseling in psychiatry. *Harv Rev Psychiatry.* 2006;14:109–121
17. Adkins DE, Aberg K, McClay JL, et al. Genomewide pharmacogenomic study of metabolic side effects to antipsychotic drugs. *Mol Psychiatry.* 2011;16(3):321–332

18. Evers K. Personalized medicine in psychiatry: ethical challenges and opportunities. *Dialogues Clin Neurosci.* 2009;11:427–434

19. Khoury MJ, Bertram L, Boffetta P, et al. Genome-wide association studies, field synopses, and the development of the knowledge base on genetic variation and human diseases. *Am J Epidemiol.* 2009;170:269–279

20. Hirschhorn JN. Genomewide association studies—illuminating biologic pathways. *N Engl J Med.* 2009;360:1699–1701

21. Goldstein DB. Common genetic variation and human traits. *N Engl J Med.* 2009;360:1696–1698

22. Kraft P, Wacholder S, Cornelis MC, et al. Beyond odds ratios—communicating disease risk based on genetic profiles. *Nat Rev Genet.* 2009;10:264–269

23. Kraft P, Hunter DJ. Genetic risk prediction—are we there yet? *N Engl J Med.* 2009;360:1701–1703

24. Tizard B. Intercountry adoption: a review of the evidence. *J Child Psychol Psychiatry.* 1991;32:743–756

25. von Borczyskowski A, Hjern A, Lindblad F, Vinnerljung B. Suicidal behaviour in national and international adult adoptees: a Swedish cohort study. *Soc Psychiatry Psychiatr Epidemiol.* 2006;41:95–102

26. Hjern A, Lindblad F, Vinnerljung B. Suicide, psychiatric illness, and social maladjustment in intercountry adoptees in Sweden: a cohort study. *Lancet.* 2002;360:443–448

27. Versluis-den Bieman HJ, Verhulst FC. Self-reported and parent reported problems in adolescent international adoptees. *J Child Psychol Psychiatry.* 1995;36:1411–1428

28. Goldney RD, Donald M, Sawyer MG, Kosky RJ, Priest S. Emotional health of Indonesian adoptees living in Australian families. *Aust N Z J Psychiatry.* 1996;30:534–539

29. Juffer F, van IJzendoorn MH. Behavior problems and mental health referrals of international adoptees: a meta-analysis. *JAMA.* 2005;293:2501–2515

30. Bimmel N, Juffer F, van IJzendoorn MH, Bakermans-Kranenburg MJ. Problem behavior of internationally adopted adolescents: a review and meta-analysis. *Harv Rev Psychiatry.* 2003;11:64–77

31. Harf A, Taieb O, Moro MR. Externalizing behaviour problems of internationally adopted adolescents: a review. *Encephale.* 2007;33:270–276

32. Fensbo C. Mental and behavioural outcome of inter-ethnic adoptees: a review of the literature. *Eur Child Adolesc Psychiatry.* 2004;13:55–63

33. Hutchison KE. Substance use disorders: realizing the promise of pharmacogenomics and personalized medicine. *Annu Rev Clin Psychol.* 2010;6:577–589

34. Kendler KS. Overview: a current perspective on twin studies of schizophrenia. *Am J Psychiatry.* 1983;140:1413–1425

35. Cardno AG, Marshall EJ, Coid B, et al. Heritability estimates for psychotic disorders: the Maudsley twin psychosis series. *Arch Gen Psych.* 1999;56:162–168

36. Grozeva D, Kirov G, Ivanov D, et al. Rare copy number variants: a point of rarity in genetic risk for bipolar disorder and schizophrenia. *Arch Gen Psychiatry.* 2010;67:318–327

37. Fanous AH, Kendler KS. Genetics of clinical features and subtypes of schizophrenia: a review of the recent literature. *Curr Psychiatry Rep.* 2008;10:164–170

38. Need AC, Ge D, Weale ME, et al. A genome-wide investigation of SNPs and CNVs in schizophrenia. *PLoS Genet.* 2009;5:e1000373

39. Owen MJ, Williams HJ, O'Donovan MC. Schizophrenia genetics: advancing on two fronts. *Curr Opin Genet Dev.* 2009;19:266–270

40. Barnett JH, Smoller JW. The genetics of bipolar disorder. *Neuroscience.* 2009;164:331–343

41. Goodwin GM, Anderson I, Arango C, et al. ECNP consensus meeting. Bipolar depression. Nice, March 2007. *Eur Neuropsychopharmacol.* 2008;18:535–549

42. Liu Y, Blackwood DH, Caesar S, et al. Meta-analysis of genome-wide association data of bipolar disorder and major depressive disorder. *Mol Psychiatry.* 2011;16(1):2–4

43. Shyn SI, Hamilton SP. The genetics of major depression: moving beyond the monoamine hypothesis. *Psychiatr Clin North Am.* 2010;33:125–140

44. Sullivan PF, Neale MC, Kendler KS. Genetic epidemiology of major depression: review and meta-analysis. *Am J Psychiatry.* 2000;157:1552–1562

45. Rice F, Harold G, Thapar A. The genetic aetiology of childhood depression: a review. *J Child Psychol Psychiatry.* 2002;43:65–79

46. Kendler KS, Karkowski-Shuman L. Stressful life events and genetic liability to major depression: genetic control of exposure to the environment? *Psychol Med.* 1997;27:539–547

47. Rice F, Harold GT, Shelton KH, Thapar A. Family conflict interacts with genetic liability in predicting childhood and adolescent depression. *J Am Acad Child Adolesc Psychiatry.* 2006;45:841–848

48. Slap G, Goodman E, Huang B. Adoption as a risk factor for attempted suicide during adolescence. *Pediatrics.* 2001;108:E30

49. Kasckow J, Liu N, Haas GL, Phillips MR. Case-control study of the relationship of depressive symptoms to suicide in a community-based sample of individuals with schizophrenia in China. *Schizophr Res.* 2010;122(1-3):226–231

50. Brent DA, Mann JJ. Family genetic studies, suicide, and suicidal behavior. *Am J Med Genet C Semin Med Genet.* 2005;133C:13–24

51. Schulsinger F, Kety SS, Rosenthal D, Wender PH. A family study of suicide. In: Schou M, Stromgren E, eds. *Origin, Prevention and Treatment of Affective Disorders.* London, United Kingdom: Academic Press; 1979:277–287

52. Runeson BS. History of suicidal behaviour in the families of young suicides. *Acta Psychiatr Scand.* 1998;98:497–501

53. Baldessarini RJ, Hennen J. Genetics of suicide: an overview. *Harv Rev Psychiatry.* 2004;12:1–13

54. Brent DA, Melhem N. Familial transmission of suicidal behavior. *Psychiatr Clin North Am.* 2008;31:157–177

55. McGirr A, Alda M, Seguin M, Cabot S, Lesage A, Turecki G. Familial aggregation of suicide explained by cluster B traits: a three-group family study of suicide controlling for major depressive disorder. *Am J Psychiatry.* 2009;166:1124–1134

56. Borowsky IW, Ireland M, Resnick MD. Adolescent suicide attempts: risks and protectors. *Pediatrics.* 2001;107:485–493

57. Gater R, Tansella M, Korten A, Tiemens BG, Mavreas VG, Olatawura MO. Sex differences in the prevalence and detection of depressive and anxiety disorders in general health care settings: report from the World Health Organization Collaborative Study on Psychological Problems in General Health Care. *Arch Gen Psychiatry.* 1998;55:405–413

58. Hettema JM, Neale MC, Kendler KS. A review and meta-analysis of the genetic epidemiology of anxiety disorders. *Am J Psychiatry.* 2001;158:1568–1578

59. Kessler RC, McGonagle KA, Zhao S, et al. Lifetime and 12-month prevalence of DSM-III-R psychiatric disorders in the United States. Results from the National Comorbidity Survey. *Arch Gen Psychiatry.* 1994;51:8–19

60. Hettema JM, Prescott CA, Myers JM, Neale MC, Kendler KS. The structure of genetic and environmental risk factors for anxiety disorders in men and women. *Arch Gen Psychiatry.* 2005;62:182–189

61. Bienvenu OJ, Hettema JM, Neale MC, Prescott CA, Kendler KS. Low extraversion and high neuroticism as indices of genetic and environmental risk for social phobia, agoraphobia, and animal phobia. *Am J Psychiatry.* 2007;164:1714–1721

62. Cadoret RJ, Yates WR, Troughton E, Woodworth G, Stewart MA. Adoption study demonstrating two genetic pathways to drug abuse. *Arch Gen Psychiatry.* 1995;52:42–52

63. Sher KJ, Dick DM, Crabbe JC, Hutchison KE, O'Malley SS, Heath AC. Consilient research approaches in studying gene x environment interactions in alcohol research. *Addict Biol.* 2010;15:200–216

64. Sartor CE, Agrawal A, Lynskey MT, Bucholz KK, Heath AC. Genetic and environmental influences on the rate of progression to alcohol dependence in young women. *Alcohol Clin Exp Res.* 2008;32:632–638

65. Li MD, Burmeister M. New insights into the genetics of addiction. *Nat Rev Genet.* 2009;10:225–231

66. True WR, Xian H, Scherrer JF, et al. Common genetic vulnerability for nicotine and alcohol dependence in men. *Arch Gen Psychiatry.* 1999;56:655–661

67. Agrawal A, Sartor CE, Lynskey MT, et al. Evidence for an interaction between age at first drink and genetic influences on DSM-IV alcohol dependence symptoms. *Alcohol Clin Exp Res.* 2009;33:2047–2056

68. Michel A, Mormont C, Legros JJ. A psycho-endocrinological overview of transsexualism. *Eur J Endocrinol.* 2001;145:365–376

69. Bakker A, van Kesteren PJ, Gooren LJ, Bezemer PD. The prevalence of transsexualism in the Netherlands. *Acta Psychiatr Scand.* 1993;87:237–238

70. Möller B, Schreier H, Li A, Romer G. Gender identity disorder in children and adolescents. *Curr Probl Pediatr Adolesc Health Care.* 2009;39:117–143

71. Coolidge FL, Thede LL, Young SE. The heritability of gender identity disorder in a child and adolescent twin sample. *Behav Genet.* 2002;32:251–257

72. Knafo A, Iervolino AC, Plomin R. Masculine girls and feminine boys: genetic and environmental contributions to atypical gender development in early childhood. *J Pers Soc Psychol.* 2005;88:400–412

73. Iervolino AC, Hines M, Golombok SE, Rust J, Plomin R. Genetic and environmental influences on sex-typed behavior during the preschool years. *Child Dev.* 2005;76:826–840

74. van Beijsterveldt CE, Hudziak JJ, Boomsma DI. Genetic and environmental influences on cross-gender behavior and relation to behavior problems: a study of Dutch twins at ages 7 and 10 years. *Arch Sex Behav.* 2006;35:647–658

75. Hyde C, Kenna JC. A male MZ twin pair, concordant for transsexualism, discordant for schizophrenia. *Acta Psychiatr Scand.* 1977;56:265–275

76. Garden GM, Rothery DJ. A female monozygotic twin pair discordant for transsexualism. Some theoretical implications. *Br J Psychiatry.* 1992;161:852–854

77. Sadeghi M, Fakhraj A. Transsexualism in female monozygotic twins: a case report. *Aust N Z J Psychiatry.* 2000;34:862–864

78. Segal NL. Twins and transsexualism: an update and a preview; research reviews: conjoined twins, angiographic lesions, single versus double embryo transfer; headlines: school placement legislation, Junior Taekwondo Olympics, prosthetic ears, murder victim. *Twin Res Hum Genet.* 2007;10:894–897

79. Bentz EK, Hefler LA, Kaufmann U, Huber JC, Kolbus A, Tempfer CB. A polymorphism of the CYP17 gene related to sex steroid metabolism is associated with female-to-male but not male-to-female transsexualism. *Fertil Steril.* 2008;90(1):56–59

80. Bosinski HA, Peter M, Bonatz G, et al. A higher rate of hyperandrogenic disorders in female-to-male transsexuals. *Psychoneuroendocrinology.* 1997;22:361–380

81. Hines M, Johnston KJ, Golombok S, Rust J, Stevens M, Golding J. Prenatal stress and gender role behavior in girls and boys: a longitudinal, population study. *Horm Behav.* 2002;42:126–134

82. Bentz EK, Schneeberger C, Hefler LA, et al. A common polymorphism of the SRD5A2 gene and transsexualism. *Reprod Sci.* 2007;14:705–709

83. Hare L, Bernard P, Sanchez FJ, et al. Androgen receptor repeat length polymorphism associated with male-to-female transsexualism. *Biol Psychiatry.* 2009;65:93–96

84. Buhrich N, Barr R, Lam-Po-Tang PR. Two transsexuals with 47-XYY karyotype. *Br J Psychiatry.* 1978;133:77–81

85. Taneja N, Ammini AC, Mohapatra I, Saxena S, Kucheria K. A transsexual male with 47,XYY karyotype. *Br J Psychiatry.* 1992;161:698–699

86. Turan MT, Eşel E, Dündar M, et al. Female-to-male transsexual with 47,XXX karyotype. *Biol Psychiatry.* 2000;48:1116–1117

87. Mouaffak F, Gallarda T, Baup N, Olie JP, Krebs MO. Gender identity disorders and bipolar disorder associated with the ring Y chromosome. *Am J Psychiatry.* 2007;164:1122–1123

88. Elsea SH, Girirajan S. Smith-magenis syndrome. *Eur J Hum Genet.* 2008;16:412–421

89. Gothelf D, Frisch A, Michaelovsky E, Weizman A, Shprintzen RJ. Velo-cardio-facial syndrome. *J Ment Health Res Intellect Disabil.* 2009;2:149–167

90. Pelc K, Cheron G, Dan B. Behavior and neuropsychiatric manifestations in Angelman syndrome. *Neuropsychiatr Dis Treat.* 2008;4:577–584

91. Cassidy SB, Driscoll DJ. Prader-Willi syndrome. *Eur J Hum Genet.* 2009;17:3–13

92. Pober BR. Williams-Beuren syndrome. *N Engl J Med.* 2010;362:239–252

93. Verhoeven WM, Tuinier S, Kuijpers HJ, Egger JI, Brunner HG. Psychiatric profile in Rubinstein-Taybi syndrome. A review and case report. *Psychopathology.* 2010;43:63–68

94. Bracken P, Coll P. Homocystinuria and schizophrenia. Literature review and case report. *J Nerv Ment Dis.* 1985;173:51–55

95. Gentile JK, Ten Hoedt AE, Bosch AM. Psychosocial aspects of PKU: hidden disabilities—a review. *Mol Genet Metab.* 2010;99:S64–S67

96. Mihaljevic-Peles A, Jakovljevic M, Milicevic Z, Kracun I. Low arylsulphatase A activity in the development of psychiatric disorders. *Neuropsychobiology.* 2001;43:75–78

97. Nyhan WL. Lesch-Nyhan disease. *Nucleosides Nucleotides Nucleic Acids.* 2008;27:559–563

98. Tierney E, Nwokoro NA, Kelley RI. Behavioral phenotype of RSH/Smith-Lemli-Opitz syndrome. *Ment Retard Dev Disabil Res Rev.* 2000;6(2):131–134

99. Hartshorne TS, Hefner MA, Davenport SLH. Behavior in CHARGE syndrome: introduction to the special topic. *Am J Med Genet.* 2005;133A:228–231

100. Hagerman RJ, Berry-Kravis E, Kaufmann WE, et al. Advances in the treatment of fragile X syndrome. *Pediatrics.* 2009;123:378–390

101. Vignoli A, Fabio RA, La Briola F, et al. Correlations between neurophysiological, behavioral, and cognitive function in Rett syndrome. *Epilepsy Behav.* 2010;17(4):489–496

102. Graham JM Jr, Visootsak J, Dykens E, et al. Behavior of 10 patients with FG syndrome (Opitz-Kaveggia syndrome) and the p.R961W mutation in the MED12 gene. *Am J Med Genet A.* 2008;146A:3011–3017

103. Christopoulos P, Deligeoroglou E, Laggari V, Christogiorgos S, Creatsas G. Psychological and behavioural aspects of patients with Turner syndrome from childhood to adulthood: a review of the clinical literature. *J Psychosom Obstet Gynaecol.* 2008;29:45–51

104. Visootsak J, Graham JM Jr. Social function in multiple X and Y chromosome disorders: XXY, XYY, XXYY, XXXY. *Dev Disabil Res Rev.* 2009;15(4):328–332

105. Tsuang D, Faraone SV, Tsuang MT. Psychiatric genetic counseling. In: Bloom FE, Kupfer DJ, eds. *Back to Psychopharmacology—the Fourth Generation of Progress.* 4th ed. Baltimore, MD: Lippincott Williams & Wilkins; 1995

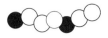

CHAPTER 7

The Neurobiology of Risk and Resilience in Adopted Children

Prachi E. Shah, MD, MS

Adoption is defined as the permanent legal placement of a child who is abandoned, relinquished, or orphaned within a family of relatives (kinship adoption) or an unrelated family (non-kinship adoption) (see chapters 1 and 2).[1] Children who are adopted often come from vulnerable backgrounds characterized by caregiver inconsistency and varying degrees of biological and psychosocial risk.[2] Adoption is a powerful intervention characterized by a radical environmental change with a child typically moving from an environment of early adversity to one of a family. Although many adoptees demonstrate remarkable developmental and behavioral resilience and catch-up post-adoption,[1,3,4] developmental outcomes among adopted children remain highly variable.[5,6] These differences in developmental and behavioral outcomes for adoptees raise the question about individual differences in adaptation post-adoption—why do some children demonstrate almost complete recovery, whereas other children manifest continued vulnerabilities post-adoption? What are the factors leading to ongoing developmental risk in children who are adopted, and furthermore, what are the factors that promote resilience? This chapter attempts to highlight the risk factors associated with specific exposures, but clearly this is only part of the story.

Research highlighting the varied outcomes of children who are adopted supports a well-known principle of developmental psychology—namely, that early experience has a profound effect on early human development, and within the context of environmental experience, there are certain periods during development when experiences have a more significant effect than others.[7] These "sensitive periods" of development are times during which the individual is more vulnerable to the effects of developmental risk factors and more susceptible to the effects of intervention.[8] The timing, dose, and duration of risk factors during this sensitive period of development and the individual's differential susceptibility to environmental influences[9] can contribute to the different developmental trajectories of children who are adopted.

To better conceptualize how risk and resilience are conferred onto children with a history of adoption, it is helpful to have a better understanding of how early experience influences the developing brain. The degree to which the developing brain is vulnerable to external influences is dependent on the dose, duration, timing, and nature of the insult. Conversely, in the postnatal caregiving environment, the degree of recovery from early injury is determined by the degree to which an optimized postnatal environment can remediate the effects of early injury. Certainly there are some developmental vulnerabilities that can be largely minimized when children are placed in a nurturing postnatal environment; yet there are some vulnerabilities that may be refractory to complete recovery, based on the nature, timing, and duration of the insult. In considering the developmental vulnerabilities of children with a history of adoption, whether domestically, internationally, privately, or from child protective services, it is helpful to consider the timing and types of developmental risk adopted children may encounter in terms of the prenatal, perinatal, and postnatal influences. Risk factors that may affect a child's development often include a combination of prenatal, perinatal, and postnatal experiences, and thus it is often difficult to disentangle the effects of prenatal substance exposure, malnutrition, neglect, abuse, multiple placements, or institutional deprivation from the context of social dysfunction (eg, poverty, institutional care, parental addiction, impaired parenting, history of mental illness or learning disabilities) in which these risk factors occur.[10] Nonetheless, to have a better understanding of the developmental risk factors conferred onto adoptees, it is helpful to consider the risk factors in terms of their developmental timing, ie, prenatal, perinatal, and postnatal insults.

Prenatal Risk Factors

One of the challenges in quantifying developmental risk in adoptees, especially those adopted internationally, is that often the prenatal history is unknown or limited at best. Complete medical histories, documenting details known to influence subsequent development, including the quality of prenatal care, family history of genetic disorders, history of alcohol and substance use, history of domestic violence, history of maternal nutrition, and exposure to teratogens, are often unavailable.[10] Each of these risk factors are known to confer developmental and behavioral risk onto the developing fetus and often co-occur. Research describing the discrete effect on later child development of several prenatal risk factors, including maternal stress, poor maternal nutrition, exposure to teratogens, and history of alcohol and substance abuse, is highlighted herein.

Maternal Stress

Considering the context of a child's adoption, circumstances contributing to that adoption are often fraught with difficulties. At the very least, children who are ultimately placed for adoption often come from biological families who are unable or unwilling to provide for them.[11] Conditions of poverty and psychosocial adversity associated with children who are adopted are common.[12] Contextualizing the early environment of the adopted child in terms of the intrauterine environment, prenatal conditions leading to a child's adoption are often situations of high maternal stress that are transmitted through the intrauterine environment to the developing fetus. The effects of stress on the developing fetus and on later child development have been well described in animal and human models.[13–16] In animal models, prenatal stress has been associated with delayed motor and mental development,[17] impaired behavioral adaptation,[17,18] and intrauterine growth restriction.[13] In humans, prenatal stress has been associated with preterm birth and low birth weight,[19] impaired mental and motor development, decreased attention regulation, and more difficult temperament in infancy,[16,20] as well as increased risk of disorders of attention, schizophrenia, depression, and drug abuse later in life.[15,18] The mechanism by which prenatal stress is thought to affect offspring is not entirely understood but is thought to be related to hyper-activation of the maternal hypothalamic-pituitary-adrenal (HPA) axis and excessive exposure of the fetus to maternal glucocorticoids.[21,22] See Chapter 10, The Long-term Consequences of Child Maltreatment in Adopted Children, on page 193 for additional details.

Cortisol, the primary glucocorticoid in humans, is a stress-responsive hormone arising from the HPA axis. Though most maternal cortisol is inactivated by placental enzymes,[23] a small amount of maternal cortisol can pass through the placenta to the fetus, thereby affecting fetal cortisol concentrations.[21] Though the mechanisms are not entirely clear, limited but consistent evidence suggests that the exposure to maternal stress hormones results in downregulation of fetal glucocorticoid receptors and alteration of receptor sensitivity, thereby leading to altered fetal HPA axis regulation.[24] Prenatal glucocorticoid exposure is thought to affect the development of the neural areas of the limbic systems involved in the regulation of fear and behavioral inhibition,[20] resulting in increased fussiness and negative affect in infancy,[25] heightened behavioral inhibition or fearfulness in response to novelty, and impaired cortisol regulation early in childhood. Thus, it appears that exposure to maternal stress and resultant exposure to prenatal glucocorticoids has consequences on infants and children through the development of behaviorally inhibited or fearful temperament.[20] Further discussion of developmental and the HPA axis can be found in Chapter 10 (page 193).

Maternal Nutrition

Poor maternal nutrition is a risk factor for, but by no means uniformly correlated with, poor fetal growth, preterm birth, and impaired brain development, all of which can lead to adverse birth outcomes.[19,26] Maternal malnutrition exerts its effects during the period of rapid brain development and periods of early neural organizational processes such as neurogenesis, cell migration, and cell differentiation.[27] Animal studies examining maternal malnutrition have demonstrated an association between maternal malnutrition and lifelong impairments in learning and attention, which may be considered the equivalent of "minimal brain dysfunction" in humans.[28] In humans, malnutrition during pregnancy has been related to challenging behaviors that are thought to arise from the effects of undernutrition on the prefrontal cortex.[29] Maternal malnutrition also impedes myelin synthesis[30] and alters the morphology and distribution of dendritic spines on neurons, resulting in a reduced ability of the brain to adapt to internal and external changes, thereby impeding the process of brain plasticity[27] and subsequent brain development.[28] One of the consequences of maternal malnutrition is that it may not always occur in isolation. Maternal undernutrition may coexist with alcohol misuse, thereby conferring a double risk on the developing fetus.[27]

Teratogen Exposure

Teratogens are known prenatal exposures that can cause an embryo or fetus to develop abnormally. The teratogenic effects of any specific agent on the fetus are highly variable and depend on the gestational timing of the exposure as well as the dose, route, and nature of the agent itself.[31] Teratogen exposure is often difficult to ascertain because of limited perinatal and family history, and congenital malformations resulting from teratogen exposure are often underdiagnosed before adoptive placement.[32]

Alcohol Use

The effects of intrauterine alcohol exposure on later child development have been widely studied and are highly variable. The range of anomalies attributed to prenatal alcohol exposure can range from mild dysmorphology and learning and behavior problems to meeting full criteria for a diagnosis of fetal alcohol syndrome, characterized by growth deficiency, central nervous system (CNS) damage, and dysmorphic facial features.[10] The range of developmental anomalies and disabilities resulting from intrauterine alcohol exposure are described broadly as *fetal alcohol spectrum disorders*,[33] which is thought to affect as many as 1 per 100 births worldwide.[34] Alcohol is a known teratogen that affects multiple organ systems during gestation, especially the CNS, including neuronal architecture, neuronal migration, and synaptogenesis.[10] Specifically, alcohol is thought to exert its teratogenic effects by interfering with nerve cell development, increasing the formation of free radicals and altering biochemical signals within cells and expression of genes, resulting in impaired nerve cell development.[33] The teratogenic effects on the developing fetus and the effect on later development are highly variable and depend on maternal factors, including the dose, duration, and timing of intrauterine alcohol exposure,[35] with greatest impairments seen with binge patterns of prenatal alcohol exposure (ie, ≥5 drinks/exposure),[36] as well as fetal factors, including the degree of alcohol metabolism at the fetal level, determined by fetal alcohol dehydrogenase activity.[37]

A history of maternal alcohol consumption is often difficult to quantify from adoption records, and the exact amount, type, and timing of alcohol use during pregnancy may be difficult to ascertain.[10] Beyond neurodevelopmental disabilities resulting from the effect of alcohol on the developing brain, other congenital defects include vision problems (refractive errors, strabismus, optic nerve hypoplasia); hearing problems (conductive and sensorineural hearing loss); cleft palate; cardiac, renal, and orthopedic impairment; as well as the dysmorphic features that characterize fetal alcohol syndrome (thin upper lip, smooth philtrum, and small palpebral fissure lengths).[33,38] Neurodevelopmental outcomes are variable and diverse, including cognitive impairment with IQ ranging from borderline to mental retardation, neuromotor deficits, attention problems, hyperactivity, difficulties with learning and working memory, and deficits in receptive and expressive language and reading comprehension.[39] In addition, children with intrauterine exposure to alcohol often demonstrate fine and gross motor deficits, deficits in motor planning, and impairments in visual spatial functioning, which can persist into adolescence.[40]

One notable challenge to identification is that children with prenatal exposure to alcohol can have a completely normal facial phenotype but still be at risk for learning and behavior problems later in life. However, because of the comorbidity of many intrauterine risk factors, it is often difficult to differentiate the effect of alcohol from other genetic and environmental factors, including concomitant substance use.[10] (For more on the effect of alcohol on prenatal and postnatal development, see Chapter 5, Prenatal Substance Exposure: Alcohol and Other Substances—Implications for Adoption, on page 97).

Substance Use

Intrauterine exposure to substances including heroin or methadone, tobacco, marijuana, cocaine, and methamphetamines may also affect later development. For more information, see Chapter 5 (page 97).

Opiates

With respect to international adoption, the most common prenatal opiate exposure is heroin, especially in Eastern Europe and the former Soviet Union.[10] Though prenatal opiate exposure is not associated with any congenital malformations, the majority of infants with a history of prenatal narcotic exposure demonstrate symptoms of withdrawal early in the newborn period[41] and have an increased risk of intrauterine growth restriction and preterm birth.[42] Early reported developmental consequences of prenatal exposure to opiates include attention problems, hyperactivity, sleep disturbances, and memory and perceptual difficulties[10]; however, later studies revealed that infant prenatal exposure to opiates was not associated with mental, motor, or behavioral deficits after controlling for neonatal and environmental risk factors.[43]

Tobacco

Intrauterine exposure to tobacco is one of the most common prenatal exposures in domestic and international adoptees, and teratogenic effects are well described.[44] Tobacco smoke contains numerous substances, including lead, cyanide, and cadmium, known to be harmful to the fetus.[45] Nicotine freely crosses the placenta and has direct and indirect effects on neurodevelopment, and intrauterine hypoxia, mediated by carbon monoxide and decreased uterine blood flow, results in growth impairment and intrauterine growth restriction.[10] The developmental and behavioral sequelae of prenatal tobacco exposure contribute to impairments in infancy and later childhood. In infancy, prenatal tobacco exposure has been associated with lower arousal, decreased suck, decreased autonomic regulation, decreased orientation to stimuli, greater negative affect, and decreased ability to sooth.[46,47] In early childhood, prenatal tobacco exposure has been associated with deficits in learning and memory, impaired eye-hand coordination, increased impulsivity, increased externalizing behavior problems, delays in language, and an increased risk of cognitive impairment.[46,48] It is not clear whether these developmental vulnerabilities can be modified in the context of the post-adoptive environment or the degree to which an optimized caregiving environment can obviate these early risks.[46]

Marijuana

Marijuana is a commonly used illicit substance among pregnant women, but evidence of prenatal exposure to marijuana is often unreported in adoption records. The active substance in marijuana, delta-9-tetrahydrocannabinol, rapidly crosses the placenta and can remain in the body for up to 30 days, thereby increasing fetal exposure.[10] The effects of prenatal marijuana use on later cognition, behavior, and development are difficult to disentangle from the effects of other substances often used concomitantly. Prenatal marijuana exposure has been shown to have mild effects on cognition, learning, and memory and greater effects on behavior, with levels of impulsivity associated with marijuana exposure.[49] In addition, prenatal marijuana exposure has been associated with impaired cognitive function early in childhood, but these effects have been shown to be modifiable by placement in an educationally enriched environment (ie, preschool).[50]

Cocaine

The effects of cocaine on child developmental outcomes have been well studied.[51-53] Cocaine and its metabolites readily cross the placenta and produce directly neurotoxic effects, increasing circulating catecholamine levels, especially norepinephrine levels; this leads to vasoconstriction, increased heart rate, and fetal hypertension, thereby placing the fetus at risk for vascular-mediated injury.[10,54] After controlling for the social risk factors commonly seen with cocaine use, significant evidence suggests a limited effect of prenatal cocaine exposure on growth, cognitive ability, academic achievement, and language functioning.[55] However, prenatal cocaine exposure does contribute to alternations in brain structure and function, which are largely manifest as deficits in attention and self-regulation.[52] Many of the developmental effects of prenatal cocaine exposure appear to be moderated by the quality of the caregiving environment.[55]

Methamphetamine

Methamphetamine abuse is increasing domestically and abroad. The effects of methamphetamine on later development are not entirely known, but amphetamines are thought to exert neurotoxic effects on subcortical brain structures.[10] Structurally, methamphetamine use in pregnancy has been linked to fetal growth restriction and cardiac and cleft anomalies. Neurodevelopmentally, infants with prenatal exposure to methamphetamines demonstrate relatively decreased arousal, increased stress, and poor quality of movement.[56] There are limited data about long-term behavioral and developmental sequelae of methamphetamine-exposed children, but associations with aggressive behavior, hyperactivity, attention problems, visual motor integration problems, and deficits in working memory have been reported.[10] Similar to other prenatal exposures, methamphetamine use during pregnancy is often a characteristic of a chaotic prenatal and later caregiving environment. It is not clear if the effects of methamphetamine on later development are modifiable once a child transitions into an optimal caregiving environment.

Other Teratogens

In addition to the teratogenic effects of alcohol and substance use, other drugs and medications can increase the risk of congenital anomalies. A more complete reference of teratogenic effects of drugs is available.[57]

Drugs known to have teratogenic effect in humans at therapeutic doses include angiotensin-converting enzyme inhibitors, antiepileptic drugs, coumarin derivatives, diethylstilbestrol, indomethacin, lithium, methotrexate, quinine, radioiodine, retinoids, tetracycline, and thalidomide, although the effect on fetal development is largely related to timing of exposure, dose, and duration. Exposure during the period of rapid organogenesis (18–60 days postconception) is known to cause fetal growth retardation, death, or severe CNS dysfunction. Dose of exposure is also critical in causing teratogenesis. Exposures are only teratogenic if they exceed a certain threshold dose. Below that dose, damage to the embryo does not occur, but above the threshold, the severity of teratogenic effects increases in a dose-responsive fashion. Finally, duration of exposure is important, with teratogenic effects more likely seen if the exposure was chronic throughout the pregnancy rather than occurring only once or twice.[31] If available, a history of maternal exposure to teratogens is helpful in ascertaining level of developmental risk to the adoptee.

Perinatal Risk Factors: Preterm Birth

One of the biggest risk factors for abnormal neurodevelopment is the perinatal risk factor of being born prematurely. Many of the risk factors delineated previously are notable risk factors for a preterm birth, including maternal stress,[58,59] maternal history of smoking,[60] low prepregnancy weight,[19,61] history of domestic violence,[62] history of substance abuse (especially cocaine use),[63] and history of psychosocial disadvantage.[64] Determination of an adopted child's perinatal status can be difficult, as infants adopted internationally may have incomplete birth records with limited information about the child's birth weight, gestational age, neonatal complications, and interventions undertaken.[65]

For the adopted infant known to be premature, the developmental vulnerabilities of preterm infants are well described and include an increased risk of cognitive impairments[66–68]; language deficits[69,70]; deficits in executive function, visual motor skills, and working memory[71,72]; vision and hearing problems[73]; autism[74–77]; learning disabilities[68,71,73]; motor deficits[78,79]; and internalizing and externalizing behavior problems,[67,71,80] including attention deficits.[66,81–83] Although the greatest developmental deficits have been observed in infants born at lower gestational ages and lower birth weights,[73,84,85] there is emerging evidence that even infants born at higher gestational ages without ostensible neurologic injury are also at risk for later developmental delay,[86–88] learning problems,[89,90] and attention and behavioral concerns.[91,92] Each preterm child's developmental prognosis, whether adopted or not, can be difficult to predict early in life (ie, some developmental difficulties are not manifest until the child is much older). However, there are some biological risk factors associated with greater neurodevelopmental challenges later in life.

One additional consideration with respect to international adoption of preterm infants is the quality of medical care available in a child's birth country. For example, while the availability of surfactant has clearly affected the outcome of preterm infants born in developing countries over the past several decades, this is one intervention clearly not routinely available in many developing countries. As a result, consideration of possible long-term outcomes for children known or suspected to be born prematurely should include the routine medical interventions available to a child at the time of birth. For extremely premature infants, survival is quite unlikely without access to current technology, but for children who may be expected to have minimal long-term risks if cared for in a modern neonatal intensive care unit, long-term risks may be more prevalent from children from developing countries.

Biological Risk Factors for Abnormal Neurodevelopment in Preterm Infants

For the preterm adopted child whose neonatal course is known, certain details in the perinatal history can help identify risk factors for an adverse developmental prognosis.[93] Known risk factors for later abnormal neurodevelopment include lower gestational age, lower birth weight, history of chronic lung disease, abnormal findings on neuroimaging, history of sepsis, and elevated bilirubin levels.[94]

Compared with full-term infants, preterm infants demonstrate differences in brain structure and function, an increased vulnerability to neurologic injury,[73,95] and smaller cortical volumes, with greatest reductions in the areas of the sensorimotor regions, premotor cortex, basal ganglia, cerebellum, and corpus callosum. These differences in brain structure appear to contribute to long-term disturbances in cerebral development, resulting in the cognitive deficits often seen in preterm infants.[96] Furthermore, the presence of neonatal brain injury, seen more often in preterm infants born at lower gestational ages and lower birth weights, is also a significant risk factor for adverse neurodevelopmental outcomes.[75,78,97–99] Ascertaining a history of neonatal brain injury in the adopted child may be difficult because details in the medical record may be limited or absent. It is well described that evidence of perinatal brain injury (ie, interventricular hemorrhage and cystic periventricular leukomalacia) on head ultrasound is associated with an increased risk of development of cerebral palsy and intellectual disability in preterm newborns.[99] However, cranial ultrasound is often not sensitive enough to detect subtle injury to the gray and white matter and cerebellum, which has been associated with motor deficits, language impairment, and cognitive deficits and is better identified with magnetic resonance imaging.[75,96,97,100]

Additional medical conditions that may be reported for preterm infants may contribute to an increased risk for later developmental challenges. One biological risk factor associated with an increased risk of abnormal neurodevelopment is history of chronic lung disease or bronchopulmonary dysplasia (BPD). Chronic lung disease/BPD is defined as an oxygen requirement at 36 weeks of age and, outside of hemorrhagic or white matter injury, is the most significant risk factor associated with neurobehavioral problems in the preterm infant,[101] with more severe BPD serving as a risk factor for lower IQ, poorer language function, deficits in perceptual organization, and need for more special education services.[102] Other medical risk factors associated with poorer developmental outcomes for preterm infants includes a history of sepsis,[66] especially a history of maternal chorioamnionitis or infant history of sepsis, meningitis, and necrotizing enterocolitis,[103] and history of neonatal hyperbilirubinemia. Hyperbilirubinemia is a common problem in the preterm infant and is known to cause neuronal injury, even at low bilirubin concentrations.[101] Long-term developmental effects of bilirubin toxicity on preterm infants may include developmental delay[104] and hearing loss.[105] Although high levels of hyperbilirubinemia are known to be neurotoxic, the neurodevelopmental consequences of modest elevations of bilirubin levels are still unclear.[101]

In sum, there is extensive evidence that infants born preterm, especially those with a history of poor prenatal care and significant postnatal complications, are at heightened risk of later developmental and behavior problems. A thorough review of known or suspected prenatal and perinatal health is important to identify potential risk factors for abnormal development.

Postnatal Risk Factors

For the child adopted beyond the newborn period, typically from domestic foster care or internationally, there appear to be several postnatal risk factors that can affect later developmental and behavioral outcomes, including but not limited to the amount of time spent in a pathogenic caregiving environment, possible exposure to toxins (eg, lead), and nutritional factors.

Quality of the Early Caregiving Environment and Time in Pathogenic Care

It has been well described that children who have been adopted are at risk for multiple adverse outcomes, including poor growth, cognitive impairments, behavior problems, adverse social-emotional development, and differences in attachment, compared with non-adopted children.[4,106–109] However, developmental outcomes of children adopted from early pathogenic caregiving environments appear to be highly variable, with some children demonstrating apparently typical outcomes and others demonstrating pervasive impairment.[108,110,111] Similar to many of the risk factors previously described, the level of subsequent impairment appears to be related to dose (level of dysfunction in the caregiving environment) and duration (how long the child was exposed to this pathogenic environment), with the degree of developmental catch-up among adoptees related to the child's age at adoption, degree of early pathogenic care, and quality of the post-adoptive caregiving environment.[3,112] Children who were adopted at younger ages and experienced less pathogenic care and more caregiving sensitivity in the post-adoptive environment appear to demonstrate the best developmental prognosis.[113–115]

The quality of the early caregiving environment in a young child's life exerts an important influence on the child's later social-emotional development.[116] One of the most important factors that all young children need for healthy emotional development, even more than food and shelter, is the experience of caregivers who are committed to them.[117] Young children in the foster care system or who were raised in institutions have, to varying degrees, histories of early pathogenic care.

Children are typically placed in orphanages or enter the foster care system because their parents are unable to provide a safe environment or appropriate physical or emotional care for them. This can include children whose mothers tested positive for illegal substances at birth, whose parents neglected or abused them, or whose parents are incarcerated or experience psychiatric hospitalization.[118] Children who enter the foster care system have experienced at least one serious disruption in their caregiving and have often been exposed to serious disturbances in their caregiver's functioning, necessitating their removal from that caregiver's care. Similarly, effects of early environmental instability, especially neglect, maltreatment, and permanent separation from a primary caregiver, appear to have detrimental effects on brain development, especially on the organization of the prefrontal cortex, and play an important role in neuroendocrine function and related behavioral regulation.[119,120]

Children who enter the foster care system or reside in institutions are also likely to experience numerous changes in placement. Placement instability and a history of multiple caregivers are associated with immediate and long-term adverse outcomes, including difficulties with attachment and an increased risk of emotional and behavioral problems.[121] For the child in foster care, the inherent biological drive of infancy—to trust and depend on the caregiver for protection and nurturance[122]—has been violated, leading to dysregulation of behavioral and biobehavioral systems.[123,124]

For the child whose early life was spent in institutional care, caregiving inconsistency as well as physical and psychosocial deprivation are often very common. Quality of care and level of deprivation in institutions can be highly variable. In some institutions, the caregiver-child ratio can be reasonable and the level of cognitive, sensory, and language deprivation may be relatively mild. However, more commonly, institutional care is characterized by high caregiver-child ratios, poorly trained caregivers who are insensitive and unresponsive to children's needs, poor nutrition, inadequate cognitive and sensory stimulation, and a lack of individualized caregiving.[125] The effects of early pathogenic care on child development are well described and include physical and brain growth deficiencies,[126] cognitive problems,[127,128] speech and language delays,[129] social and behavior abnormalities,[130] attention and behavior problems,[130,131] disturbances of attachment,[132] and autistic-like behavior.[6]

It should be noted, however, that although psychosocial deprivation is associated with impairment across a range of developmental domains, the degree of impairment and trajectory of recovery are highly variable.[125] It appears that for children who are adopted, the duration of deprivation and pathogenic care plays an important role in the severity of impairment and potential for recovery—but the outcome for any individual child is not easily predicted. In general, children who were adopted at younger than 6 months and who spent less time in pathogenic care demonstrated the best developmental prognosis. Children institutionalized for more than 6 months of life demonstrated pervasive impairment that persisted for many years, despite placement in an optimal caregiving environment.[8] (See Chapter 11, Long-term Developmental and Behavioral Issues Following Adoption, on page 217.)

Lead

Another well-described developmental risk factor is the exposure to environmental neurotoxins, the most common of which is lead. For children who live in poverty or with high psychosocial risk, lead toxicity may follow ingestion of lead-containing paint or plaster that may be on cribs, furniture, or walls or in contaminated drinking water. Children who are adopted from other countries (eg, Asia, Africa, Eastern Europe) may have acquired lead poisoning in their home countries related to environmental exposures, especially if they come from poverty-stricken households where dilapidated housing; poor industrial and environmental controls; continued use of leaded gasoline, paint, pottery, or cosmetics; and living conditions expose children to ongoing lead contamination.[133]

The neurophysiologic mechanism for lead exposure contributing to neurodevelopmental outcomes has been copiously studied for decades. Lead readily traverses the blood-brain barrier, accumulates in the brain, and preferentially damages the prefrontal cerebral cortex, hippocampus, and cerebellum.[134] The pathogenesis of lead toxicity is not entirely known but is thought to derive from 2 different basic mechanisms—interference with neurotransmission at the synapse and disruption in cellular migration during critical periods of CNS development.[133] Specifically, lead appears to disrupt the organization and maintenance of neuronal connections and acts specifically at N-methyl-d-aspartate glutamate receptors, thereby affecting long-term potentiation and other forms of synaptic plasticity that are involved in learning and memory.[135]

The consequences of lead toxicity are varied and include cognitive losses, aggression, hyperactivity, impulsivity, inattention, and learning failure.[133] More specifically, neurocognitive deficits associated with lead toxicity have been reported in almost all major domains of function, including verbal and performance IQ, academic skills such as reading and mathematics, visual-spatial skills, problem-solving skills, executive function, fine and gross motor skills, memory, and language skills.[133,136] Although neurologic deficits have been well documented with high lead levels,[135] it appears that cognitive and behavioral deficits are also noted at lower lead levels, which were once thought to be safe.[137,138] Furthermore, it appears that the neurodevelopmental and behavioral sequelae related to elevated lead levels, including attention problems,[133] aggression,[137] antisocial behavior,[139] and neurocognitive deficits, are pervasive and demonstrate minimal improvement despite correction of blood lead levels.[140–142]

Nutrition and Growth

Another determinant of later neurodevelopmental outcomes for adoptees is their pre-adoptive nutritional status. It is well described that international adoptees, especially those who spend their first few years of life in institutional care, demonstrate signs of malnutrition, nutrient deficiency,[143] and aberrant growth and development pre-adoption.[5,131] Psychosocial growth failure is the most common medical problem identified in international adoptees,[129,144] with pre-adoptive nutritional status highly correlated with development at time of adoption.[1,5,144] These growth deficits appear to be universal for children raised in institutions, regardless of country of origin.[11,129,145,146] It is estimated that young children lose 1 month of linear growth for every 2 to 3 months in institutional care[147]; however, remarkable catch-up growth has been well described on removal from their pathogenic environment.[1,5,11,131,145] Duration of time in institutional care appears to influence degree of catch-up growth, with infants adopted at 6 months and younger (ie, infants who spent the least amount of time in a pathogenic caregiving environment) demonstrating the best-catch up growth.[11] The differential recovery in growth parameters raises questions about developmental risk and malleability in adoptees—to what degree do early developmental risks confer permanent injury on the developing organism, and to what degree are the effects of those early risks modifiable by the quality of the post-adoptive environment? For more information, see Chapter 12, Long-term Growth and Puberty Concerns for Adopted Children, on page 239.

Recovery and Resilience in Adopted Children

The Role of Resilience

The variable outcomes of children after adoption appear to relate in part to the degree of pre-adoptive risk the child experienced (ie, prenatal biological risk and degree of postnatal pathogenic care). However, there is greater evidence that the influence of pre-adoptive risk factors on subsequent neurodevelopment outcomes is largely moderated by environmental experiences.[148] This raises the question about the capacity for resilience in children who experienced early adversity. *Resilience* is defined broadly as the capacity of a system to withstand or recover from significant disturbances and is often conceptualized as positive adaptation during or following adversities that have the potential to harm development.[149] Resilience for children is only evident later in life but is demonstrated by the following outcomes: (1) at-risk individuals show better-than-expected outcomes; (2) positive adaptation is maintained despite the occurrence of stressful experiences; and (3) there is a good recovery from trauma.[150] For the child who is adopted, resilience translates to relative improvements in cognitive and behavioral functioning measured at some period after adoption given pre-adoptive neurodevelopmental and environmental risks.[149]

Importantly and unfortunately, there appears to be a limit to the level of resilience demonstrated in children who are adopted from challenging circumstances. For children who were exposed early in life to parental abuse or neglect, adoption is highly advantageous. However, when the environment is profoundly pathogenic, as has been demonstrated with severe early institutional deprivation, the limits of resilience can be reached, after which the enduring biological effects of deprivation cannot be reversed.[151]

The origins of resilience for any child have been heavily debated, with ongoing discussion about resilience as a trait, process, outcome, or pattern of development. The predominant theory is that resilience is impacted by interactions across multiple domains of development with positive attachment relationships, quality caregiving environments, and supportive family interactions modulating genetic vulnerabilities predisposing an individual to long-term emotional challenges.[149]

Quality of Caregiving

There is significant and continually mounting evidence of the potential for corrective experiences in the post-adoptive environment and how the effects of early risk factors on later outcomes can be moderated by environmental experiences.[148] For example, low birth weight is a well-described risk factor for attention problems in school-aged children but not when children have a history of warm and supportive caregiving relationships.[152] In addition, the association between perinatal complications and later development of aggressive behavior is demonstrated when children are raised in environments of persistent psychosocial adversity but obviated when children are raised in a sensitive, nurturing caregiving environment.[153] This raises questions about specific qualities of the caregiving environment needed to optimize an adoptive child's developmental, emotional, and psychosocial adaptation. It appears that the post-adoptive environments that promote resilience in adoptees are high in warmth, structure, and parental sensitivity and characterized by a high degree of psychologic investment in the child. Early pathogenic care has been associated with early physiological and behavioral dysregulation.[118] However, behavioral and physiological recovery has been demonstrated on placement in family environments that are characterized by a high level of caregiver commitment and psychologic investment in the child.[120,154]

How can adoptive parents best provide this restorative caregiving environment? It can be challenging to read and respond to the cues of the adopted child because, as a result of the history of inconsistent caregiving, foster and adoptive infants often behave in ways that fail to elicit nurturance from their new caregivers.[155] In response, adoptive parents must respond not to the cues that are *given* but rather to the cues that are *intended.*[156] Adoptive parents must learn to reinterpret a child's rejecting signals and provide nurturance to the child, even though the child may not appear to need nurturance. It is through the experience of contingent, responsive caregiving that all children, but especially adoptees with challenging pre-adoptive environments, learn the capacity to develop organized strategies for coping with negative affect. In addition, caregivers need to provide a predictable environment for the child and a world that is particularly responsive to the child's signals.[155]

Differential Susceptibility to Environmental Risk

There is evidence suggesting that biological vulnerability to behavior problems can be modified by the quality of caregiving in animals and humans[157–159] and that the children who benefit the most from a supportive caregiving environment are those who demonstrated the greatest biological predisposition and behavioral dysregulation.[9,160,161] This research raises the prospect that developmental plasticity and recovery is a function of nurture as much as nature.[162] This provides encouragement in planning for post-adoptive environments for adoptees because it suggests that although early adversity may confer heightened risk for later difficulties, the most vulnerable children may also be the most susceptible to the effects of positive post-adoptive experiences.

Conclusion

Children who are adopted are at heightened risk of developmental and behavioral problems because of their pre-adoptive exposures to a range of prenatal, perinatal, or postnatal insults. On transition to their post-adoptive environment, children should be immediately evaluated and provided with intervention for signs of atypical nutrition, growth, development, and behavior, as well as for chronic medical problems that are known to affect behavior and development. Interventions with post-adoptive families should focus on optimizing the quality of post-adoptive care. This should include provision of developmental and behavioral services to address challenges, coupled with support and intervention for caregivers to assist them in learning how to provide responsive, nurturing, and contingent care. Adoptive parents should ideally be supported by professionals and family-friendly policies to provide corrective attachment experiences and consistent caregiving for all children, especially those who have had experiences of early adverse rearing, in hopes of optimizing their adaptation in the post-adoptive environment.

References

1. van IJzendoorn MH, Juffer F. The Emanuel Miller Memorial Lecture 2006: adoption as intervention. Meta-analytic evidence for massive catch-up and plasticity in physical, socio-emotional, and cognitive development. *J Child Psychol Psychiatry.* 2006;47(12):1228–1245
2. Zamostny KP, O'Brien KM, Baden AL, Wiley MOL. The practice of adoption: history, trends, and social context. *Couns Psychol.* 2003;31(6):651–678
3. van IJzendoorn MH, Juffer F. Adoption is a successful natural intervention enhancing adopted children's IQ and school performance. *Curr Dir Psychol Sci.* 2005;14(6):326–330

4. van IJzendoorn MH, Juffer F, Poelhuis CW. Adoption and cognitive development: a meta-analytic comparison of adopted and nonadopted children's IQ and school performance. *Psychol Bull.* 2005;131(2):301–316

5. Rutter M. Developmental catch-up, and deficit, following adoption after severe global early privation. English and Romanian Adoptees (ERA) Study Team. *J Child Psychol Psychiatry.* 1998;39(4):465–476

6. Rutter M, Andersen-Wood L, Beckett C, et al. Quasi-autistic patterns following severe early global privation. English and Romanian Adoptees (ERA) Study Team. *J Child Psychol Psychiatry.* 1999;40(4):537–549

7. Fox NA, Rutter, M. Introduction to the special section on the effects of early experience on development. *Child Dev.* 2010;81(1):23–27

8. Kreppner JM, Rutter M, Beckett C, et al. Normality and impairment following profound early institutional deprivation: a longitudinal follow-up into early adolescence. *Dev Psychol.* 2007;43(4):931–946

9. Belsky J, Bakersman-Kranenburg, MJ, van IJzendoorn MH. For better *and* for worse: differential susceptibility to environmental influences. *Curr Dir Psychol Sci.* 2007;16(6):300–304

10. Davies JK, Bledsoe JM. Prenatal alcohol and drug exposures in adoption. *Pediatr Clin North Am.* 2005;52:1369–1393

11. Johnson D. Adoption and the effect on children's development. *Early Hum Dev.* 2002;68(1):39–54

12. Payne-Price AC. Etic variations on fosterage and adoption. *Anthropol Q.* 1981;54(3):134–145

13. Lesage J, Del-Favero F, Leonhardt M, et al. Prenatal stress induces intrauterine growth restriction and programmes glucose intolerance and feeding behaviour disturbances in the aged rat. *J Endocrinol.* 2004;181(2):291–296

14. Barros VG, Berger MA, Martijena ID, et al. Early adoption modifies the effects of prenatal stress on dopamine and glutamate receptors in adult rat brain. *J Neurosci Res.* 2004;76(4):488–496

15. Huizink AC, Mulder EJH, Buitelaar JK. Prenatal stress and risk for psychopathology: specific effects or induction of general susceptibility? *Psychol Bull.* 2004;130(1):115–142

16. Buitelaar JK, Huizink AC, Mulder EJ, de Medina PGR, Visser GHA. Prenatal stress and cognitive development and temperament in infants. *Neurobiology Aging.* 2003;24(Suppl 1):S53–S60

17. Weinstock M. Does prenatal stress impair coping and regulation of hypothalamic-pituitary-adrenal axis? *Neurosci Biobehav Rev.* 1997;21(1):1–10

18. Weinstock M. The potential influence of maternal stress hormones on development and mental health of the offspring. *Brain Behav Immun.* 2005;19(4):296–308

19. Hobel CJ. Stress and preterm birth. *Clinical Obstet Gynecol.* 2004;47(4):856–880

20. Davis EP, Glynn LM, Schetter CD, Hobel C, Chicz-Demet A, Sandman CA. Prenatal exposure to maternal depression and cortisol influences infant temperament. *J Am Acad Child Adol Psychiatry.* 2007;46(6):737–746

21. Gitau R, Cameron A, Fisk N, Glover V. Fetal exposure to maternal cortisol. *Lancet.* 1998;352(9129):707–708

22. Davis EP, Sandman CA. Prenatal psychobiological predictors of anxiety risk in preadolescent children. *Psychoneuroendocrinology.* 2012;37(8):1224–1233

23. Benedicktsson R, Calder AA, Edwards CR, Seckl JR. Placental 11 beta-hydroxysteroid dehydrogenase: a key regulator of fetal glucocorticoid exposure. *Clin Endocrinol (Oxf).* 1997;46(2):161–166

24. McEwen B. The neurobiology of stress: from serendipity to clinical relevance. *Brain Res.* 2000;886(1–2):172–189

25. de Weerth C, Buitelaar JK. Physiological stress reactivity in human pregnancy-a review. *Neurosci Biobehav Rev.* 2005;29(2):295–312

26. Kramer M. Intrauterine growth and gestational duration determinants. *Pediatrics.* 1987; 80(4):502–522

27. Guerrini I, Thomson AD, Gurling HD. The importance of alcohol misuse, malnutrition and genetic susceptibility on brain growth and plasticity. *Neurosci Biobehav Rev.* 2007;31(2):212–220

28. Morgane PJ, Austin-LaFrance R, Bronzino J, et al. Prenatal malnutrition and development of the brain. *Neurosci Biobehav Rev.* 1993;17:91–128

29. Raine A. Annotation: the role of prefrontal deficits, low autonomic arousal, and early health factors in the development of antisocial and aggressive behavior in children. *J Child Psychol Psychiatry.* 2002;43:417–434

30. Montanha-Rojas EA, Ferreira AA, Tenorio F, Barradas PC. Myelin basic protein accumulation is impaired in a model of protein deficiency during development. *Nutr Neurosci.* 2005;8:49–56

31. Polifka JE, Friedman JM. Medical genetics: 1. Clinical teratology in the age of genomics. *CMAJ.* 2002;167(3):265–273

32. Frank DA, Graham JM Jr, Smith DW. Adoptive children in a dysmorphology clinic: implications for evaluation of children before adoption. *Pediatrics.* 1981;68(5):744–745

33. National Center on Birth Defects and Developmental Disabilities, Centers for Disease Control and Prevention. *Fetal Alcohol Syndrome: Guidelines for Referral and Diagnosis.* Atlanta, GA: Department of Health and Human Services; 2004

34. Sampson PD, Streissguth AP, Bookstein FL, et al. Incidence of fetal alcohol syndrome and prevalence of alcohol-related neurodevelopmental disorder. *Teratology.* 1997;56(5):317–326

35. Goldschmidt L, Richardson GA, Stoffer DS, Geva D, Day NL. Prenatal alcohol exposure and academic achievement at age six: a nonlinear fit. *Alcohol Clin Exp Res.* 1996;20(4):763–770

36. Bailey BN, Delaney-Black V, Covington CY, et al. Prenatal exposure to binge drinking and cognitive and behavioral outcomes at age 7 years. *Am J Obstet Gynecol.* 2004;191(3):1037–1043

37. Stoler JM, Ryan LM, Holmes LB. Alcohol dehydrogenase 2 genotypes, maternal alcohol use, and infant outcome. *J Pediatr.* 2002;141(6):780–785

38. Martínez-Frías ML, Bermejo E, Rodríguez-Pinilla E, Frías JL. Risk for congenital anomalies associated with different sporadic and daily doses of alcohol consumption during pregnancy: a case-control study. *Birth Defects Res A Clin Mol Teratol.* 2004;70(4):194–200

39. Mattson SN, Riley EP. A review of the neurobehavioral deficits in children with fetal alcohol syndrome or prenatal exposure to alcohol. *Alcohol Clin Exp Res.* 1998;22(2):279–294

40. Olson HC, Feldman JJ, Streissguth AP, Sampson PD, Bookstein FL. Neuropsychological deficits in adolescents with fetal alcohol syndrome: clinical findings. *Alcohol Clin Exp Res.* 1998;22(9):1998–2012

41. Burgos AE, Burke Jr BL. Neonatal abstinence syndrome. *Neoreviews.* 2009;10(5):e222–e229

42. Liu AJW, Sithamparanathan S, Jones MP, Cook CM, Nanan R. Growth restriction in pregnancies of opioid-dependent mothers. *Arch Dis Child Fetal Neonatal Ed.* 2010;95:F258–F262

43. Messinger DS, Bauer CR, Das A, et al. The maternal lifestyle study: cognitive, motor, and behavioral outcomes of cocaine-exposed and opiate-exposed infants through three years of age. *Pediatrics.* 2004;113(6):1677–1685

44. Fried PA. Prenatal exposure to tobacco and marijuana: effects during pregnancy, infancy, and early childhood. *Clin Obstet Gynecol.* 1993;36(2):319–337

45. Lee M. Marihuana and tobacco use in pregnancy. *Obstet Gynecol Clin North Am.* 1998;25(1):65–83

46. Olds D. Tobacco exposure and impaired development: a review of the evidence. *Ment Retard Dev Disabil Res Rev.* 1997;3(3):257–269

47. Schuetze P, Eiden RD. The association between prenatal exposure to cigarettes and infant and maternal negative affect. *Infant Behav Dev.* 2007;30(3):387–398

48. Cornelius MD, Ryan CM, Day NL, Goldschmidt L, Willford JA. Prenatal tobacco effects on neuropsychological outcomes among preadolescents. *J Dev Behav Pediatr.* 2001;22(4):217–225

49. Richardson GA, Ryan C, Willford J, Day NL, Goldschmidt L. Prenatal alcohol and marijuana exposure: effects on neuropsychological outcomes at 10 years. *Neurotoxicol Teratol.* 2002;24(3):309–320

50. Day NL, Richardson GA, Goldschmidt L, et al. Effect of prenatal marijuana exposure on the cognitive development of offspring at age three. *Neurotoxicol Teratol.* 1994;16(2):169–175

51. Bada HS, Das A, Bauer CR, et al. Impact of prenatal cocaine exposure on child behavior problems through school age. *Pediatrics.* 2007;119(2):e348–e359

52. Ackerman JP, Riggins T, Black MM. A review of the effects of prenatal cocaine exposure among school-aged children. *Pediatrics.* 2010;125(3):554–565

53. Frank DA, Augustyn M, Knight WG, Pell T, Zuckerman B. Growth, development, and behavior in early childhood following prenatal cocaine exposure: a systematic review. *JAMA.* 2001;285(12):1613–1625

54. Gingras JL, Weese-Mayer DE, Hume Jr RF, O'Donnell KJ. Cocaine and development: mechanisms of fetal toxicity and neonatal consequences of prenatal cocaine exposure. *Early Hum Dev.* 1992;31(1):1–24

55. Singer LT, Minnes S, Short E, et al. Cognitive outcomes of preschool children with prenatal cocaine exposure. *JAMA.* 2004;291(20):2448–2456

56. Smith LM, LaGasse LL, Derauf C, et al. Prenatal methamphetamine use and neonatal neurobehavioral outcome. *Neurotoxicol Teratol.* 2008;30(1):20–28

57. Friedman JM. *Teratogenic Effects of Drugs: A Resource for Clinicians (TERIS).* Baltimore, MD: Johns Hopkins University Press; 2000

58. Dole N, Savitz DA, Hertz-Picciotto I, Siega-Riz AM, McMahon MJ, Buekens P. Maternal stress and preterm birth. *Am J Epidemiol.* 2003;157(1):14–24

59. Goldenberg RL, Culhane JF, Iams JD, Romero R. Epidemiology and causes of preterm birth. *Lancet.* 2008;371(9606):75–84

60. Kyrklund-Blomberg NB, Granath F, Cnattingius S. Maternal smoking and causes of very preterm birth. *Acta Obstet Gynecol Scand.* 2005;84(6):572–577

61. Hendler I, Goldenberg RL, Mercer BM, et al. The Preterm Prediction Study: association between maternal body mass index and spontaneous and indicated preterm birth. *Am J Obstet Gynecol.* 2005;192(3):882–886

62. Neggers Y, Goldenberg R, Cliver S, Hauth J. Effects of domestic violence on preterm birth and low birth weight. *Acta Obstet Gynecol Scand.* 2004;83(5):455–460

63. Kelly RH, Russo J, Holt VL, et al. Psychiatric and substance use disorders as risk factors for low birth weight and preterm delivery. *Obstet Gynecol.* 2002;100(2):297–304

64. Smith LK, Draper ES, Manktelow BN, Dorling JS, Field DJ. Socio-economic inequalities in very preterm birth rates. *Arch Dis Child Fetal Neonatal Ed.* 2007;92(1):F11–F14

65. Smith-Garcia T, Brown JS. The health of children adopted from India. *J Community Health.* 1989;14(4):227–241

66. Bhutta A, Cleves MA, Casey PH, Cradock MM, Anand KJS. Cognitive and behavioral outcomes of school aged children who were born preterm. *JAMA.* 2002;288(6):728–737

67. Johnson S. Cognitive and behavioral outcomes following very preterm birth. *Semin Fetal Neonatal Med.* 2007;12(5):363–373

68. Marlow N. Neurocognitive outcome after very preterm birth. *Arch Dis Child Fetal Neonatal Ed.* 2004;89(3):F224–228

69. Wolke D, Samara M, Bracewell M, Marlow N. Specific language difficulties and school achievement in children born at 25 weeks of gestation or less. *J Pediatr.* 2008;152(2):256–262

70. Luu TM, Vohr BR, Schneider KC, et al. Trajectories of receptive language development from 3 to 12 years of age for very preterm children. *Pediatrics.* 2009;124(1):333–341

71. Salt A, Redshaw M. Neurodevelopmental follow-up after preterm birth: follow up after two years. *Early Hum Dev.* 2006;82:185–197

72. Fawke J. Neurological outcomes following preterm birth. *Semin Fetal Neonatal Med.* 2007; 12(5):374–382

73. Allen MC. Neurodevelopmental outcomes of preterm infants. *Curr Opin Neurol.* 2008; 21(2):123–128

74. Limperopoulos C, Bassan H, Sullivan NR, et al. Positive screening for autism in ex-preterm infants: prevalence and risk factors. *Pediatrics.* 2008;121(4):758–765

75. Limperopoulos C, Bassan H, Gauvreau K, et al. Does cerebellar injury in premature infants contribute to the high prevalence of long-term cognitive, learning, and behavioral disability in survivors? *Pediatrics.* 2007;120(3):584–593

76. Hack M, Taylor HG, Schluchter M, Andreias L, Drotar D, Klein N. Behavioral outcomes of extremely low birth weight children at age 8 years. *J Dev Behav Pediatr.* 2009;30(2):122–130

77. Kuban KC, O'Shea TM, Allred EN, Tager-Flusberg H, Goldstein DJ, Leviton A. Positive screening on the Modified Checklist for Autism in Toddlers (M-CHAT) in extremely low gestational age newborns. *J Pediatr.* 2009;154(4):535–540

78. Woodward LJ, Anderson PJ, Austin NC, Howard K, Inder TE. Neonatal MRI to predict neurodevelopmental outcomes in preterm infants. *N Engl J Med.* 2006;355(7):685–694

79. Marlow N, Hennessy EM, Bracewell MA, Wolke D, for the EPICure Study Group. Motor and executive function at 6 years of age after extremely preterm birth. *Pediatrics.* 2007;120(4):793–804

80. Reijneveld SA, de Kleine MJ, van Baar AL, et al. Behavioural and emotional problems in very preterm and very low birthweight infants at age 5 years. *Arch Dis Child Fetal Neonatal Ed.* 2006;91:F423–F428

81. Foulder-Hughes LA, Cooker RW. Motor, cognitive and behavioural disorders in children born very preterm. *Dev Med Child Neurol.* 2003;45:97–103

82. Wolke D. Psychological development of prematurely born children. *Arch Dis Child.* 1998; 78(6):567–570

83. Hack M, Youngstrom EA, Cartar L, Schlucter M, Taylor HG, Flannery D. Behavioral outcomes and evidence of psychopathology among very low birthweight infants at age 20 years. *Pediatrics.* 2004;114(4):932–940

84. Kelly YJ, Nazroo JY, McMunn A, Boreham R, Marmot M. Birthweight and behavior problems in children: a modifiable effect? *Int J Epidemiol.* 2001;2001(30):88–94

85. Wood N, Marlow N, Costeloe K, Gibson AT, Wilkinson AR. Neurological and developmental disability after extremely preterm birth. *N Engl J Med.* 2000;343(6):378–384

86. Adams-Chapman I. Neurodevelopmental outcome of the late preterm infant. *Clin Perinatol.* 2006;33(4):947–964

87. Reuner G, Hassenpflug A, Pietz J, Philippi H. Long-term development of low-risk low birth weight preterm born infants: neurodevelopmental aspects from childhood to late adolescence. *Early Hum Dev.* 2009;85(7):409–413

88. Morse SB, Zheng H, Tang Y, Roth J. Early school-age outcomes of late preterm infants. *Pediatrics.* 2009;123(4):e622–e629

89. Kirkegaard I, Obel C, Hedegaard M, Henriksen TB. Gestational age and birth weight in relation to school performance of 10-year-old children: a follow-up study of children born after 32 completed weeks. *Pediatrics.* 2006;118(4):1600–1606

90. Chyi LJ, Lee HC, Hintz SR, Gould JB, Sutcliffe TL. School outcomes of late preterm infants: special needs and challenges for infants born at 32 to 36 weeks gestation. *J Pediatr.* 2008;153(1):25–31

91. Huddy CL, Johnson A, Hope PL. Educational and behavioural problems in babies of 32–35 weeks gestation. *Arch Dis Child Fetal Neonatal Ed.* 2001;85(1):F23–F28

92. Gray RF, Indurkhya A, McCormick MC. Prevalence, stability, and predictors of clinically significant behavior problems in low birth weight children at 3, 5, and 8 years of age. *Pediatrics.* 2004;114(3):736–743

93. Msall ME, Buck GM, Rogers BT, Merke D, Catanzaro NL, Zorn WA. Risk factors for major neurodevelopmental impairments and need for special education resources in extremely premature infants. *J Pediatr.* 1991;119(4):606–614

94. Hack M, Wilson-Costello D, Friedman H, Taylor GH, Schluchter M, Fanaroff AA. Neuro-development and predictors of outcomes of children with birth weights of less than 1000 g: 1992–1995. *Arch Pediatr Adolesc Med.* 2000;154(7):725–731

95. Inder TE, Warfield SK, Wang H, Huppi PS, Volpe JJ. Abnormal cerebral structure is present at term in premature infants. *Pediatrics.* 2005;115(2):286–294

96. Peterson BS, Vohr B, Staib LH, et al. Regional brain volume abnormalities and long-term cognitive outcome in preterm infants. *JAMA.* 2000;284(15):1939–1947

97. Miller S, Ferriero D, Leonard C, et al. Early brain injury in premature newborns detected with magnetic resonance imaging is associated with adverse early neurodevelopmental outcome. *J Pediatr.* 2005;147(5):609–616

98. Hack M, Taylor HG. Perinatal brain injury in preterm infants and later neurobehavioral function. *JAMA.* 2000;284(15):1973–1974

99. Holling EE, Leviton A. Characteristics of cranial ultrasound white-matter echolucencies that predict disability: a review. *Dev Med Child Neurol.* 1999;41(2):136–139

100. Mirmiran M, Barnes PD, Keller K, et al. Neonatal brain magnetic resonance imaging before discharge is better than serial cranial ultrasound in predicting cerebral palsy in very low birth weight preterm infants. *Pediatrics.* 2004;114(4):992–998

101. Perlman JM. Neurobehavioral deficits in premature graduates of intensive care—potential medical and neonatal environmental risk factors. *Pediatrics.* 2001;108(6):1339–1348

102. Short EJ, Kirchner HL, Asaad GR, et al. Developmental sequelae in preterm infants having a diagnosis of bronchopulmonary dysplasia: analysis using a severity-based classification system. *Arch Pediatr Adolesc Med.* 2007;161(11):1082–1087

103. Adams-Chapman I, Stoll BJ. Neonatal infection and long-term neurodevelopmental outcome in the preterm infant. *Curr Opin Infect Dis.* 2006;19(3):290–297

104. van de Bor M, van Zeben-van der Aa TM, Verloove-Vanhorick SP, Brand R, Ruys JH. Hyperbilirubinemia in preterm infants and neurodevelopmental outcome at 2 years of age: results of a national collaborative survey. *Pediatrics.* 1989;83(6):915–920

105. Anagnostakis D, Petmezakis J, Papazissis G, Messaritakis J, Matsaniotis N. Hearing loss in low-birth-weight infants. *Am J Dis Child.* 1982;136(7):602–604

106. Vorria P, Papaligoura Z, Sarafidou J, et al. The development of adopted children after institutional care: a follow-up study. *J Child Psychol Psychiatry.* 2006;47(12):1246–1253

107. Juffer F, van IJzendoorn MH. Behavior problems and mental health referrals of international adoptees: a meta-analysis. *JAMA.* 2005;293(20):2501–2515

108. van IJzendoorn MH, Bakermans-Kranenburg MJ, Juffer F. Plasticity of growth in height, weight, and head circumference: meta-analytic evidence of massive catch-up after international adoption. *J Dev Behav Pediatr.* 2007;28(4):334–343

109. Dobrova-Krol NA, van IJzendoorn MH, Bakermans-Kranenburg MJ, Cyr C, Juffer F. Physical growth delays and stress dysregulation in stunted and non-stunted Ukrainian institution-reared children. *Infant Behav Dev.* 2008;31:539–553

110. Ringeisen H, Casanueva C, Urato M, Cross T. Special health care needs among children in the child welfare system. *Pediatrics.* 2008;122(1):e232–e241

111. Bimmel N, Juffer F, van IJzendoorn MH, Bakermans-Kranenburg MJ. Problem behavior of inter-nationally adopted adolescents: a review and meta-analysis. *Harv Rev Psychiatry.* 2003;11(2):64–77

112. Jaffari-Bimmel N, Juffer F, van IJzendoorn MH, Bakermans-Kranenburg MJ, Mooijaart A. Social development from infancy to adolescence: longitudinal and concurrent factors in an adoption sample. *Dev Psychol.* 2006;42(6):1143–1153

113. Kreppner JM, Rutter M, Beckett C, et al. Normality and impairment following profound early institutional deprivation: a longitudinal follow-up into early adolescence. *Dev Psychol.* 2007;43(4):931–946

114. Rutter M, O'Connor TG. Are there biological programming effects for psychological development? Findings from a study of Romanian adoptees. *Dev Psychol.* 2004;40(1):81–94

115. Beckett C, Bredenkamp D, Castle J, O'Connor TG, Rutter M, Groothues C. Behavior patterns associated with institutional deprivation: a study of children adopted from Romania. *J Dev Behav Pediatr.* 2002;23(5):297–303

116. Sroufe LA. Infant-caregiver attachment and patterns of adaptation in preschool: the roots of maladaptation and competence. In: Perlmutter M, ed. *The Minnesota Symposia on Child Psychology Vol.16. Development and Policy Concerning Children with Special Needs.* Hillsdale, NJ: Lawrence Erlbaum Associates; 1983

117. Dozier M. Challenges of foster care. *Attach Hum Dev.* 2005;7(1):27–30

118. Dozier M, Albus K, Fisher PA, Sepulveda S. Interventions for foster parents: implications for developmental theory. *Dev Psychopathol.* 2002;14(4):843–860

119. Lewis EE, Dozier M, Ackerman J, Sepulveda-Kozakowski S. The effect of placement instability on adopted children's inhibitory control abilities and oppositional behavior. *Dev Psychol.* 2007;43(6):1415–1427

120. Fisher PA, Gunnar MR, Chamberlain P, Reid JB. Preventive intervention for maltreated preschool children: impact on children's behavior, neuroendocrine activity, and foster parent functioning. *J Am Acad Child Adolesc Psychiatry.* 2000;39(11):1356–1364

121. Newton RR, Litrownik AJ, Landsverk JA. Children and youth in foster care: disentangling the relationship between problem behaviors and number of placements. *Child Abuse Negl.* 2000; 24(10):1363–1374

122. Bowlby J. *Attachment and Loss, Vol 1 (Attachment).* New York, NY: Basic Books; 1969

123. Dozier M, Manni M, Gordon MK, et al. Foster children's diurnal production of cortisol: an exploratory study. *Child Maltreat.* 2006;11(2):189–197

124. Tarullo AR, Gunnar MR. Child maltreatment and the developing HPA axis. *Horm Behav.* 2006; 50(4):632–639

125. Nelson CA. A neurobiological perspective on early human deprivation. *Child Dev Perspect.* 2007; 1(1):13–18

126. Johnson DE. Medical and developmental sequelae of early childhood institutionalization in Eastern European adoptees. In: Nelson CA, ed. *The Effects of Early Adversity on Neurobehavioral Development.* Mahwah, NJ: Lawrence Erlbaum Associates; 2000:113–162

127. Rutter M, Beckett C, Castle J, et al. Effects of profound early institutional deprivation: an overview of findings from a UK longitudinal study of Romanian adoptees. *Eur J Dev Psychol.* 2007;4(3):332–350

128. O'Connor TG, Rutter M, Beckett C, Keaveney L, Kreppner JM. The effects of global severe privation on cognitive competence: extension and longitudinal follow-up. English and Romanian Study Team. *Child Dev.* 2000;71(2):376–390

129. Albers LH, Johnson DE, Hostetter MK, Iverson S, Miller LC. Health of children adopted from the former Soviet Union and Eastern Europe. Comparison with preadoptive medical records. *JAMA.* 1997;278(11):922–924

130. Rutter ML, Kreppner JM, O'Connor TG. Specificity and heterogeneity in children's responses to profound institutional privation. *Br J Psychiatry.* 2001;179(2):97–103

131. MacLean K. The impact of institutionalization on child development. *Dev Psychopathol.* 2003; 15(4):853–854

132. Zeanah CH, Smyke AT, Dumitrescu A. Attachment disturbances in young children. II: indiscriminate behavior and institutional care. *J Am Acad Child Adolesc Psychiatry.* 2002;41(8):983–989

133. Woolf A, Goldman R, Bellinger D. Update on the clinical management of childhood lead poisoning. *Pediatric Clin North Am.* 2007;54(2):271–294

134. Marchetti C. Molecular targets of lead in brain neurotoxicity. *Neurotoxicol Res.* 2003;4(3):221–236

135. Bellinger DC. Interpreting the literature on lead and child development: the neglected role of the "experimental system." *Neurotoxicol Teratol.* 1995;17(3):201–212

136. Needleman H. Lead poisoning. *Annu Rev Med.* 2004;55:209–222

137. Sciarillo WG, Alexander G, Farrell KP. Lead exposure and child behavior. *Am J Public Health.* 1992;82(10):1356–1360

138. Lanphear BP, Hornung R, Khoury J, et al. Low-level environmental lead exposure and children's intellectual function: an international pooled analysis. *Environ Health Perspect.* 2005;113(7):894–899

139. Dietrich KN, Ris MD, Succop PA, Berger OG, Bornschein RL. Early exposure to lead and juvenile delinquency. *Neurotoxicol Teratol.* 2001;23(6):511–518

140. Ris MD, Dietrich KN, Succop PA, Berger OG, Bornschein RL. Early exposure to lead and neuropsychological outcome in adolescence. *J Int Neuropsychol Soc.* 2004;10(2):261–270

141. Fergusson DM, Horwood LJ, Lynskey MT. Early dentine lead levels and educational outcomes at 18 years. *J Child Psychol Psychiatry.* 1997;38(4):471–478

142. Tong S, Baghurst PA, Sawyer MG, Burns J, McMichael AJ. Declining blood lead levels and changes in cognitive function during childhood: the Port Pirie Cohort Study. *JAMA.* 1998;280(22):1915–1919

143. Fuglestad A, Lehmann A, Kroupina M, et al. Iron deficiency in international adoptees from Eastern Europe. *J Pediatr.* 2008;153(2):272–277

144. Miller LC. Initial assessment of growth, development, and the effects of institutionalization in internationally adopted children. *Pediatr Ann.* 2000;29(4):224–232

145. Gunnar MR, Bruce J, Grotevant HD. International adoption of institutionally reared children: research and policy. *Dev Psychopathol.* 2000;12(4):677–693

146. Miller L, Chan W, Comfort K, Tirella L. Health of children adopted from Guatemala: comparison of orphanage and foster care. *Pediatrics.* 2005;115(6):e710–e717

147. Johnson DE. The impact of orphanage rearing on growth and development. In: Nelson CA, ed. *The Effects of Early Adversity on Neurobehavioral Development.* Mahwah, NJ: Lawrence Erlbaum Associates; 2000:113–162

148. Jaffee SR. Sensitive, stimulating caregiving predicts cognitive and behavioral resilience in neurodevelopmentally at-risk infants. *Dev Psychopathol.* 2007;19(3):631–647

149. Masten AS. Resilience in developing systems: progress and promise as the fourth wave rises. *Dev Psychopathol.* 2007;19(3):921–930

150. Luthar SS, Cicchetti D, Becker B. The construct of resilience: a critical evaluation and guidelines for future work. *Child Dev.* 2000;71(3):543–562

151. Rutter M. Resilience, competence, and coping. *Child Abuse Negl.* 2007;31(3):205–209

152. Laucht M, Esser G, Schmidt MH. Developmental outcome of infants born with biological and psychosocial risks. *J Child Psychol Psychiatry.* 1997;38(7):843–853

153. Raine A. Biosocial studies of antisocial and violent behavior in children and adults: a review. *J Abnorm Child Psychol.* 2002;30(4):311–326

154. Lindhiem O, Dozier M. Caregiver commitment to foster children: the role of child behavior. *Child Abuse Negl.* 2007;31(4):361–374

155. Dozier M, Higley E, Albus KE, Nutter A. Intervening with foster infants' caregivers: targeting three critical needs. *Infant Ment Health J.* 2002;23(5):541–554

156. Steele M, Hodges J, Kaniuk J, Steele H. Mental representation and change: developing attachment relationships in an adoption context. *Psychoanal Inq.* 2010;30(1):25–40

157. Kaufman J, Yang BZ, Douglas-Palumberi H, et al. Social supports and serotonin transporter gene moderate depression in maltreated children. *Proc Natl Acad Sci U S A.* 2004;101(49):17316–17321

158. Bakermans-Kranenburg MJ, van IJzendoorn MH. Gene-environment interaction of the dopamine D4 receptor (DRD4) and observed maternal insensitivity predicting externalizing behavior in preschoolers. *Dev Psychobiol.* 2006;48:406–409

159. Belsky J, Hsieh K, Crnic K. Mothering, fathering and infant negativity as antecedents of boys' externalizing problems and inhibition at 3 years: differential susceptibility to rearing experience? *Dev Psychopathol.* 1998;10(2):301–319

160. Klein Velderman M, Bakersman-Kranenburg MJ, Juffer F, van IJzendoorn MH. Effects of attachment-based interventions on maternal sensitivity and infant attachment: differential susceptibility of highly reactive infants. *J Fam Psychol.* 2006;20(2):266–274

161. Belsky J. Differential susceptibility to rearing influence: an evolutionary hypothesis and some evidence. In: Ellis BB, David F, eds. *Origins of the Social Mind: Evolutionary Psychology and Child Development.* New York, NY: Guilford Press; 2005:139–163

162. Belsky J, Pluess M. The nature (and nurture?) of plasticity in early human development. *Perspect Psychol Sci.* 2009;4(4):345–351

CHAPTER 8

Post-adoptive Evaluation for the Health Care Professional

Elaine E. Schulte, MD, MPH, FAAP, and Sarah H. Springer, MD, FAAP

Pediatricians and other health care professionals are in a unique position to help a family prepare to welcome a child into its home. While ideally all of the information known about a child should be available to the family prior to adoption, the unfortunate reality is that this is often not the case. Whether the information is not released to the family by the US social welfare system or is just not available for an abandoned child from abroad, the family is often left not knowing exactly what happened in the child's life before adoption. The parents and health care team are in a position of uncertainty. The initial evaluation of the child following a domestic or an international adoption is critical to address the child's unknown health and developmental issues. While evaluations are addressed separately, there is considerable overlap with the post-adoption life of the child, regardless of where the child was before adoption. By understanding the unique circumstances that these children bring into a family, the health care team can quickly identify areas of concern and aid in a smooth transition for the child.

Domestic Adoption

Unlike in the past, when only completely healthy newborns were considered to be "adoptable," today's domestic adoptions may include older children, children with significant complex medical or behavioral needs, or even sibling groups. While healthy infants with no identifiable special needs are still being placed with adoptive families, it is far more common for children to come into their adoptive families with complex histories and traumatic life experiences. Pediatricians and other members of the health care team must be ready to address the special needs of these children and must be skilled in helping families with particular challenges overcome obstacles.

The initial health screening for a child newly adopted from within the United States will vary depending on each child's unique history. Some details may be difficult or impossible to obtain, but the child's agency, caseworker, or attorney should work with the adopting parents to help fill in details. Court-appointed special advocate volunteers and foster parents may also be able to fill in details for adopting parents. Obtaining consents for the release of historical information can unfortunately be a challenge, although these same professionals should work with adopting parents to secure appropriate consents as well as the desired information. Pediatricians should collaborate with adopting parents and these adoption professionals to help determine which information might be relevant for each individual child (Box 8-1). Ideally, all of this information should be available to prospective parents before they make final decisions about whether to adopt a particular child so that they can learn about the child's potential needs and adequately assess their ability to meet these needs over the long term (see Chapter 4, Pre-adoption Considerations for Pediatricians, on page 73).

Medical and dental screening, follow-up of chronic conditions, and ongoing preventive care plans should be based on the details of the historical information gathered for each individual child. Chronic medical conditions should be managed as they would be for any other child, albeit with recognition that new adoptive parents may need more education and support as they learn to manage their new child's health needs.

Written documentation of immunizations should be used to verify past vaccinations. If no records are available, the child should be re-immunized according to the catch-up schedule published by the American Academy of Pediatrics (www.aapredbook.org/site/resources/izschedules.xhtml).[1] Children with unknown or definite exposure risks should be screened for tuberculosis, HIV, hepatitis B, hepatitis C, syphilis, and other sexually transmitted infections. Even apparently healthy newborns should be screened unless documentation of the birth mother's late prenatal testing is available.

Nutritional status should be carefully evaluated for each newly adopted child. Many children may be at risk for iron and calcium deficiency, from past dietary inadequacies, and some exhibit growth stunting as a result of chronic adversity. In contrast, many children in the child welfare system today are obese, resulting from a combination of inactivity and diets high in sugar and fat. Screening for anemia, rickets, or hyperlipidemia may be in order depending on the child's age, known personal and birth family history, and physical examination. Newly adopted children should also be screened for lead exposure.

Careful attention to developmental and educational needs is also in order. Many younger children will qualify for early intervention (EI) assessments based on risk factors for delay, and many will qualify for ongoing support. Special educational needs are common among older children because many have experienced frequent disruptions in their education as well as medical and social adversities that may

Box 8-1. Useful Information for an Adoptive Family

- Prenatal and birth history
  - Prenatal care
  - Prenatal nutrition
  - Infectious exposures and treatment history
    - ❖ Blood-borne viruses
    - ❖ Syphilis and other sexually transmitted infections
    - ❖ Congenital infections such as toxoplasmosis, rubella, cytomegalovirus, herpes simplex virus
  - Drug, alcohol, tobacco use
    - ❖ Details, eg, what was used, how often, how much
  - Delivery details
  - Neonatal complications and treatment details
  - Newborn metabolic and hearing screening results
- General past medical history
  - Significant illnesses, injuries, hospitalizations, surgeries
  - Growth records
  - Immunization records
  - Allergies
  - Current medications and treatments
  - Infectious exposure risks
    - ❖ Tuberculosis
    - ❖ Blood-borne viruses such as hepatitis
    - ❖ Sexually transmitted infections
  - Dental history
- Birth family medical history
  - Including substance abuse and mental health details
- Mental health history
  - Past and current diagnoses and treatments
  - History of suicidal or violent behaviors
- Detailed history of abuse, neglect, traumatic experiences, placement changes
- Relationship histories
  - Important ongoing relationships
    - ❖ Birth parents, biological siblings, grandparents
    - ❖ Foster families
    - ❖ Friends
  - Important losses or traumatic relationships
- Educational history
  - Learning disabilities or special needs
  - Supports in place
  - Grade retention

have negatively affected learning capacity. Hearing and vision should be carefully assessed using age-appropriate screening. Pediatricians and adoptive parents should monitor a child's educational needs closely over time because the effects of early adversity may not be seen until many years later as academic rigor increases.

Similarly, pediatricians should pay careful attention to the mental health of adopted children because birth family histories of mental illness, as well as traumatic life experiences prior to adoption, leave adopted children at high risk for short- and long-term mental health struggles. Children adopted from foster care should have a comprehensive mental health evaluation by a pediatric mental health care professional if no such assessment was done prior to placement, and existing care plans should be reviewed and updated as a child adjusts to a new family. Parents and pediatricians should continue over time to monitor for long-term sequelae of early adversity.

Ongoing health care for adopted children should follow all usual health maintenance guidelines plus additional surveillance and consideration for long-term consequences and risks of a child's early history.

International Adoption

Why Screen?

Children who are internationally adopted are at risk of nutritional deficiencies, medical and dental conditions and diseases, and developmental delays related to their pre-adoption environment. Some children have been living in adequate foster care homes, but most have resided in institutional settings where there have been limits in staffing, hygiene, nutrition, medical care, and environmental stimulation.

For a variety of reasons, parents may be under false impressions of their newly adopted child's health and may refuse or not seek post-adoption screening. Medical records from certain countries typically describe a child as being "normal" or "adoptable." Records may also contain unfamiliar medical terminology that parents interpret as insignificant. Laboratory data from the country of origin may also indicate that the child is "healthy." It is useful to remind parents (and adoption agencies) that there may be no standardization of laboratory tests from abroad or any quality control of these tests. Even if results are accurate, the possibility of transmission of any number of infectious diseases between the time of the laboratory test and the timing of arrival in the child's new home cannot be ruled out.

Before leaving the country of origin, the child must have a medical examination performed by a panel physician who is a US Department of State–designated medical doctor who performs medical examinations overseas for immigrants (including international adoptees). The extent of this examination is often variable among countries and is generally concerned with completing legal requirements for screening for certain communicable diseases and examination for serious physical or mental defects that would prevent issue of a permanent residency visa. It is typically not a comprehensive assessment of a child's health.

US international adoption clinics have screened thousands of children over the last few decades. Data from these clinics demonstrate that at least half of all internationally adopted children will have some medical diagnosis that may or may not be known at the time of arrival. This may include many completely asymptomatic children with an infectious disease (eg, *Giardia)*. Because children come from a variety of developing countries where the epidemiology of infectious diseases changes or is unknown, a full investigation is warranted. Clinical data also demonstrate that between 50% and 90% of children who are internationally adopted have some degree of developmental delays at the time of arrival.[2–7] For all these reasons, post-adoption screening is essential for the internationally adopted child.

When to Screen

After international adoption, routine screening for infectious diseases, environmental risks, and vision and hearing difficulties are early priorities for the child's post-adoptive health care. Unless the child is acutely ill or has known special needs or medical problems, an office visit is recommended within 3 weeks of the child's arrival in the new home.[8] While many parents (and adoption agencies) wish to have the child evaluated immediately, this type of visit is often impractical and frustrating for all involved. The parents and child will be exhausted from long travel or fresh transition. Parents will not be able to provide a detailed history about feeding, sleeping, behavior, developmental milestones, or daily schedule because none of these has been established or observed in the new home for a significant period. Additionally, parents will not have time to formulate important questions about their child's health and development.

After the first screening visit, a follow-up visit should be planned 4 to 6 weeks later. At minimum, this will allow the pediatrician to review all post-adoption laboratory work and confirm the initiation and timeline for catch-up of delayed immunizations. Occasionally the laboratory is unable to obtain the necessary volume of blood to perform all requested tests, and these should be reordered. Stool specimen collection may have been overlooked or felt to be unnecessary by parents. If the pediatrician has obtained immunization titers, these should be reviewed and appropriate immunizations should be administered. Parents should be given a catch-up schedule based on current *Red Book* recommendations (www.aapredbook.org/site/resources/izschedules.xhtml),[1] and the pediatrician will want to document this in the patient's chart to assist other office personnel in delivering timely immunizations. The final and most important benefit of a 4- to 6-week visit is the opportunity to obtain more specific information from parents about the child's experiences in a new home. At this time, most parents will be able to provide more detailed information about the child's developmental, behavioral, and transitional progress and will more likely be able to be receptive to the pediatrician's anticipatory guidance.

Screening in the Office

Post-adoption screening visits typically are long, complicated office visits. When possible, the pediatrician may wish to schedule this visit at the end of a morning session. Given that most children who are internationally adopted are younger than 3 years, a morning visit may be more conducive to the child's schedule. Parents should bring copies of all medical and immunizations records. While the focus of the visit is on the medical needs of the child, pediatricians may find that the majority of the time is spent answering parent questions and addressing their concerns, particularly if they are first-time parents or have not had a pre-adoption consultation. Common initial medical findings and concerns include congenital conditions, nutritional deficiencies, growth retardation, acute infectious diseases, deficient immunizations, and developmental delays. Dental problems are also common due to the lack of dental care in most countries of origin. Pediatricians should reinforce the importance of a dental examination during this first post-adoption consultation.

Red Book *Medical Evaluation of Internationally Adopted Children for Infectious Diseases*[8]

Infectious diseases are among the most common medical diagnoses identified in international adoptees after arrival in the United States. Children may be asymptomatic, and therefore the diagnoses must be made by screening tests in addition to history and physical examination. Suggested screening tests for infectious diseases are listed in Box 8-2.[8] Blood work for HIV, hepatitis B, and hepatitis C should be repeated 6 months after arrival.

Immunizations

Providing age-appropriate immunizations is essential for all children, particularly a child who is internationally adopted who may not have received any protection against vaccine-preventable diseases. Vaccines given in other countries are often stored incorrectly or given at the wrong time. It is important to understand that the internationally adopted child may have never received any vaccination despite evidence of an immunization record.

To determine which immunizations are needed, pediatricians must first assess any existing immunization record and then may choose to evaluate a child's immunologic response to certain immunizations. This evaluation may come at the parents' request, be based on a desire to reduce the overall number of injections, or satisfy a requirement for child care or school entry. The quality of immunization records and serologic evidence of immunity varies by country of origin.

Box 8-2. Screening Tests for Infectious Diseases in International Adoptees[8]

Hepatitis B virus serologic testing: hepatitis B surface antigen

Hepatitis C virus serologic testing

Syphilis serologic testing: nontreponemal test (rapid plasma reagin, Venereal Disease Research Laboratories, or automated reagin test); treponemal test (microhemagglutination test for *Treponema pallidum;* fluorescent treponemal antibody absorption; *T pallidum* particle agglutination)

HIV 1 and 2 serologic testing

Complete blood cell count with red blood cell indices and differential

Stool examination for ova and parasites (3 specimens) with specific request for *Giardia intestinalis* and *Cryptosporidium* species testing

Tuberculin skin test

In children from countries with endemic infection: *Trypanosoma cruzi* serologic testing

In children with eosinophilia (absolute eosinophil count exceeding 450 cells/mm^3) and negative stool ova and parasite examinations: *Strongyloides* species serologic testing; *Schistosoma* species serologic testing (for sub-Saharan African, Southeast Asian, and certain Latin American adoptees)

Serologic testing for lymphatic filariasis (for children >2 years from endemic countries)

Pediatricians are encouraged to study any existing record carefully, paying close attention to the type of vaccine, dates and methods of administration, and intervals between doses. Titers can be checked, or alternatively, these children should be revaccinated. Most vaccines may be repeated safely.[8]

Vaccination records from Korea, India, Guatemala, Colombia, and the Americas may be more reliable, and some clinicians may be more willing to accept these records. A more cautious approach may again be to check antibody titers and accept the records after verification of immunity. For young children from other countries, it is often very reasonable to check antibody titers and proceed according to the results. Holding off on immunizations until these titers have been obtained may be a reasonable approach for the family and practitioner.

Children from developing countries are not immunized routinely with varicella, rubella, *Haemophilus influenzae* type b, and conjugated pneumococcal vaccines. These vaccines should be considered for age-appropriate internationally adopted children. A useful resource to assist with vaccine catch-up[1] can be found at www.aapredbook.org/site/resources/izschedules.xhtml.

Thyroid

Thyroid function tests and blood lead levels should be obtained on all new international adoptees. One study of Chinese adoptees demonstrated that 10% had abnormal thyroid function tests at the time of arrival.[6] Each child should be screened initially with a thyroid-stimulating hormone (TSH) test and free thyroxine test. If these are normal on arrival, no further evaluation should be needed. Many international adoptees may be coming from regions of the world that have iodine deficiency. These children may be expected to have a slightly elevated TSH level initially but usually have a normal free thyroxine level. Time may be given with improved nutrition to see if this normalizes. It has been the authors' observation that if TSH is elevated secondary to poor nutrition and iodine deficiency, TSH values often return to normal by 3 months post-adoption. If at 3 months TSH levels have not improved or if the free thyroxine is abnormal at any time, an endocrine evaluation and possible treatment should be considered.

Lead

Environmental lead exposure continues to be a ubiquitous health problem in many parts of the developing world. Several surveys of children seen in international adoption clinics reveal that blood lead levels in children who are internationally adopted are frequently above the US threshold of 10 mcg/dL.[6,9] For children with blood lead levels high enough to warrant source investigation, investigators should consider that lead exposure may have occurred before arrival into the child's new country in addition to considering sources of lead exposure in the current environment.

Hearing

Conductive and sensorineural hearing loss occur in internationally adopted children at a rate that justifies formal audiologic screening for all international adoptees. The lack of a detailed family history or accurate past medical history may not allow determination of a specific etiology of hearing impairment. Children may have a history of frequent upper respiratory tract infections, chronic otitis media, use of ototoxic topical medications, or bacterial, viral, protozoal, or spirochetal infections. Screening for certain infections (eg, cytomegalovirus, herpes, parvovirus B19, toxoplasmosis, syphilis) may not be definitive but may offer some explanation for parents. High-resolution computed tomography or magnetic resonance imaging may be indicated to better delineate possible abnormal ear anatomy, when hearing loss is present. In addition, a pediatric otolaryngologist can be helpful in further elucidating an underlying etiology of hearing loss.

Hearing can be assessed using a variety of methodologies, depending on the age of the child and willingness to cooperate. Children younger than 3 years should be referred to a reliable hearing center, where they may undergo otoacoustic emission testing, auditory brain stem response, behavioral observation audiometry, or visual reinforcement audiometry. For older children, assessment within the primary care pediatrician's office is an option, but children with questionable test results should be referred to a hearing center.

Regardless of a child's adoption history, the presence of permanent or chronic transient hearing loss during the first years of life has the potential to compromise a child's speech and language acquisition. All internationally adopted children who are slow to acquire language skills should have a hearing assessment. The age of the child and degree of the speech and language delay will determine the timing of the assessment. Most adoption providers agree that early evaluation and intervention is preferred.

Vision

Parents should be questioned about their child's vision at the initial post-adoption screening visit and each subsequent visit, and an eye examination should be performed. Common findings may include crossed eyes and tearing. Many children of Asian descent, as well as some children from Eastern Europe, have widely spaced eyes with flat nasal bridges. One eye may appear to "disappear" behind the labial fold (pseudostrabismus). The most useful test of alignment is the cover test. At any age, a person with misaligned eyes will use the stronger eye, allowing the weaker eye to drift. Some children, especially those who are very young, cannot cooperate for reliable cover testing. In these cases, the corneal light reflex can be used. If the eyes are straight, the reflection of the light will fall near the center of each pupil.[10] Previously institutionalized children are more likely to have strabismus (occurring in 10%–25% of internationally adopted children). Children of Asian descent may also have an epiblepharon; this is an extra fold of skin along the upper or lower eyelid margin that may cause in-turning of the lower lid and eyelashes, resulting in irritation and tearing. These usually resolve spontaneously. All previously institutionalized international adoptees should be examined by a pediatric ophthalmologist within the first few months of arrival.[11,12]

Nutrition and Growth Assessment

Growth impairment in institutionalized children should not come as a surprise to primary care pediatricians, as it makes intuitive sense and has been well described by a number of authors.[5–7] As part of the physical examination, all children need to have an accurate length, height, weight (unclothed), and head circumference measurement. Growth parameters should be plotted on standard Centers for Disease Control and Prevention or World Health Organization growth charts to determine growth percentiles. (Use of country-specific growth charts is not recommended because these may not be standardized and are not derived from institutionalized children's measurements.) Most children grow rapidly during the first months in their new home, crossing percentiles on the height, weight, and head circumference curves, and will frequently begin to follow a curve within the normal range within 9 to 12 months after arrival. Some children, particularly older children who endured malnutrition and deprivation for longer periods, may continue to make catch-up growth for years after adoption. With the exception of the rare child who was very well nourished at arrival and continues to grow appropriately along the same curve, a child who is not exhibiting catch-up growth after international adoption should be evaluated for other conditions that might cause growth failure. (For more information, see Chapter 12, Long-term Growth and Puberty Concerns for Adopted Children, on page 239.)

Sometimes the degree of growth delay can be quite alarming to parents (and primary care pediatricians), and when there is an assigned birthday, parents frequently assume that a child may really be significantly younger even though more often, the opposite is true. Making decisions about changing a child's birthday should be delayed until at least a year after the adoption, when catch-up growth and development can be taken into account.[13] Bone-age testing is almost never helpful earlier than a year after a child's adoption because malnutrition and deprivation typically cause a delay in the child's bone age. It is only after malnutrition and other stressors have resolved that a bone-age film may be helpful. Given the wide range in standard deviations for a bone-age assessment, ranging from several months up to a year, its ultimate usefulness is of some question. Bone-age assessment should therefore be just one of many factors ultimately used to assess and modify a child's age.

Most often, concerns about age discrepancies resolve as children catch up in growth and development. When significant concerns persist a year or more after adoption, it may be reasonable to consider legally changing a child's birth date. Before making such a change, parents and pediatricians should carefully consider what will be gained—or lost—for the child involved. For children with significant developmental disabilities, a later birthday (ie, making the child younger) may provide the child with more time to receive educational support services. A child who is quite small and socially immature might fit in better with school classmates of a younger age. Keep in mind that a child assigned a younger birth date may be a "second grader" who begins to go through puberty long before peers. Changing the date of birth may, however, worsen the situation. Artificially reducing the extent of a child's delays by changing the child's birthday may provide a family a false sense of security, thus delaying needed intervention. It may also make a child less likely to qualify for needed services. Prior to initiating these changes, the team may need to be expanded to include other members, such as social workers, child psychologists, and education specialists. While the family may focus on short-term benefits, this decision should often be made very slowly and cautiously and in general should be avoided unless overly compelling reasons are found.

Other Nutritional Issues

Pediatricians should obtain a complete blood cell count to evaluate for anemia and other blood disorders. Hemoglobin electrophoresis may be needed for children at risk for hemoglobinopathies based on regional and genetic factors. Among micronutrient deficiencies, iron, zinc, and vitamin D are likely to be the most common, and levels are justified at the time of arrival. If low levels are documented, careful follow-up and perhaps supplementation are advised, as diet alone may not be sufficient for repletion.

Developmental Assessment

Developmental delays in gross motor skills, fine motor skills, cognition, and language are all common for the internationally adopted child at arrival.[2-7] The amount of recovery appears to be dependent on many factors, including the duration of time a child may have spent in an institution. The likelihood of long-term developmental, behavioral, and academic problems has been shown to increase with the age of the child at the time of adoption.[14,15] However, delays in specific areas of development may be partially or completely reversible following adoption, and numerous authors have suggested that the rate of development exceeds the rate of normal development over a period of years. The primary care pediatrician should remember that developmental and behavioral issues may have multiple causes, including genetic, prenatal exposures, and individual experiences with early neglect or abuse. Because each child's experience is unique, it is impossible to predict a child's long-term outcome at an initial meeting.

After a child's international adoption, primary care pediatricians should perform a baseline screening of a child's development soon after the child's arrival and repeat screenings at follow-up visits. These ideally should be done at least 2 to 3 times during the first year home, then at least semiannually, depending on the severity of the delay. Although many excellent screening tools exist, providers may be most familiar with the Denver II Developmental Screening Test. This test relies on children's past typical experiences and exposures, which an institutional child will not have had, and requires more time than is typically available during a routine primary care visit. More recently available measures include the Parents' Evaluation of Developmental Status (PEDS) and the Pediatric Symptom Checklist (PSC). Both instruments have high sensitivity and specificity and are easy to administer in the office. They rely on parent input, so they may not be as accurate on the first visit, given parents' unfamiliarity with the child's skills. The PEDS (www.pedstest.com) is designed for children 0 to 8 years of age. The PSC behavior screening tool (designed for any child 4 years and older) and the 35-question form can be downloaded from www.massgeneral.org/psychiatry/services/psc_home.aspx.

Developmental Delay: When to Refer to Early Intervention

The decision about whether to refer to EI programs or the school district because of developmental delays should not be a difficult one, as most children will qualify for services and parents are typically very motivated to support their child's ongoing development. Almost 90% of children who spent more than one year in an institution will be delayed in at least one area of development at the time of arrival in their new families.[2] Prior studies of growth and cognitive development determined that after adoption, many institutionalized children make developmental gains faster than the normal maturational curve.[16,17] However, it is impossible to predict which children will catch up and which children will have ongoing needs. For this reason, it is recommended that pediatricians refer children for evaluation and treatment of developmental delays sooner rather than later. Occasionally, parents or an EI program or school district will want to take a "wait and see" approach. Pediatricians may need to intervene on the child's behalf should a local development program or school district elect not to provide services.

After the post-adoption screening, primary care pediatricians should carefully review development progression with an emphasis on speech and language acquisition. This is critical because communication difficulties are significantly related to behavioral concerns. Not all infants and toddlers will develop English according to the same language acquisition trends that are seen in non-adopted English-speaking peers. Glennen and Masters[18] have created criteria for referral for speech and languages services based primarily on language production, age at adoption, and time elapsed since adoption (Table 8-1). (For more information, see Chapter 14, Speech and Language Outcomes After International Adoption, on page 283.)

While the formation of a family through adoption can have its own unique issues, most children do very well. By better understanding the child's past history and experiences and through systematic screening for known issues, the health care team can quickly address issues that are noted on arrival, helping in the ultimate goal of aiding the integration of the child into the new family.

Table 8-1. Suggestions for Referral to a Speech and Language Pathologist[18]

Age at Adoption	Suggested Referral Criteria
0–12 mo	Refer as if primary English speaker.
13–18 mo	Refer if not producing 50 words or 2-word phrases at 24 months.
19–24 mo	Refer if not using English by 24 months, 50 words at 28 months, or 2-word phrases at 28–30 months.
25–30 mo	Refer if not using English within several weeks at home or not speaking 50 English words or 2-word phrases by 31 months.

References

1. American Academy of Pediatrics. Scheduling immunizations. In: Pickering LK, Baker CJ, Kimberlin DW, Long SS, eds. *Red Book: 2012 Report of the Committee on Infectious Diseases*. Elk Grove Village, IL: American Academy of Pediatrics; 2012:25–32

2. Johnson DE, Dole K. International adoptions: implications for early intervention. *Infant Young Child*. 1999;11(4):34–45

3. Johnson DE, Albers L, Iverson S, et al. Health status of Eastern European orphans referred for adoption. *Pediatr Res*. 1996;39(4 Pt 2):134A

4. Ames EW, Chisholm K, Fisher L, et al. *The Development of Romanian Children Adopted to Canada*. Burnaby, BC: Human Resources Development Canada; 1997:138

5. Miller LC, Kiernan MT, Mathers MI, Klein-Gitelman M. Developmental and nutritional status of internationally adopted children. *Arch Pediatr Adolesc Med*. 1995;149(1):40–44

6. Miller LC, Hendrie N. Health of children adopted from China. *Pediatrics*. 2000;105(6):E76

7. Albers LH, Johnson DE, Hostetter MK, Iverson S, Miller LC. Health of children adopted from the former Soviet Union and Eastern Europe. Comparison with preadoptive medical records. *JAMA*. 1997;278(11):922–924

8. American Academy of Pediatrics. Medical evaluation of internationally adopted children for infectious diseases. In: Pickering LK, Baker CJ, Kimberlin DW, Long SS, eds. *Red Book: 2012 Report of the Committee on Infectious Diseases*. Elk Grove Village, IL: American Academy of Pediatrics; 2012:191–193

9. Elevated blood lead levels in internationally adopted children—United States, 1998. *MMWR*. 1998;49(5):97–100

10. Simon JW, Calhoun JH. *A Child's Eyes: A Guide to Pediatric Primary Care*. Gainesville, FL: Triad Publishing Company; 1998

11. Johnson DE. Long-term medical issues in international adoptees. *Pediatr Ann*. 2000;29(4):234–241

12. Spitz R. *The First Year of Life: A Psychoanalytic Study of Normal and Deviant Development of Object Relations*. New York, NY: International Universities Press; 1965

13. Mason P, Narad C. Long-term growth and puberty concerns in international adoptees. *Pediatr Clin North Am*. 2005;52:1351–1368

14. Johnson DE. Adoption and the effect on children's development. *Early Hum Dev*. 2002;68:39–54

15. O'Connor TG, Rutter M, Beckett C, Keaveney L, Kreppner JM. The effects of global severe privation on cognitive competence: extension and longitudinal follow-up. English and Romanian Study Team. *Child Dev*. 2000;71(2):376–390

16. Aronson J, Johnson D, Melnikova M, Alonso M. Catch-up brain growth in children adopted form Eastern Europe and Russia. Paper presented at the Ambulatory Pediatric Association Annual Conference, San Francisco, CA. May 1999

17. Morison SJ, Ames EW, Chisholm K. The development of children adopted from Romanian orphanages. *Merrill Palmer Q*. 1995;41:411–430

18. Glennen S, Masters MG. Typical and atypical language development in infants and toddlers adopted from Eastern Europe. *Am J Speech Lang Pathol*. 2002;11:417–433

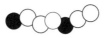

CHAPTER 9

Immediate Developmental and Behavioral Challenges Post-adoption

Laurie C. Miller, MD, FAAP

The Transition

The arrival of a new child is a dramatic moment in the life of a family, whether the child arrives by birth or adoption. Although parents have had months or even years to prepare for these moments, little can be done to prepare infant and young toddler adoptees for this momentous event. Some older children being adopted may have little or no preparation for this major life transition as well. As a result, the intersection of dreams, expectations, and realities may be difficult for everyone involved. Incredibly, most children and parents weather this remarkable change and readily unite as a family. Understandably, however, many experience some difficulties during the transition. In this chapter, several aspects of this extraordinary event in a family's history will be reviewed, including commonly seen child behaviors—especially as related to eating, sleeping, and activities of daily living—and health. The emotional stages for adoptive parents, any siblings, and the adoptive child in the immediate post-adoptive period will be discussed, along with some suggestions for adoption-friendly anticipatory guidance for families. Transition issues related to international adoption are highlighted because of the specialized issues related to pre-adoption institutionalization of children and international travel.[1] Specific features of transition for domestic adoptees are also addressed. Some of the material in this chapter may also be relevant to other situations in which custody and care of a child changes, such as entry of children into foster care, kinship adoptions, or stepfamily arrangements.

The Process of Transition

The process of transition for families varies greatly depending on the specific situation of the child. Children face this enormous change in their lives with differing degrees of resilience. This reflects innate personality characteristics as well as individual vulnerabilities, some of which derive from prenatal exposures to alcohol, illicit drugs, tobacco, maternal stress, or early life experiences. For newborn domestic adoptions, adoptive parents may attend the birth and bring the newborn directly home from the hospital, or they may receive a child who is weeks or months old and has been living in any number of possible arrangements (eg, prolonged hospitalization, birth family care, temporary foster care). In adoptions from state social service departments, a child may transition relatively seamlessly within a foster-to-adoption situation or, alternately, may have the opportunity to get acquainted gradually with adoptive parents through a series of visits while the adoption is processed. Older children may participate actively in the tempo and timing of this process, indicating when they are ready to make the transition and commitment to their new family.

Children adopted from other countries usually live in institutional care prior to placement. This may be a hospital, specialized center, or most typically, an orphanage. A small number of international adoptees are assigned to foster care shortly after birth; others enter foster care after a period of orphanage residence. Still others reside for periods with their birth families prior to entering a care arrangement. Thus, the pre-adoption experiences of children in these settings vary greatly, depending on the number of caregivers, resources and nurturing characteristics of the environment, health and nutritional status of the child, and many other factors.

Because of legal constraints and geographic distances, international adoptions usually provide little, if any, opportunity for children and adopting parents to spend meaningful time together before paperwork is finalized.[2] Although parents may have the opportunity to visit the child on several occasions prior to finalizing the adoption (most notably, in Russia and Ethiopia, where parents are required to visit the child 2 to 3 times before finalization of adoption), these visits are often spaced over many months, making it unlikely that the young child remembers the parents from one visit to the next. Adoptions from Kazakhstan (now mostly on hold) are a notable exception; the residency requirement for adopting parents makes extended stays common. This allows a child to gradually transition from orphanage care to new parents over several weeks, a decidedly less traumatic method than a sudden handover. Abrupt transfer is common in Chinese adoptions; children are brought by orphanage workers to a hotel or civil affairs office (often a lengthy bus or train ride away) and literally handed to the adoptive parents by caregivers who may not know their history and preferences. Chinese children who have been in foster care are removed from their foster families and often spend several weeks in an orphanage in preparation for adoptive placement, thus experiencing 2 major transitions during this vulnerable time. Procedures differ in other countries. For example, children adopted from South Korea are sometimes escorted to the United States by an unfamiliar person.

Understandably, such abrupt transitions are stressful for children and their parents. Adoptive parents commonly observe several unusual behaviors during this early transition. For example, some children become hyper-somnolent, sleeping more than 14 hours each night and taking lengthy and frequent naps. Others appear withdrawn, with blank affect, poor eye contact, and limited social engagement; occasionally, this may be so severe as to raise concerns about possible autism. Practitioners contacted for advice during this transition time must be extremely cautious about diagnosing autism or related disorders in a child who has just undergone a major life upheaval; this withdrawal reaction happens often enough that parents should be prepared for it and willing to wait it out. Usually the most severe symptoms disappear within a few days as the child becomes more comfortable with the new parents. Other children display extreme tantrums or violent behaviors—crying, biting, scratching, spitting, or kicking their new parents in an attempt to get away and get back to their known and beloved caregivers. Many young children exhibit true grief, sobbing inconsolably for hours or even days, with nightmares and refusal to accept comfort or affection, or poignantly standing by the hotel room door with their few belongings for hours at a time. Parents should be reassured that grieving by children for all they have lost is normal in this situation and usually reflects a prior strong and positive attachment to previous caregivers.

Along with these obvious emotional reactions, children may go on a hunger strike, refusing even a morsel of food from their new parents; regress completely in potty training; or exhibit signs of illness (eg, vomiting, diarrhea, severe constipation). Some children cling forcefully to the new parent; this is often misinterpreted as instant attachment. During this time, some children may accept one parent (even if grudgingly) while completely rejecting the second parent. Sometimes a reason for these strong preferences can be suspected (eg, the child has never seen a man with a beard before; no one in the orphanage wears glasses), but often there is no obvious reason other than the child's realization that he needs someone to take care of him—but that doesn't mean he's going to like it.

Undoubtedly, stress underlies all these reactions. During this early transition period, adoptive parents are well advised to remain calm and provide as much comfort and empathy to their child as possible. Even with language barriers and emotional extremes, young children seem (eventually) to understand and accept empathy from their new parents ("I know you are sad and miss your nannies! I'm so sorry that you had to leave them. I promise we will take good care of you and love you forever"). Usually, within a few days, the most dramatic of the transition behaviors subside and the real adjustment of the newly formed family can begin. If one parent had been strongly favored over the other, this split gradually starts to lessen, although it can take time for both parents to feel on equal footing in the child's estimation. One family's journey through these early stages is described in Box 9-1.

Box 9-1. When Lea First Came Home: A Description of an Adoption Transition

By Lea's Mother

(Notes from clinic visits are included in italics.)

When we first met our daughter, she was a healthy and alert 14-month-old with no signs of problems. She came from an orphanage in a quiet neighborhood on the outskirts of a rural town, and she had had minimal interaction with people outside the orphanage up to the time we met her. While traveling with her in China, we soon found that she was terrified of being abandoned again. She bonded quickly to my husband and preferred to be held or comforted by him. We were not able to sit her in high chairs at meals or in a stroller when we were out. We had to constantly hold her. Luckily, we had brought 2 different kinds of baby carriers (shoulder/hip harness) with us, and we used them constantly.

Clinic visit no. 1, 14 months of age: Wakens screaming at night, clings to father, sucks wrist nervously, can't figure out sippy cup, hates bath, eats everything. Examination: Looks very frightened—obvious emotional fragility, flat occiput, marked hypotonia, poor eye contact; gross motor, 10 months; fine motor, 12 months; cognition, 11 months; receptive language, 6 months; expressive language, 7 months.

In the first few weeks after being home, we noticed that when we took her out of the house, she would sit quietly in our baby carrier and not make eye contact with us. To not overwhelm her, we decided not to take her out in public for the first 2 to 3 months. The only exception to that rule was a daily walk outside in our neighborhood. I placed her in a carrier and walked on the same path and constantly point out to her what she was seeing. That was the only experiences she had outside the home. To cope with her requirement to stay home, my husband and I worked out a system of taking turns doing the grocery shopping so we still got out, although not together.

We continued to use the baby carriers when we took her out or when she got tired at the end of the day. I would often place her in the carrier and do some chores around the house so she was close to me at all times. I made sure to get eye contact with her as much as possible and stroke her arms and legs for physical input. We would play different games with her to always get eye contact with her. We played in front of the mirror, peekaboo, hide-and-seek, and many other games that would require her to look at us.

Clinic visit no. 2, 16 months of age: Still very clingy but accepting mom well. Starting to make intermittent eye contact with strangers, showing some curiosity. Doing 4 to 5 signs. Crib in parents' room. Settles herself in crib using a "blankie" for self-comfort. Initiating play—peekaboo. Loves brushing teeth; starting to like massage. Knows 2 to 3 animal sounds but not imitating words. Examination: Able to calm herself a bit. Marked hypotonia. Some vocalizations and jabber. Gross motor, 16 months; fine motor, 17 months; cognition, 17 months; receptive language, 13 months; expressive language, 12 months.

To ease the transition to a new family home life, my husband had taken a short leave from work after returning from China. We were concerned about how she would cope with him leaving on a daily basis when he had to go back to work, so we practiced the routine of him leaving a couple of times for an hour or so, while he still was at home from work. The day came when he had to go back to work, and together we created an elaborate good-bye ceremony every morning. He would say good-bye, we would all hug, and we waved and watched him go into his car and drive away. When he came back from work, we made a big deal out of greeting him too. We stayed with that routine for almost a year, until she didn't need it any longer.

Our daughter was at first very scared of taking baths, as we learned when we tried to put her down in the bathtub in the hotel room the day after meeting her. When we came home, we changed our strategy and placed a small bucket of water on the floor in the bathroom. Every night we would all play with the water and get her used to a few toys and bubbles. After just a few days, she put one hand in the tub by herself. We finally transferred the bucket to the bathtub after 2½ months. Shortly thereafter she took her first bath in the regular tub.

Even though she was able to hold her bottle at 14 months, we decided not to allow her. Instead we regressed her bottle-feeding to give her some of the close physical contact and stimulation she had missed out on in the orphanage. I would sit in a rocker, holding her and holding the bottle for her. At first she wouldn't allow us to hold her lying down, but after a couple of days she gave in to us. I would talk and sing to her and rock her while she was feeding. At mealtimes she sat in a high chair and ate with us. We allowed her to explore her foods with her fingers and hands. She quickly showed interest in regular food, although we kept her on the bottle in the morning and at nap time and bedtime.

Within the first couple of weeks of being home, we created a photo book for our daughter with 8" x 10" photos of each step of her day. We took pictures of her getting up, having her diaper changed, eating breakfast, saying good-bye to Daddy, napping, eating lunch, playing, Daddy returning home from work, brushing her teeth, taking a bath, and going to sleep. We read the book to her every day, explaining each step to her. It didn't take long for her to recognize the photos and start to understand the new routine in her life. She even created a sign for brushing her teeth by putting her index finger in her mouth when she saw the picture of herself doing it. We started to use that sign for brushing teeth, and she understood that.

Clinic visit no. 3, 18 months of age: Remains panicky at home if mom not in view. Follows her everywhere. Doing better with strangers and other people but still has times of pure panic (recent doctor visit). Knows 40 signs, puts 2 together. Fearful of haircuts, nail clipping. Hates noises (eg, hair dryer, vacuum, motorcycles, airplanes). Hears noises before others notice them. Very upset if held horizontally. Wakes distressed during naps, but overall sleeping well. Examination: Playful and engaging; becomes distressed but able to "get it together" for her physical. Hypotonia improving. Gross motor, 16 months; fine motor, 20 months; cognition, 19 months; receptive language, 22 months; expressive language, 16 months. Sensory processing questionnaire completed by mother revealed definite differences in all areas. Referred for sensory therapy.

To ease her language transition, we taught her baby sign language. We started out with just 3 signs: more, milk, and all done. Within a month she started using these signs, and slowly we taught her more signs. Signing allowed her to express her basic needs and alleviate some frustration in her new daily life. By constantly naming things around her, we showed her what things and their names were. At lunchtime, I would sit with her and point out all the things around us. When she started to understand and recognize words, it became a game for her to point to the correct things, and she was rewarded with lots of cheering and applause. Within 6 months of arriving home, she was using up to 50 baby signs (we found Web sites with video of signs on the Internet). When she started to be more expressive in her language, the signs slowly disappeared, although now, a year and a half later, she will still use a couple of them if I don't understand her right away.

Box 9-1. When Lea First Came Home: A Description of an Adoption Transition, continued

Her gross motor skills were not very strong when she first came home. Within a week at home, she started to walk, although she was unable to crawl. She had spent most of her time in a walker in the orphanage, and she was not used to spending time on the floor. To help her learn to crawl, I threw pillows and blankets on the floor and made her crawl over them to get to toys or me on the other side. At the playground I assisted her crawling up straight ladders so she would strengthen both sides equally.

Clinic visit no. 4, 21 months of age: Seems happier overall but still has occasional panic episodes— thought pharmacist was doctor and had major meltdown. Still has increased sensitivity to sounds but somewhat less panicky. Hasn't started sensory therapy yet. Examination: Clings desperately to mom, holding her blankie, unable to cooperate at all with examination. Gross motor, 23 months; fine motor, 24 months; cognition, 26 months; receptive language, 22 months; expressive language, 22 months.

The first 4 to 5 months, we had a visitor rule that all family and friends were asked to respect: We allowed only 1 to 2 people visiting us at a time. When visitors came to our house, we would hold her until she felt comfortable to get down herself. Only if she invited interaction with our guests would we allow them to get close to her. Also, we asked all friends to bring us food when they came to visit. The first couple of months were a lot of work for us all to adjust to each other, so it was a relief to have many prepared meals available. People even came to our house and cooked for us!

Clinic visit no. 5, 27 months of age: Doing great! Able to travel with parents and accept changes in routine. Getting sensory therapy and mom doing a lot of desensitization activities at home. In playgroup, tolerates separation from mom. Tolerates sounds. Co-sleeping. Able to calm self. Unable to tolerate mom being on the phone, otherwise no big behavior problems. Examination: Completely cooperative and responsive. Gross motor, 27 months; fine motor, 24 months; cognition, 31 months; receptive language, 36 months; expressive language, 28 months.

In short, the first couple of months were a steep learning curve for my husband and me. When one thing didn't seem to work, we tried something different. And sometimes one thing would only work for a while. It was important for us to get a feel for what our daughter needed and what worked best for her. We sought advice all around us from other adoptive parents and the medical field. It was a hard time to adjust as first-time parents, but we knew our hard work would be rewarded in the long run. Now a year and a half later, she has overcome most of the challenges she first had. I don't think our work will ever be completely done with her, but I am confident that she is on the right path to reach her true potential as a happy and well-balanced little girl.

Infant and Toddler Adoption

Some domestically adopted children are placed as older infants or toddlers. Few young infants (<6 months of age) are placed in international adoptions, mostly due to ingrained bureaucratic delays in the system of adoptive placement: the average age of an international adoptee is approximately 14 months at placement.[1] By this age, experience has taught children the degree to which their environment is safe, trustworthy, and responsive. This understanding accompanies children to their new adoptive home, where the actual situation typically differs considerably from their previous experiences. It takes time for children to come to trust the realities of their new environment. Children also often bring to their new homes a definite strong sense of how things are done, so when this changes, there may be confusion and distress. The most obvious examples of this are the common behavioral problems observed in newly adopted infants and toddlers. Distress with feeding, bathing, and diapering are quite common, as the child protests that "this is not how I'm used to doing this." Frequent sensory processing problems (especially tactile hypersensitivity) exacerbate problems with these activities, as some children are not used to or comfortable with being touched, moved, or handled in certain ways. New adoptive parents need to understand that from the child's point of view, everything they do will be "wrong" and it will take time to get it "right."

Older Children

Different issues arise with children who are older at the time of adoption. Older children should be prepared as much as possible for this major life change. Ideally, a caregiver explains in detail what is going to happen and is willing to repeat this information in an age-appropriate manner as often as needed for the child to process. Availability of photo albums and other visual aids from the adoptive family can aid this process ("Here's a picture of your new bedroom waiting for you; here's your new sister; here's the family dog"). Parents should prepare several copies of such material (in case of loss); for international adoptions, providing a version translated into the local language is helpful and respectful. When parents arrive to first meet the child, it is helpful if they wear the same clothes as in the photos; this can help the child make the connection between the book and the new people before her.

Whether placed internationally or domestically, older adoptees often grieve the loss of their friends, foster siblings, schools, and other familiar parts of their lives. Some children have had ongoing contact with birth relatives; if possible, this should continue. International adoptees may be very frustrated at their lack of ability to communicate with new family members; having a bilingual interpreter available (even by phone) during the early days after placement can greatly reduce problems and decrease stress for everyone. Children who have experienced difficulties with their birth families (eg, abuse) often have anxieties about again being placed in a family. For some of these children, the orphanage or group home may have represented safety and security. It takes time for children to accept that their new family is safe and secure.

Preparing a Life Book

For children who have experienced changes and disruptions in early life, a *life book* may be a valuable asset to ease this latest transition. Adoptive parents can prepare this as a loving gift for their new child. It should contain photos and (appropriate) information detailing the child's early life experiences. It is important for children to have a record of where they were at different ages and who cared for them.

Family Travel

Parents adopting internationally must prepare themselves for the physical and emotional demands of an adoption trip. For parents not familiar with international travel, a visit to a travel medicine clinic[3,4] is invaluable to update their vaccines and review basic hygiene recommendations and travel precautions.[5,6] This should be done far in advance of the expected travel date because many vaccines (notably hepatitis B) require a series of immunizations over time (if necessary, the hepatitis B vaccine can be administered using an accelerated schedule[7]). Up-to-date and reliable destination-specific information about needed vaccines and other health issues is widely available on the Internet.[8,9]

Sometimes, other children in the family accompany their parents on an international adoption trip. Traveling children should be up to date on their vaccines[10]; their parents should be knowledgeable about how to minimize health risks for the children. Young travelers need close supervision in areas of traffic safety, mosquito precautions, water and food hygiene, and encounters with animals (eg, street dogs).[11] Adequate supplies of any medications needed by family members should be brought with them in carry-on luggage. Some travel clinics may also dispense ciprofloxacin and various other antibiotics depending on the destination; recommendations for child travelers include ciprofloxacin for children older than 16 years and azithromycin for younger travelers.[10]

A general rule of thumb is that the number of traveling adults should equal or preferably exceed the number of children (including the new adoptee). This insures adequate resources if a child or adult becomes ill or requires extra attention during the trip.

The Early Days After Placement

The early days after placement can be a very emotional time. The family must adjust to a new member, and the adopted child must adjust to new caregivers and a completely new household culture. Changes include diet, behavioral expectations for every aspect of life, discipline, beliefs and values, and even sense of humor. Not surprisingly, in the face of this major transition, many children show behavioral symptoms.[12] The frequency of behavioral symptoms related to feeding, sleeping, and self-stimulation/self-soothing among a group of international adoptees is shown in Table 9-1.

Table 9-1. Behavioral Symptoms in Newly Arrived Internationally Adopted Children (<3 Years; N=387)[13]

Eating disturbances • Stuffs food in cheeks • Food anxiety • Weak muscles of mastication • Ravenous or insatiable appetite	35
Sleeping problems • Frequent night terrors and nightmares • Excessive crying • Nap/sleep disturbances • Unable to separate at bedtime	41
Self-stimulatory/self-soothing behaviors • Rocking • Head shaking • Hair twisting • Withdrawal	22
Children with problems in 2 areas	10
Children with problems in all 3 areas	3

Feeding

The infant or young child must adapt to unfamiliar feeding practices in the new environment. Many young children from orphanages have never eaten solid food or been fed from a spoon. Orphanages commonly use bottles with large holes cut in the nipples to speed feeding in infancy, and children must use pharyngeal muscles to prevent choking, rather than exercising the muscles of mastication. Parents may need to try several brands and shapes of nipple to find one that is acceptable. At any age, new textures and tastes may be challenging.[14,15] If the child is malnourished (as is common among international adoptees), parental anxiety may exacerbate feeding disturbances. Some children are insatiable or ravenous. Others exhibit extreme anxiety when they see food being prepared but not yet available to them. Stuffing cheeks and hoarding or hiding food are also common. These behaviors usually diminish with time. Parents should understand the origins of such behaviors, which include lack of development of a true feeding/satiety cycle, frequent true hunger, and sensory processing disorders. It is best to allow free access to food for the insatiable eater. The child must learn to regulate and recognize his own hunger and satiety and also literally internalize the message that the new environment has unlimited food available (food availability can be seen by a previously hungry child as a proxy for love). Providing such children with their own supply of food (lunch box or other private container) can greatly reduce anxiety and the need to stuff themselves at mealtimes. Less commonly, children, often those who are malnourished, appear to have limited or no interest in food. These children present a considerable challenge to their parents, who are understandably anxious at their seeming inability to feed a malnourished child. Doctors also become frustrated at the child's poor progress with growth. There is no universal explanation for this lack of interest in food; in some cases, this undoubtedly derives from the child's discovery in orphanage care that refusal to eat brought extra attention. In other cases, medical conditions may interfere with the child's appetite (eg, gastroesophageal reflux, temporary lactose intolerance related to parasitism, extensive dental caries). Medical evaluation of such children is recommended to rule out obvious organic conditions, but behavioral consultants and feeding teams are often necessary to improve feeding patterns. Parents of such children need support and understanding for at least several months post-adoption.

Young children often enjoy their bottles for some time after arrival home; there is no urgency to wean children to toddler (sippy) cups. The bottle may be comforting and offer bonding opportunities for parent and child. In addition, using a bottle to drink may provide needed exercise for oral-facial muscles of mastication and speech. Bottle-feeding a young child in front of a mirror reinforces the loving care of the parent as the child views himself in mom's or dad's arms on her or his lap. This can be a helpful bridge for children who may have difficulty with the intimacy of eye contact.

Parents often ask about the need to maintain familiar foods for the child. For older children, this is an especially welcoming gesture, even if done only occasionally. As part of the transition, parents can inquire about the child's favorite foods and later provide these in their home. Regardless of age, over time most children transition well to the new foods offered in the family. However, a number of children steadfastly refuse milk. Kefir or yogurt-type drinks may taste more familiar; these can be gradually diluted with milk. Alternatively, flavorings (eg, chocolate, strawberry) may be added to milk until the child becomes accustomed to the taste.

Sleeping

Sleep disturbances are common in newly arrived international adoptees for a range of reasons including, but not limited to, changes in time zone and sleeping environment (ie, sleeping alone or with others; sleeping in a crib or bed or on the floor). Nightmares, night terrors, refusal to separate from parents, and other sleep problems are common in children adopted from orphanages. Children may seem happy and well-adjusted during the day, but at night they become needy, sad, and tearful. Falling asleep may be particularly hard for children who have experienced losses with other transitions. Parents of a new adoptee must realize that the origins of sleep disturbances are rooted in anxiety and insecurity, not manipulative behavior that can develop in toddlers who have learned to use the nighttime routine as a time to run the show. The latter should be treated very differently. In her book *Toddler Adoption: The Weaver's Craft,* Mary Hopkins-Best wisely suggests that parents reframe their newly adopted toddler's demands for parental attention during the night as an opportunity to promote bonding.[16] Co-sleeping or other supportive arrangements often diminish sleep disturbances for new adoptees and other family members.

Toileting

Many orphanages introduce early toilet training, which may actually be scheduled toileting. Young toddlers may be toileted on a very rigid schedule. After adoption, most young children regress to diapers. Again, toilet training should not be demanded or expected from a newly adopted toddler. Parents can use the physical care of diaper changing as a time to bond with their child (again, doing this in front of a mirror reinforces parental caring). It is noteworthy, however, that some children become agitated when placed supine for diaper changes. One possible explanation is that this position reminds children of being placed in their cribs, where they had long waits until the next time they received attention from their caregivers. If children are excessively upset when supine during diaper changes, changing diapers with the child standing may be helpful.

Bowel elimination patterns are often disrupted in new adoptees. Diarrhea (unrelated to intestinal infection) and constipation are common; stress is often suspected as a cause.

Bathing

At first, some children become distraught with baths. The sensory stimulation of water all over their skin may be overwhelming for a stressed child who has never learned that bath time can be pleasant. The change in bath routine from prior custom may alarm some children. Watching a sibling bathe or starting with slow, gentle sponge baths can help some children get used to bathing.

Self-stimulatory/Self-soothing Behaviors

In a recent survey, more than 20% of newly arrived internationally adopted toddlers were noted to have self-stimulatory or self-soothing behaviors. These include such behaviors as rocking, head banging, hair twisting, and ear pulling. Some children momentarily withdraw or space out, sometimes raising the question of a seizure disorder; in others, stereotypical movements raise concerns about autism.[17] These behaviors often persist after children arrive in their adoptive homes, although in most children, these behaviors lessen with time. Parents can greatly reduce the intensity and frequency of these behaviors for many children by providing sensory stimulating activities (eg, rocking with the child, massage).

Play and Development

Play is often difficult in the early days after adoption. Children are easily over-whelmed by their new world. Many children are highly sensory seeking—under-standable after living in a monotonous, limited environment. Children often appear to have very brief or fragmented attention spans and are highly distractible. Parents may need to demonstrate how to play with some toys, as many children seem to lack any understanding about how to engage with toys beyond flinging or drop-ping them. Patient modeling of and opportunities for interactive play (eg, rolling a ball back and forth, taking turns building a tower) are not typically done by orphanage caregivers.

Development delays are commonly observed in newly adopted children.[12,18–21] Children residing in orphanages have many potential reasons for developmental delays, including lack of nurturing physical contact, lack of opportunities to explore and interact, prolonged swaddling, ill health, malnutrition, and micronutrient deficiencies.[1] In addition, the stress of transition leads many children to regress in their developmental abilities. This is the usual explanation of a child who is reported to be unable to sit independently at adoption but able to walk independently 2 weeks later. However, rapid recovery of developmental milestones is typical. While reveling in their child's catch-up, parents must remain aware of needed changes in childproofing and safety.

Health

Fortunately, most children remain healthy through the transition to their new families. However, parents who travel to other countries to adopt may wish to bring medical supplies for their new child. A suggested list is shown in Box 9-2; most of these items are available for purchase over the counter in the children's countries of origin. Before administering antibiotics, parents should seek medical advice, preferably from local doctors who can examine the child. In addition to orphanage

---

Box 9-2. Basic Supplies for Traveling Parents[22]

Adjust as appropriate for child's age.

Alcohol wipes	Dosage syringe
Antibacterial wipes	Insect repellent
Antibiotic ointment	Permethrin (eg, Elimite)
Antihistamine	Sunscreen
Antipyretic	Waterless soap gel
Diaper rash cream (as age appropriate)	

staff physicians, adoption facilitators often have medical contacts. Large hotels often have physicians on call. The US embassy or consulate will provide the names of local physicians and also assist with emergencies. The American Academy of Pediatrics online directory at www.healthychildren.org/findapediatrician is searchable by country of residence[23]; providing these names to traveling parents in advance can be reassuring. Parents may also be comforted by being able to contact their child's future pediatrician; this can easily be accomplished via e-mail. Setting this up in advance is helpful for the travelers and the pediatrician.

Travel

International adoptees must not only adapt to their entirely new lives but also must adjust to the unfamiliar challenges of travel. Many of these children have never left the orphanage grounds; thus, car, train, and air travel are completely new. Not surprisingly, some children have motion sickness or prolonged distress. Older children should be prepared in their own language for the various stages of travel. Picture books can help with communication for all ages of children. Helpful resources on air travel with children are available on the Internet.

Medical Care After Arrival in the United States or After Domestic Placement

After arrival home, children should be seen by their pediatrician within 3 to 4 weeks if healthy or immediately if ill. This early visit is valuable to document growth measurements and any obvious abnormal physical findings, as well as to reassure parents about the child's basic health. A referral to early intervention services can be made at this visit if a child has profound deficits or parents need instructions on how to promote developmental progress in their child. Because children need time to transition and typically make significant progress simply by being placed in a nurturing environment, practitioners can often wait 2 to 3 months before having the child engage with therapists. Unless the child is ill, needle exposures (eg, blood tests, tuberculin test, vaccinations) and other painful procedures should be avoided at this visit. These can be accomplished along with a more detailed developmental assessment at a second visit several weeks later with less trauma for the child. Usually, a minimum of 1 to 2 hours is needed to complete the examination portion of the assessment. Dental evaluations are advisable for children with teeth, as many have multiple cavities and other dental problems. A standardized medical assessment for infectious diseases and other health problems is useful.[10,24–29]

Family Adjustment

After adoption, the entire adoptive family must readjust to the new member and their new roles. Siblings have a new identity in the family hierarchy (eg, moving from being the youngest to being the youngest *girl)*. As with the arrival of birth siblings, older children may resent the arrival of an adopted sibling. This situation can be especially challenging when the new arrival is not a newborn but rather a mobile, active toddler or school-aged child. The sibling may be frustrated at the new arrival's inability to communicate or participate in reciprocal play. The new child's mobility, dexterity, and lack of awareness of boundaries may allow him to get into everything with no respect for his sibling's possessions or personal space. The pediatrician can provide helpful guidance related to sibling adjustments and expected difficulties depending on ages, personalities, and overall family composition.

Parent adjustment should also be monitored by the pediatrician. Most new adoptive parents are thrilled and excited with their new children. However, post-adoption depression is increasingly recognized among new adoptive parents. These adoptive parents usually feel deep shame about their feelings and may be reluctant to discuss this unless directly questioned. Sleep deprivation, attachment difficulties, and unexpected medical, developmental, or behavioral problems may all contribute to post-adoption depression. Open-ended questions (eg, "Is this new child what you expected? Is everything going as you imagined? How are you feeling about the process and your child? How would you describe your new child?") allow parents to express ambivalent feelings. Pediatricians should also be aware of local resources for family support.

Attachment

Adoptive parents often do not realize that their attachment to their new child—and the child's attachment to them—takes time and is affected by thousands of reciprocal interactions over many weeks, months, and years. Without this realization, parents feel guilty or ashamed that they did not instantly attach to their new child. Instant attachment is a myth; many children cling to a new parent, but this is not the same as sharing a deep emotional connection. Providing physical care for the child (eg, feeding, bathing, diapering, putting to bed) and spending time together are the basic building blocks of attachment. These activities should be reserved for parents in the immediate post-adoptive period until attachment with primary caregivers is solidly established. Well-meaning relatives and friends who wish to help the new parents should do so by offering to perform household chores rather than child care. Parents will need to proactively discuss their efforts to promote attachment and decrease "stranger seeking" with well-intended adults who may be coming to visit. It is important for parents to be the source of this care as much as possible in the early weeks after adoption. Children who have had multiple caregivers and gone through this major life transition will be reassured by this routine and will gradually understand that the parents can be relied on to provide this care. Extended family who will be involved in the life of the child on a regular basis should not be excluded from visiting, as these attachments are also important to foster. However, physical caring of the child should be exclusively provided by the parents in the initial adjustment period.

Parental Leave

With these facts in mind, parents must be realistic about child care arrangements for a newly adopted child. Parents adopting internationally may have used up leave time during necessary travel. However, it is important for all new adoptees to have a solid sense of their parents and family before entering a child care situation. For children who have never lived in a family, it is vital to learn about the consistency of parents and depth of their commitment. While it is ideal for a parent to remain home full time with the newly adopted child for at least 3 months (and preferably longer), children can still make a positive transition with thoughtful planning about child care arrangements.

References

1. Miller LC. *Handbook of International Adoption Medicine.* New York, NY: Oxford University Press; 2005
2. US Department of State Bureau of Consular Affairs. Intercountry adoption. http://adoption.state. gov. Accessed February 12, 2014
3. Centers for Disease Control and Prevention. Traveler's health: destinations. http://wwwnc.cdc.gov/ travel/destinations/list. Accessed February 12, 2014
4. American Society of Tropical Medicine and Hygiene. Tropical and travel medicine consultant directory. http://www.astmh.org/source/clinicaldirectory. Accessed February 12, 2014
5. Chen LH, Barnett ED, Wilson ME. Preventing infectious diseases during and after international adoption. *Ann Intern Med.* 2003;139(5 Pt 1):371–378
6. Ryan ET, Wilson ME, Kain KC. Illness after international travel. *N Engl J Med.* 2002;347: 505–516
7. Bock HL, Loscher T, Scheiermann N, et al. Accelerated schedule for hepatitis B immunization. *J Travel Med.* 1995;2(4):213–217
8. Centers for Disease Control and Prevention. *CDC Health Information for International Travel 2014: The Yellow Book.* http://wwwnc.cdc.gov/travel/yellowbook/2014/table-of-contents. Accessed February 12, 2014
9. World Health Organization. International travel and health. http://www.who.int/ith. Accessed February 12, 2014
10. American Academy of Pediatrics Committee on Infectious Diseases. *Red Book: 2012 Report of the Committee on Infectious Diseases.* Pickering LK, ed. Elk Grove Village, IL: American Academy of Pediatrics; 2012
11. Hostetter MK. Epidemiology of travel-related morbidity and mortality in children. *Pediatr Rev.* 1999;20(7):228–233
12. Faber S. Behavioral sequelae of orphanage life. *Pediatr Ann.* 2000;29(4):242–248
13. Tirella LG, Miller LC. Self-regulation in newly arrived international adoptees. *Phys Occup Ther Pediatr.* 2011;31(3):301–314
14. Cermak S, Groza V. Sensory processing problems in post-institutionalized children: implications for social workers. *Child Adol Soc Work J.* 1998;15(1):5–37
15. Cermak SA, Daunhauer LA. Sensory processing in the post-institutionalized child. *Am J Occup Ther.* 1997;51(7):500–507

16. Hopkins-Best M. *Toddler Adoption: The Weaver's Craft*. Indianapolis, IN: Perspectives Press; 1997

17. Rutter M, Andersen-Wood L, Beckett C, et al. Quasi-autistic patterns following severe global privation. English and Romanian Adoptees (ERA) Study Team. *J Child Psychol Psychiatry.* 1999;40(4):537–549

18. Cermak SA. The effects of deprivation on processing, play, and praxis. In: Bundy AC, Lane SJ, Murray EA, eds. *Sensory Integration*. Philadelphia, PA: FA Davis Co; 2002

19. Miller LC. Initial assessment of growth, development, and the effects of institutionalization in internationally adopted children. *Pediatr Ann.* 2000;29(4):224–232

20. Miller LC, Kiernan MT, Mathers MI, Klein-Gitelman M. Developmental and nutritional status of internationally adopted children. *Arch Pediatr Adolesc Med.* 1995;149(1):40–44

21. O'Connor TG, Rutter M, Beckett C, Keaveney L, Kreppner JM. The effects of global severe privation on cognitive competence: extension and longitudinal follow-up. English and Romanian Adoptees Study Team. *Child Dev.* 2000;71(2):376–390

22. Borchers DA. Adoption medical travel guide. http://www.adoptivefamilies.com/pdf/TravelMed.pdf. Accessed February 12, 2014

23. American Academy of Pediatrics. Find a pediatrician or pediatric specialist. http://www.healthychildren.org/findapediatrician. Accessed February 12, 2014

24. Aronson J. Medical evaluation and infectious considerations on arrival. *Pediatr Ann.* 2000;29(4):218–223

25. Hostetter MK, Iverson S, Thomas W, McKenzie D, Dole K, Johnson DE. Medical evaluation of internationally adopted children [see comments]. *N Engl J Med.* 1991;325(7):479–485

26. Jenista JA. Medical issues in international adoption. *Pediatr Ann.* 2000;29:204–252

27. Miller LC. Caring for internationally adopted children [editorial; comment] [see comments]. *N Engl J Med.* 1999;341(20):1539–1540

28. Nicholson AJ, Francis BM, Mulholland EK, Moulden AL, Oberklaid F. Health screening of international adoptees. Evaluation of a hospital based clinic [see comments]. *Med J Aust.* 1992;156(6):377–379

29. Jones VF; American Academy of Pediatrics Committee on Early Childhood, Adoption and Dependent Care. Comprehensive health evaluation of the newly adopted child. *Pediatrics.* 2012;129(1):e214–e223

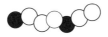

CHAPTER 10

The Long-term Consequences of Child Maltreatment in Adopted Children

Katherine P. Deye, MD, FAAP, and Kent P. Hymel, MD, FAAP

An unfortunate truth is that many of the children adopted from institutional settings or the foster care system in the United States have experienced severe, chronic, or repetitive child abuse or neglect. The adverse consequences of their experiences can continue long after their maltreatment ends. Adult survivors of child maltreatment frequently manifest significant health harms that can be causally linked to their previous abuse. Adoptive and foster care children deserve and require active vigilance, screening and interventions for these long-term health harms. In this chapter, we will discuss the effect of trauma on the child and relate it to what is known about living in foster care and institutional care settings.

Overview of Child Maltreatment

What constitutes a neglectful or abusive act toward a child? The federal Child Abuse Prevention and Treatment Act (42 USC §5106g), amended later by the Keeping Children and Families Safe Act of 2003 and again in 2010 (www.govtrack. us/congress/bills/111/s3817), defines the minimum sets of acts or behaviors that constitute abuse or neglect. State laws and statutes defining child maltreatment are derived largely from these federal definitions. At a minimum, child abuse and neglect is defined as "any recent act or failure to act on the part of a parent or caretaker, which results in death, serious physical or emotional harm, sexual abuse or exploitation, or an act or failure to act which presents an imminent risk of serious harm…."[1]

Children who are adopted from public agencies initially enter the foster care system during or following an investigation by child protective services into alleged maltreatment. An estimated 899,000 children were the victims of substantiated maltreatment in the United States in 2005, including 1,460 child fatalities.[2]

Approximately 1 in 5 child victims (21.7%) of maltreatment was placed in foster care as the result of an investigation.[2] Data from 2005 show that the mean length of stay for children in foster care is 28.6 months.[3] The primary goal for children in foster care is family reunification. However, in 2005, this goal was achieved in only 54% of the cases, and 18% of children (approximately 51,000) were ultimately adopted.[3]

The National Child Abuse and Neglect Data System (NCANDS) was established by the US Department of Health and Human Services to capture information annually from child protective service agencies about reported and substantiated cases of child maltreatment. Data from the 2005 NCANDS survey demonstrated that neglect is the most common form of substantiated child maltreatment, representing 62.8% of reported cases.[2] The remaining substantiated cases of abuse included 16.6% of victims who were physically abused, 9.3% who were sexually abused, 7.1% who were psychologically maltreated, and 2% who were medically neglected (the percentages total more than 100% because some children experienced more than one type of maltreatment).[2]

There is evidence that many children experience repetitive episodes of maltreatment. Studies of young children with acute, inflicted head injury demonstrate that 45% have evidence of prior head injury by computed tomography (CT) or magnetic resonance imaging (MRI) at the time of their diagnosis.[4] Approximately 1 in 5 children suffers from multiple forms of victimization, or "poly-victimization." In a nationally representative sample of more than 2,000 children aged 2 to 17 years, children experiencing 4 or more different kinds of victimization in a single year ("poly-victims") comprised 22% of the sample.[5] These poly-victims manifested higher scores of anxiety than all other groups of children, even children who were repetitively exposed to a single type of victimization.

The NCANDS data from 2005 also demonstrated that recognized and reported maltreatment was more common in a variety of subpopulations. Girls were more likely to be victims of maltreatment than boys—50.7% vs. 47.3% of victims.[2] African American children, American Indian or Alaska Native children, and Pacific Islander children had the highest rates of victimization at 19.5, 16.5, and 16.1 per 1,000 children, respectively.[2] White and Hispanic children had rates of 10.8 and 10.7 per 1,000 children, respectively, and Asian children had the lowest rate of 2.5 per 1,000 children.[2] Young children had the highest rate of victimization—16.5 per 1,000 children birth to 3 years of age and 13.5 per 1,000 children 4 to 7 years of age.[2]

Finally, a 2005 study suggests the extent to which official reports underestimate the rate of child maltreatment.[6] Telephone interviews of mothers revealed that for every one case of substantiated physical abuse, mothers reported approximately 40 instances meeting the definition of physical abuse that went undetected. For child sexual abuse, the mothers reported a rate of victimization 15 times higher than is reflected in official reports. Estimates reported by the Centers for Disease Control and Prevention (CDC) suggest approximately 15% of American adults recall having been physically abused as children.[7]

International Adoption

The extent to which children who are adopted internationally experience maltreatment prior to their adoption is unknown. Countries from which children may be adopted often employ institutionalized care for children with complex social situations. The time that children spend in foreign orphanages and institutions prior to adoption might expose some of these children to profound deprivation and neglect.

To help clarify the experience of institutionalized children, Gunnar and colleagues[8] defined 3 levels of privation that can have an effect on a child's health and well-being.

> "At the most basic level, there are needs for adequate nutrition, hygiene and medical care. The extent to which these basic needs are met may fluctuate with the political and economic conditions within the country. At the next level, it is important to consider the need for stimulation and the opportunity to act upon the environment in ways that support motor, cognitive, language and social development. Finally, there is a need for stable interpersonal relationships and the opportunity to develop an attachment relationship with a consistent caregiver."[8]

These 3 levels of privation can have significant interplay. As Weitzman and Albers observe,[9] adequate growth of a child in an institution implies adequate nutrition as well as additional caregiving beyond feeding. Ultimately, they conclude, the degree of privation a child suffered before adoption is "essentially impossible to determine but may be significant."[9]

Risk Factors for Abuse

Child maltreatment affects all socioeconomic, ethnic, racial, and religious groups. Assorted risk factors for child maltreatment, including certain child and caregiver characteristics, have been identified. However, the presence of one or more of these risk factors within a particular child's environment does not mean that this child will be abused in the future or has been abused in the past. As Goldman and colleagues caution, although several researchers have shown a link between poverty and child maltreatment, the majority of families living in poverty do not harm their children.[10]

While no child is responsible for the maltreatment that he or she may endure, research has delineated certain characteristics that may increase a child's risk of maltreatment. The Boys Town National Research Hospital demonstrated that children with disabilities are 1.8 times more likely to be neglected, 1.6 times more likely to be physically abused, and 2.2 times more likely to be sexually abused than children without disabilities.[11] Factors that can contribute to this increased risk include a child with a disability's potential difficulty with communication and increased dependency for care throughout their lifetime, which obviates a sense of privacy and accustoms the child to having adults touch his or her body.[12] Children with difficult temperaments or behavior problems such as attention-deficit/hyperactivity disorder (ADHD) are at increased risk for child maltreatment,[13] especially if combined with certain caregiver characteristics such as poor coping skills, poor ability to empathize with a child, or difficulty controlling emotions.[10]

Child characteristics also affect the form of abuse that is likely to occur or be recognized. While adolescents are at greater risk of sexual abuse than younger children, infants and small children are at greater risk for physical abuse[2] because they are dependent on adults for almost total care and are less able to gauge their environment for signs of danger, escape from harm's way, or defend themselves.

Caregiver characteristics that are associated with an increased risk of child maltreatment include young age, a history of childhood maltreatment, parental substance abuse, depression or other mental illness, unrealistic expectations about normal child development, lack of parenting skills, poor impulse control, emotional immaturity, low self-esteem, and poor coping skills.[10] Family risk factors for child maltreatment include marital conflict and domestic abuse, social isolation, single parenthood, multiple children in the household, and unemployment and financial stress.[10] Finally, community factors that are associated with an increased risk of child maltreatment include a high crime rate, poverty, and high unemployment rate.[10]

Biological Responses to Stress

Throughout the course of everyday life, people encounter a number of stressful events. Mammals have evolved a number of biological responses that allow them to respond to and modulate stressful experiences, chief among them the hypothalamic-pituitary-adrenal (HPA) axis and autonomic nervous system. The central nervous system receives environmental information through the various sensory receptive organs. Information about a detected threat is relayed through the limbic system, converges in the amygdala, and culminates in the activation of the HPA axis and sympathetic nervous system.[14] This stress response system, mediated through cortisol and catecholamine, effects behavioral and physiological changes that increase an organism's chance for survival, including increased arousal, alertness, and vigilance; improved cognition; focused attention; inhibition of appetite; and increased cardiovascular tone, respiratory rate, and metabolism. Cortisol's role in this process has been the focus of intensive research. Glucocorticoids are essential for life, but when present in excessive amounts, they can have deleterious effects on an organism's health, particularly on the developing brain.

Hypothalamic-Pituitary-Adrenal Axis Dysfunction

The HPA axis is not fully developed at birth. During the first year of life, the axis matures and is able to refine its response to perceived threats.[15] For example, as a typical infant encounters recurring stressors, an elevation in measured cortisol levels is no longer observed when the stressor is reencountered. This has been demonstrated in typical children receiving multiple immunizations administered over the first year of life.[16] This phenomenon of blunted cortisol response to mildly stressful situations (eg, first day of school) appears to extend into the toddler and preschool age groups as well.[17] Tarullo and Gunnar observe that the mechanisms that serve to diminish the cortisol response may protect the brain from the potentially injurious effects of elevated adrenocortical steroids.[16]

This maturation of the HPA axis appears to be under the strong influence of caregiver behavior. Caldji and colleagues[18] demonstrated that a mother rat's care of her offspring during infancy alters their neural pathways that mediate fearfulness. As adults, the offspring of mothers that exhibited high levels of licking/grooming behaviors and arched-back nursing (more attentive behavior) showed substantially reduced fearfulness and anxiety in response to novel situations compared with controls. A similar phenomenon has been observed in humans as well. Nachmias and colleagues[19] showed that when a sensitively responding parent accompanied toddlers in novel situations, the children did not demonstrate elevations in salivary cortisol levels.

In contrast, for maltreated children, the caregiver is an unreliable, unpredictable, and occasionally violent source of support.[16] Toddlers who are unable to use their caregivers as a coping resource may be particularly vulnerable to stress because their HPA axis may not mature as in normal children. Gunnar and Donzella observed that toddlers deprived of responsive caregiving produce increases in cortisol in response to stress similar to younger infants.[15]

Further evidence of the dysregulation of the HPA axis in children who have been maltreated and neglected comes from analysis of their patterns of salivary cortisol levels throughout the day. Normally, cortisol levels demonstrate an early morning peak after a child awakens and decrease gradually throughout the course of the day. Tarullo and Gunnar[16] observed that toddlers living in orphanages in Romania have lower early morning peak cortisol levels but fail to demonstrate the expected declines in cortisol levels over the course of the day.[20] Among toddlers in foster care, 38% showed a diminished morning peak cortisol level that further diminished little over the course of the day.[21] Fries and colleagues[22] hypothesized that this "hypocortisolism" is a protective response dampening chronic HPA axis activity in response to initially high levels of circulating glucocorticoids and thereby reducing the damaging effects of these compounds.

On the other hand, children who have experienced maltreatment can also experience elevations in cortisol levels (for review, see De Bellis et al[23]). In Dozier et al's study of toddlers in foster care, 18% demonstrated high levels of salivary cortisol,[21] and De Bellis and colleagues[23] demonstrated elevated 24-hour urine-free cortisol levels in prepubertal maltreated children with post-traumatic stress disorder (PTSD) compared with typically treated children. It has been hypothesized by several researchers that these seemingly contradictory findings in maltreated children—atypically high and low levels of cortisol production—reflect changes to the HPA axis over time. Initially high levels of cortisol may induce a down-regulation of the HPA response in an attempt to minimize the hazardous effects of a more chronic glucocorticoid exposure.[22] As Dozier and Peloso[24] caution, although this hypothesis "makes intuitive sense, a strong case for this cannot yet be made," and further investigations are warranted to develop a fuller picture.

Neuroanatomic Changes Seen in Response to Stress

> "Our brains are sculpted by our early experiences. Maltreatment is a
> chisel that shapes a brain to contend with strife, but at the cost of
> deep, enduring wounds."[25]

When a child is maltreated, the heightened stress response and elevated serum cortisol levels afford the child the ability to contend with a threatening environment and enable survival. During infancy and early childhood, when brain growth and development are most active, cortisol can exact powerful changes. Early exposure to maltreatment has been shown to ultimately change the brain's anatomy. Teicher and colleagues[26] propose a cascade of alterations within the developing brain in which exposure to severe stress initiates changes on a molecular level and culminates in behavioral and neuropsychiatric consequences.

The initial molecular brain alterations were illuminated by a study by Caldji and colleagues[18] of rat pups. Those pups that experienced more neglectful maternal behaviors (less licking/grooming and arched-back nursing) demonstrated decreased receptor density of multiple neurotransmitters. These changes diminish inhibition of the amygdala, the brain structure involved in the perception of and response to fear-evoking stimuli. The decreased neurotransmitter receptor density also appeared to dampen the feedback inhibition of the locus coeruleus, the midbrain structure that mediates sympathetic outflow. Maternal inattention also decreases the glucocorticoid receptor density in the hippocampus, thereby inhibiting negative feedback control of the production of cortisol and increasing stress production of corticosterone.[27] Early experience, therefore, determines central nervous system responses to stress, as mediated by the HPA axis and sympathetic nervous system. The molecular changes wrought by excessive cortisol exposure enhance the brain's fight-or-flight response, vigilance, and anxiety.

The second step in Teicher's proposed cascade of alterations within the brain that follows early exposure to maltreatment involves the cellular effects of corticosteroids. Glucocorticoids exert powerful effects on cell division,[28] differentiation, and myelination[29] and influence the number of connections between neurons,[30] all processes critical to brain development and growth. Glucocorticoids administered during early life reduce DNA content and brain weight in rats[31] and in extreme conditions have been demonstrated to have a direct neurotoxic effect.[32] These glucocorticoid effects may require the presence of additional factors. Teicher and colleagues[26] hypothesize that the absence of these observed sequelae in children administered high doses of glucocorticoids for the treatment of childhood asthma or inflammatory conditions is caused by failure to activate other arms of the stress response system, such as the sympathetic nervous system and vasopressin.

The third step in the cascade reflects the variable sensitivity of different brain regions to the effects of cortisol. Teicher et al observed that the regions of the brain most vulnerable to the effects of excess cortisol and maltreatment are those that "develop slowly during the postnatal period, have a high density of glucocorticoid receptors, and continue to generate new neurons after birth."[33] Along with the amygdala, these at-risk regions include the hippocampus, corpus callosum, cerebellum, and prefrontal cortex.

The hippocampus, which plays a central role in memory and emotion regulation, is particularly vulnerable because of a prolonged postnatal development and high concentration of glucocorticoid receptors. In a longitudinal prospective study of children with a history of maltreatment, elevated serum cortisol levels and the presence of PTSD symptoms predicted a reduction in hippocampal volume from baseline over a 12- to 18-month period.[34] This suggests that stress induces damage in the hippocampus, which in turn plays a critical role in the development of anxiety disorders.[35]

The myelinated corpus callosum is another brain region thought to be vulnerable to the effects of early maltreatment. As noted previously, glucocorticoids are known to disrupt the process of myelination. De Bellis and colleagues demonstrated that maltreated children diagnosed with PTSD had smaller corpus callosum volumes on MRI imaging than matched controls, and the difference was most pronounced in male patients.[36] However, it is not clear whether these differences were caused by the effects of maltreatment or existed only in the population of maltreated children who developed PTSD. Teicher and colleagues[37] demonstrated that early traumatic experience, rather than psychiatric illness, was associated with a reduction in corpus callosum size. Specifically, the corpus callosum in boys appeared most sensitive to the effects of neglect, whereas that of girls appeared most sensitive to the effects of sexual abuse. Attenuated corpus callosum development may lead to disturbances in the transfer of information between the cerebral hemispheres.

Because its postnatal development is protracted, the cerebellum is also expected to be sensitive to elevated stress hormone levels. Maltreated children with PTSD were recently shown to have smaller cerebellar volumes than non-maltreated children with generalized anxiety disorder and normal controls. The size of the cerebellum correlated negatively to duration of the maltreatment—the more maltreatment the child endured, the larger the reduction in cerebellar size.[38] Studies of preterm infants who suffered hemorrhagic cerebellar injury suggest that this area of the brain plays a wider role in a child's neurodevelopment than previously known. Important not only for postural, attentional, and emotional balance, the cerebellum appears to play a role in compensating for and regulating emotional instability. When compared with age-matched controls, infants who had suffered damage to the cerebellum from hemorrhagic injury demonstrated significantly lower mean scores on all tested measures, including severe motor difficulties, delayed expressive and receptive language, cognitive deficits, increased scores on autism screening tests, and an increased tendency to display internalizing behavior problems (eg, anxiety, depression).[39] This study suggests that the cerebellum plays a significant role in the cognitive, communicative, and social domains.

Finally, the prefrontal cortex is vulnerable. Its development is the most delayed of any brain region, beginning in adolescence and continuing into adulthood, and the region has a high density of glucocorticoid receptors.[40] It has been hypothesized that in neglected children, chronic amygdala activation impairs the development of the prefrontal cortex.[41] De Bellis and colleagues have shown that maltreated children and adolescents with PTSD displayed a magnetic resonance spectroscopy profile suggestive of neuronal loss in the anterior cingulated region of the medial prefrontal cortex.[42] The prefrontal cortex is involved in higher executive functions such as planned behaviors, decision-making, working memory, and attention.[43] For example, damage to the prefrontal cortex in humans leads to a tendency to prefer immediate small rewards over delayed, more efficient rewards when making decisions.[44] Thus, changes to the prefrontal cortex induced by severe stress and excessive catecholamine may lead to problems with age-related acquisition of behavioral and emotional regulation, manifesting as inattention, inability to focus, impulsive behaviors,[41] and poor academic achievement.

As Teicher summarizes: "If an individual is born into a malevolent and stress-filled world, it is crucial for his survival and reproductive success to maintain a state of vigilance and suspiciousness that enables him to readily detect danger."[45] All of the observed neuroanatomic changes seen through this prism can be interpreted as beneficial adaptations for a maltreated child. Heightened arousal responses and aggressive defenses, wrought by changes in the amygdala, cerebellum, and limbic system, dovetail with hippocampal changes that augment the corticosteroid response to perceived threat.

Behavioral and Developmental Sequelae

The Allostatic Load

Though protective in an abusive environment, in a more benign environment, the neuroanatomic changes described previously can prove maladaptive. The persistence of these fear-related neurophysiologic alterations may affect emotional, behavioral, cognitive, and social functioning. McEwen describes the concept of allostasis as the active stress response adaptations to daily events that are essential for an organism's homeostasis and survival.[46] Over the long term, these changes exact a heavy price or *allostatic load*—the cumulative cost to the body incurred by stress response through which serious pathophysiology can occur.

The allostatic load of child maltreatment is behavioral and developmental impairment. While some of these resulting impairments were briefly discussed in the previous section, the white paper of the National Child Traumatic Stress Network Complex Trauma Task Force prepared by Cook et al[47] provides an excellent summary of the effects of maltreatment and framework for understanding their origins. They organize the behavioral and developmental consequences of maltreatment into the following categories: attachment, biology, affect regulation, dissociation, behavioral regulation, cognition, and self-concept. Each of these effects is likely to have its origin in the anatomic or functional changes in the brains of children who have been maltreated. Adoptive parents require help to understand, recognize, and cope with each of these potential consequences of child abuse or neglect.

Attachment

Caregiver-child relationships characterized by maltreatment impair child development. As young children grow, they negotiate and ultimately master developmental tasks with the help of their caregivers. Bowlby first identified the fundamental importance of the child-caregiver or "attachment" relationship more than 50 years ago.[48] When infants experience distressful sensations such as hunger, fright, discomfort, or uncertainty, they rely on their caregivers to calm these sensations and provide reassurance and protection. Through such interactions, infants begin to learn and incorporate soothing strategies that allow them to gradually tolerate some distress. Their early interactions with caregivers and the world around them facilitate communication of their needs through rudimentary language acquisition.

Consistent, sensitive caregiving provides a secure base from which an infant or young child is able to venture out, explore her environment, and return to her caregiver for comfort, safety, or help when necessary. Through these early interactions, a child develops working models or internalized concepts of self and others. Thus, "through these models, children's affects, cognitions, and expectations about future interactions are organized and carried forward into subsequent relationships."[49]

The quality and tenor of this relationship reverberates throughout an individual's life. If a child experiences loving, attentive, and consistent caregiving, she is likely to face life's challenges with a sense of confidence and self-worth. When caregiving is responsive and nurturing, the resulting attachment pattern is termed secure and is found in 55% to 60% of the general population. If a child experiences erratic, disinterested, or violent caregiving, she is likely to feel unlovable, incompetent, and overwhelmed by stressful situations. Patterns of parental caregiving that are insufficient to meet the developmental needs of the child lead to a class of attachment patterns termed insecure. Insecure attachment patterns are reported in approximately 80% of maltreated children[20] and can be classified as avoidant, ambivalent, or disorganized.[50]

An *avoidant* attachment pattern has been described in children whose parents are predominantly rejecting or dismissive.[47] Children raised in these environments learn to "disregard their emotions…relationships and even their own bodies"[47] and may exhibit an avoidance of closeness and emotional connection that can generalize to relationships with other adults and peers.

An *ambivalent* attachment pattern is thought to form in response to caregivers who provide inconsistent validation in a predictable pattern.[47] To cope, these children may disengage when adults are acting in an excessively friendly or a critical manner.[47] They can display extreme distress when separated from a parent or caregiver but do not seem reassured or comforted by the return of the parent. "Instead, during reunion, these babies vacillate abruptly between angry, frustrated resistance to contact…and clinging, dependent, contact-maintaining behavior."[51]

A *disorganized* attachment pattern reflects "…a complex and severe type of disruption of all of the core biopsychosocial competencies."[47] A chaotic environment and an unpredictable caregiving relationship can overwhelm a child's coping mechanisms. These children are unable to self-regulate emotions and display altered help seeking. Younger children manifest the disorganized attachment pattern as "erratic behavior in relation to caregivers (alternatively clingy, aggressive and dismissive)."[47] Older children and adolescents manifest disorganized attachment as "primitive survival-based relational working models that are rigid, extreme and thematically focused…on either helplessness or coercive control."[47,52] When these children have experiences that overwhelm, traumatize, or frighten them, they become disorganized and chaotic because they have not developed the ability to self-soothe or the language that enables them to process the experience or ask for help.

Biology

Victims of maltreatment can behave "irrationally." According to Cook and colleagues, the developmental tasks of early childhood can be described as a transition from a "right hemispheric dominance (feeling and sensing) to that of the left hemisphere (language, abstract reasoning, and long-range planning),"[47] with coordination and communication between the hemispheres mediated by the corpus callosum.[47,53] Early maltreatment can damage the corpus callosum.[36,37] Unable to integrate analytical inputs from their left hemisphere, their right hemispheric, emotion-based capacities predominate. They become disorganized and have a tendency to react with rage, confusion, aggression, and helplessness.[47]

Damage to the prefrontal cortex induced by abuse and neglect can cause deficits of executive functioning. As Cook et al observe,[47] there are 3 features of executive functioning that are necessary for an individual's successful transition to adulthood, including "(i) conscious self-awareness and genuine involvement with other persons; (ii) the ability to assess the valence and meaning of complex emotional experiences; and (iii) the ability to determine a course of action based on learning from past experiences and an inner frame of reference informed by understanding others persons' different perspectives."[47] Deficits of executive functioning, including poor abstract reasoning, impulse control, and decision-making, coupled with difficulties forming relationships, likely contribute to the observed irrationality and have been linked to later substance abuse, eating disorders, personality disorders, promiscuity, and interpersonal violence.[47,54–58]

Affect Regulation

Maltreated children frequently manifest problems with mood regulation. Mood regulation involves the ability to correctly recognize the emotion one is experiencing, communicate how one feels in an appropriate manner, and moderate unpleasant emotions with self-soothing techniques learned through interactions with attentive caregivers. Abused and neglected children are not able to use the attachment relationship to learn techniques that help them moderate emotional distress to handle or manage their feelings. Because they can have difficulty identifying and labeling their emotional experiences,[47] their patterns of emotional expression tend to be more restricted, erratic, and disruptive. They can "present as emotionally labile, with extreme responses to minor stressors, with rapid escalation and difficulty self-soothing."[47] Some abused children eventually resort to maladaptive coping strategies to help manage overwhelming feelings, such as dissociation, avoidance of emotionally charged experiences, or substance abuse.[47]

Throughout their lifetimes, individuals who have experienced childhood maltreatment are at greater risk for developing mood disorders such as depression.[59,60] Wise and colleagues[60] report that compared with non-abused adults, the relative risk of depression is 2.4 times higher for those with a history of physical abuse, 1.8 times higher for those with a history of sexual abuse, and 3.3 times higher for those with a history of both types of abuse. Other studies have shown that among adults sexually abused as children, the odds of attempted suicide are 2 to 4 times higher among women and 4 to 11 times higher among men compared with adults not reporting any history of childhood sexual abuse and controlling for other adversities.[61] As Cook et al observe,[47] a history of childhood maltreatment predisposes to early onset of affective disorders,[62] more episodes, longer duration, and less response to standard treatment.[63]

Dissociation

Children who have been maltreated can resort to dissociation as a defensive or coping mechanism. The American Psychiatric Association defines dissociation as "a disruption in the usually integrated functions of consciousness, memory, identity, or perception."[64] An episode of brief dissociation, or detachment from one's experiences and surroundings, can be a normal phenomenon occurring during daily life, exemplified by daydreams. However, dissociative phenomena also serve as a maladaptive coping strategy used by repetitively traumatized children in an attempt to protect themselves psychologically by holding overwhelmingly traumatic experiences at arm's length.[65] Cook and colleagues state that the spectrum of dissociative phenomena that can be observed in maltreated children can range from depersonalization to more pervasive dissociative disorders that represent severe deficits in the development of self-integration.[47,66] The Child Dissociative Checklist developed by Putnam and colleagues lists the following behaviors as suggestive of dissociation in children: unusual forgetfulness, a poor sense of time, difficulty learning from experience, frequent daydreaming or trance states, having vivid imaginary companions, sleepwalking, and abrupt changes in demeanor, access to knowledge, and age-appropriate behavior.[67] Traumatized children initially use dissociation to distance themselves from overwhelmingly painful experiences. Continued use of dissociation as a defense mechanism can lead to "difficulties with behavioral management, affect regulation, and self-concept."[47]

Behavioral Regulation

Maltreated children can exhibit difficulties regulating their behavior. When children are cared for within an insecure attachment relationship, they are unable to learn and internalize self-soothing strategies and are uncertain about the reliability and predictability of the world. These children may also be hypervigilant for predictors of threat in the environment (eg, maltreatment) and therefore are predisposed to interpret situations with a more menacing overlay. For example, when children who were physically abused are shown photographs of faces manipulated to show various emotions, they report detecting anger for a longer period than control children.[68]

Some maltreated children are described as displaying *under-controlled* behavior patterns.[47] These children may be easily set off or triggered by seemingly innocuous stimuli, display explosive emotions, are hyperactive, and have difficulty calming down. They display poor impulse control, are frequently aggressive toward others, and have difficulty understanding and complying with rules. Ford and colleagues[69] demonstrated that a history of physical and sexual maltreatment is associated with the development of oppositional defiant disorder (ODD) and, to a lesser extent, ADHD.

Conversely, children who have been maltreated may display *overcontrolled* behavior patterns.[47] They attempt to control many aspects of their lives, from inflexible routines to compulsive compliance with adult requests.[52] According to Cook and colleagues, "over-control is a strategy that may counteract feelings of helplessness and lack of power that are often a daily struggle for chronically traumatized children."[47]

Cognition

Young victims of chronic maltreatment can manifest cognitive deficits. The caregiving relationship provides a child with security as he begins to explore the surrounding world and discover his ability to effect changes through actions. The caregiver provides the language and interactions necessary to interpret and understand the environment. This learning process forms the "basic cognitive building blocks of later life."[47] The effects of maltreatment on cognitive development can be seen throughout a child's lifetime, beginning in infancy and culminating in adulthood. It is important to remember, however, that cognitive development may reflect other factors such as nutritional status or neurologic injury. One study that speaks eloquently to the effect of maltreatment on a child's cognitive potential found that children adopted from institutions before age 2 years had a mean IQ of 100, which is average for the general population. Children adopted between ages 2 and 6 years had a mean IQ of 80, which is a borderline normal IQ. Finally, non-adopted adolescents in institutions at age 16 years had a mean IQ of approximately 50, which is classified as moderate to severe mental retardation.[70]

Infants and toddlers who are maltreated have lower Bayley Scales of Infant Development scores,[71,72] a measure of cognitive functioning, even when controlling for the effects of socioeconomic status. Neglect appears to be the subtype of maltreatment that has the most profound effect on cognitive development.[72] These children also demonstrate delays in receptive and expressive language development.[73,74] Language difficulties may portend future aggression and conduct disorders in maltreated children,[75] possibly reflecting frustration from an inability to communicate effectively.

Adequate school performance is an important developmental milestone, and many factors contribute to academic success in addition to cognitive ability[47]—attention, interpersonal functioning, and frustration tolerance, to name a few. The child's brain must be in a state of attentive calm to learn and incorporate new information, a rare occurrence in children who have been maltreated.[76] A history of maltreatment is consistently associated with below average standardized achievement test scores, frequent repeated grades, low cumulative grade point averages, referrals for special education services, and significant social and behavior problems in class.[77–82] Finally, Perez and Widom[78] showed that the cognitive sequelae of early childhood maltreatment persist into early adulthood. When compared with controls matched for age, sex, race, socioeconomic status, and neighborhood, individuals with a history of substantiated early childhood maltreatment demonstrated significantly lower IQ, reading ability, and completed years in school.

Self-concept

Maltreatment can make a child feel unworthy. A child's experiences, observations, and beliefs about the world, mediated through the attachment relationship, eventually become incorporated into the fabric of a child's self-concept. According to Cook and colleagues,[47] "responsive, sensitive care giving and positive early life experiences allow children to develop a model of self as generally worthy and competent…children who perceive themselves as powerless or incompetent… expect others to reject and despise them." Compounding this is the powerful sense of shame that accompanies maltreatment.

The abused child, irrespective of the form of parental maltreatment, is left to conclude that the pain he feels at the hands of the parent is his fault, deserved because of the way he is. This conclusion may well be supported, even insisted on, by the parent overtly stating that his or her treatment of the child is "for his own good." The child's overriding need to believe that his parents care about him drives him to conclude that there is something fundamentally wrong with him and thus to experience a pervasive, and often lifelong, sense of shame.[83]

A possible early manifestation of low self-esteem is demonstrated when toddlers looked at themselves in the mirror after blue rouge had been surreptitiously applied to their noses. Non-maltreated toddlers reacted positively when they saw themselves in the mirror, whereas maltreated children reacted negatively or neutrally.[84] As maltreated children grow older, their low self-esteem and sense of incompetence persist and continue into adulthood.[72,85,86]

To summarize, the allostatic load of child maltreatment has been linked to neurodevelopmental, functional, emotional, and behavioral deficits that can greatly challenge new adoptive parents.

The Adverse Childhood Experiences Study

Health Harms

Powerful observations of the long-term effects of childhood maltreatment have emerged from the Adverse Childhood Experiences (ACE) study. The study, a result of collaboration between the CDC and the Department of Preventive Medicine at Kaiser Permanente in San Diego, CA, analyzed the link between the current health status of more than 17,000 adults and their adverse childhood experiences decades earlier. They delineated the relationship between childhood experience and adult emotional and physical health as well as the leading causes of morbidity and mortality in the United States.

Study Design

To characterize the extent of childhood trauma experienced by an individual, the researchers devised an ACE score. Originally, 3 categories were used to capture various forms of child maltreatment: recurrent physical abuse, contact sexual abuse, and recurrent emotional abuse. Five categories reflected the degree of household dysfunction in the childhood home: a parent or caregiver who was an alcoholic or a drug user; a household member in prison; a household member who was chronically depressed, mentally ill, or suicidal; a mother who was treated violently; and parents who were separated, divorced, or in some way lost to the patient during childhood. Later ACE studies added 2 additional categories for chronic physical neglect and chronic emotional neglect during childhood. Exposure to one category of adverse childhood experience qualified as 1 point. When the points are tabulated, the ACE score was achieved. An ACE score of 0 meant that the person reported no exposure to any traumatic experiences. An ACE score of 10 meant that the person reported exposure to all of the traumatic experiences.

The original study population consisted of 17,000 adult, middle-class Americans who voluntarily sought comprehensive medical evaluation in the Department of Preventive Medicine at Kaiser Permanente in San Diego. Eighty percent of the population was white (including Hispanic), 10% black, and 10% Asian. The average age of the study participants was 57 years, and 75% had attended some college, while 44% had completed college. Less than half of the study population (37%) had an ACE score of 0; 1 in 14 had an ACE score of 4 or more. One in 4 study participants reported growing up in a household with an alcoholic or drug-abusing member, and 22% revealed a history of contact sexual abuse.

Findings

When the ACE researchers looked at current smokers within their study population, they found that the prevalence of smoking displayed a clear, graded relationship to reported adverse childhood experiences. There is an almost 250% increase in the likelihood that an individual with an ACE score of 6 or more is a current smoker when compared with an individual with an ACE score of 0.[87] Not unexpectedly, when the prevalence of adult chronic bronchitis and emphysema within this population is compared with reported ACE score, a strong dose-response relationship is once again observed.[88]

Despite well-publicized adverse health effects of smoking and a large public health effort aimed at eradication of tobacco use, there remain individuals within society who are willing to continue smoking and accept the long-term health risks. Tobacco does afford some powerful psychoactive benefits; namely, it aids in the modulation of anger, anxiety, and hunger. Specifically, smoking is thought to counteract stress-induced depletion of neurotransmitters in the primary reward center within the brain.[89,90] These data offer compelling evidence that adverse childhood experiences have consequences that echo into adulthood and that affected individuals use imperfect, and ultimately harmful, agents to modulate daily stressful experiences. Eventually, adverse childhood experience is transformed into organic disease and health harms.

The ACE study examined the use of other substances of abuse within the study population, such as alcohol and illicit and injection drug use, and again found a dose-response relationship between the number of adverse childhood experiences and substance abuse. For individuals whose neurobiologic stress systems have been altered by childhood maltreatment, these substances are coping devices that allow them to handle everyday stressors or an avenue to escape from emotional pain. Alcohol and heroin function to decrease heightened anxiogenic locus coeruleus and norepinephrine activity[91] associated with childhood trauma. Alcohol is also thought to serve an anxiolytic function[92] that counters the decreased GABAergic transmission within the amygdala. Dube and colleagues[54] performed an attributable risk fraction (ARF) analysis of the illicit drug use data and demonstrated that 67% of drug injection can be attributed to adverse childhood experiences. Interestingly, the graded association between childhood maltreatment and illicit drug use was stable across 4 successive birth cohorts dating back to 1900, suggesting that the effects of child maltreatment remain constant despite changing societal norms and enormous drug eradication efforts.[54] Given the frequent health complications of substance abuse—HIV, hepatitis, cirrhosis, endocarditis, and early death—these results have profound public health as well as societal implications.

In another example, the ACE studies demonstrated a graded relationship between child maltreatment and sexual health risk factors. Individuals with high ACE scores were more likely to self-report a history of sexually transmitted infection,[93] teen pregnancy,[94] and promiscuity.[95] Anda and colleagues[96] observe that rat experiments demonstrate that early stress affects the long-term expression of oxytocin, which facilitates social behaviors such as pair bonding and social attachment.[97] This evidence may provide a neurobiological foundation for the observation that adverse childhood experiences may lead to multiple sexual partners and the attendant health risks of promiscuous behavior.

The ACE studies demonstrate that individuals aren't able to get a handle on their adverse childhood experiences and use imperfect, and ultimately hazardous, solutions to self-medicate their feelings of anger, anxiety, worthlessness, and stress that are the legacy of their maltreatment. Years later, these solutions exact a heavy toll on adult health outcomes. The ACE study revealed a dose-response relationship between the number of an individual's adverse childhood experiences and his or her risk of depression,[59] obesity,[98] cancer,[98] liver disease,[98] skeletal fractures,[98] chronic lung disease,[98] ischemic heart disease,[99] and suicide.[98] Thus, the legacy of childhood maltreatment contributes considerably to many of the leading causes of death in adults.[100]

In a recent study, for the first time, cohorts of children at high risk for abuse (recruited primarily through social service agencies) were followed prospectively over an approximate 2-year period.[101] The authors demonstrated that one adverse exposure almost doubled the risk of poor overall health in childhood and 4 adverse exposures tripled the risk of illness requiring professional medical attention. The researchers failed to replicate a dose-response graded relationship between the number of adverse childhood experiences and poor childhood health outcomes similar to the adult ACE studies. This may, however, reflect selection bias, as the children in the study had already experienced substantiated maltreatment or were considered at high risk for maltreatment. However, as the authors observe, "Because the effect on the child's health becomes evident early in childhood, physicians may have a window of opportunity to intervene and prevent the long-term medical complications described in the ACE Study."[101]

Resilience

Some children appear to suffer little ill-toward effects of their childhood experiences with abuse. Masten has defined the term *resilience* as "good outcomes in spite of serious threats to adaptation or development."[102]

What enables some individuals who have experienced childhood adversity to have a positive life trajectory? Research suggests that there is interplay of child, family, and broader social network factors over the life span that explains a child's response to maltreatment.[103,104] An individual's genetic makeup may play a role in the response to maltreatment. Kim-Cohen and colleagues performed a meta-analysis of studies that showed that a boy's level of monoamine oxidase A activity, an enzyme responsible for the metabolism of various neurotransmitters, moderates the effect of childhood maltreatment on his risk for developing antisocial behavior as well as other mental health problems.[105] Personality traits thought to be protective against adversity include optimism, self-esteem, creativity, independence, and humor. The importance of family and community experiences on maltreatment outcomes is also evident. Studies have suggested that while higher IQ[106] and an easygoing temperament are protective factors, they are easily overwhelmed in the face of multiple family stressors.[103] In a population-based study of children who were abused followed prospectively over a 30-year period, Collishaw and colleagues showed that resilience was not a function of higher IQ or gender. Instead, relationships with parents, friends, and partners were the most potent predictors of adult resilience and served to mitigate the effects of childhood maltreatment.[107]

Finally, what effect does adoption have on a child's outcome? Meta-analyses indicate that adoption exerts an overwhelmingly positive effect in a child's life. On a basic level, children adopted before puberty demonstrate almost complete catch-up growth in weight and height and significant growth in head circumference, although catch-up growth in the latter category is not complete.[108] A meta-analysis[109] that compared adopted children with children who remained in institutional care or the original birth family *and* current non-adopted siblings in the adoptive family demonstrated that adopted children had higher IQ scores and higher school achievement than non-adopted siblings and institutional peers. When adopted children were compared with current siblings in adoptive families, they demonstrated a negligible difference in IQ between the 2 groups. Adopted children were found to have somewhat delayed school performance as well as a small delay in language development and increase in the number of special education referrals made. Finally, a meta-analysis of the behavioral and mental health referrals of international adoptees[110] demonstrated that the majority of these adoptees are well-adjusted, and international adoptees showed fewer behavior and mental health problems than children adopted domestically. Somewhat surprisingly, the age at adoption did not appear to predict the development of future behavior problems.

Conclusion

Many children who are adopted have likely experienced one or several forms of child maltreatment. Exposure to various forms of early childhood maltreatment is a stressful experience for young children, resulting in a heightened stress response and elevated serum cortisol levels. Cortisol has powerful effects on the growing and developing brain and alters structures within the brain during critical developmental periods. As Teicher and colleagues postulate, these changes are crucial for a child's survival because they allow a child to maintain a state of vigilance and suspiciousness and to readily detect danger in an unpredictable and violent environment that does not permit attachment to a caregiver. In a more benign environment, these brain changes can cause a child to experience attention problems, anxiety, depression, and social isolation. As maltreated children grow and develop, they experience higher rates of poor overall health, ADHD, school problems and failure, low self-esteem, and psychiatric diagnoses.

In adulthood, individuals with a history of childhood maltreatment often attempt to self-medicate their feelings of anxiety, depression, and worthlessness with food, smoking, risky sexual behaviors, alcohol, and illicit substances. As the ACE studies powerfully attest, the legacy of childhood maltreatment exacts a heavy toll on adult health outcomes and society as a whole. A nurturing, supportive home environment and intensive early interventions are key to minimizing the long-term and permanent effects of traumatic events on a maltreated child's brain.

AAP Policy Statement and Technical Report on Early Childhood Adversity and Toxic Stress

The American Academy of Pediatrics (AAP) 2012 policy statement, "Early Childhood Adversity, Toxic Stress, and the Role of the Pediatrician: Translating Developmental Science Into Lifelong Health" (http://pediatrics.aappublications.org/content/129/1/e224), discusses how pediatricians are ideally positioned to inform science-based policies and programs that prevent or mitigate the damage associated with such health-threatening adversities as poverty, maltreatment, parental depression, and exposure to violence.

The related AAP technical report, "The Lifelong Effects of Early Childhood Adversity and Toxic Stress" (http://pediatrics.aappublications.org/content/129/1/e232), discusses how the biological consequences of psychosocial adversity are as real as the damaging physical effects of poor nutrition or exposure to lead and provides a framework for understanding the long-term impact of toxic stress in children.

References

1. Child Abuse Prevention and Treatment and Adoption Reform. 42 USC §5106g. http://www.gpo.gov/fdsys/pkg/USCODE-2010-title42/html/USCODE-2010-title42-chap67-subchapI-sec5106g.htm. Accessed February 13, 2014
2. US Department of Health and Human Services Administration for Children and Families. *Child Maltreatment 2005*. Washington, DC: US Government Printing Office; 2007
3. US Department of Health and Human Services Administration for Children and Families. The AFCARS report: preliminary FY2005 estimates as of September 2006 (#13). http://www.acf.hhs.gov/programs/cb/resource/afcars-report-13. Accessed February 13, 2014
4. Ewing-Cobbs L, Kramer L, Prasad M, et al. Neuroimaging, physical, and developmental findings after inflicted and noninflicted traumatic brain injury in young children. *Pediatrics.* 1998;102:300–307
5. Finkelhor D, Ormrod RK, Turner HA. Polyvictimization and trauma in a national longitudinal cohort. *Dev Psychopathol.* 2007;19:149–166
6. Theodore AD, Chang JJ, Runyan DK, Hunter WM, Bangdiwala SI, Agans R. Epidemiologic features of the physical and sexual maltreatment of children in the Carolinas. *Pediatrics.* 2005;115:e331–e337
7. Centers for Disease Control and Prevention. Adverse childhood experiences reported by adults—five states, 2009. *MMWR.* 2010;59(49):1609–1613
8. Gunnar MR, Bruce J, Grotevant HD. International adoption of institutionally reared children: research and policy. *Dev Psychopathol.* 2000;12(4):677–693
9. Weitzman C, Albers L. Long-term developmental, behavioral, and attachment outcomes after international adoption. *Pediatr Clin North Am.* 2005;52(5):1395–1419, viii
10. Goldman J, Salus MK, Wolcott D, Kennedy KY, eds. *A Coordinated Approach to Child Abuse and Neglect: The Foundation for Practice.* Washington, DC: US Department of Health and Human Services; 2003
11. Sullivan P, Cork PM, eds. *Developmental Disabilities Training Project.* Omaha, NE: Center for Abused Children with Disabilities, Boys Town National Research Hospital, Nebraska Department of Health and Human Services; 1996

12. Hibbard RA, Desch LW; American Academy of Pediatrics Committee on Child Abuse and Neglect, Council on Children With Disabilities. Maltreatment of children with disabilities. *Pediatrics.* 2007;119:1018–1025

13. Black DA, Heyman RE, Smith-Slep AM. Risk factors for child physical abuse. *Agg Viol Behav.* 2001;6:121–188

14. LeDoux JE. Emotion circuits in the brain. *Annu Rev Neurosci.* 2000;23:155–184

15. Gunnar MR, Donzella B. Social regulation of the cortisol levels in early human development. *Psychoneuroendocrinology.* 2002;27(1–2):199–220

16. Tarullo AR, Gunnar MR. Child maltreatment and the developing HPA axis. *Horm Behav.* 2006;50(4):632–639

17. Gunnar MR, Tout K, de Haan M, Pierce S, Stansbury K. Temperament, social competence, and adrenocortical activity in preschoolers. *Dev Psychobiol.* 1997;31:65–85

18. Caldji C, Tannenbaum B, Sharma S, Francis D, Plotsky PM, Meaney MJ. Maternal care during infancy regulates the development of neural systems mediating the expression of fearfulness in the rat. *Proc Natl Acad Sci U S A.* 1998;95:5335–5340

19. Nachmias M, Gunnar M, Mangelsdorf S, Parritz RH, Buss K. Behavioral inhibition and stress reactivity: the moderating role of attachment security. *Child Dev.* 1996;67:508–522

20. Carlson M, Earls F. Psychological and neuroendocrinological sequelae of early social deprivation in institutionalized children in Romania. *Ann N Y Acad Sci.* 1997;807:419–428

21. Dozier M, Manni M, Gordon MK, et al. Foster children's diurnal production of cortisol: an exploratory study. *Child Maltreat.* 2006;11(2):189–197

22. Fries E, Hesse J, Hellhammer J, Hellhammer DH. A new view on hypocortisolism. *Psychoneuroendocrinology.* 2005;30:1010–1016

23. De Bellis MD, Baum AS, Birmaher B, et al. AE Bennett research award. Developmental traumatology. Part I: biological stress systems. *Biol Psychiatry.* 1999;45:1259–1270

24. Dozier M, Peloso E. The role of early stressors in child health and mental health outcomes. *Arch Pediatr Adolesc Med.* 2006;160:1300–1301

25. Teicher MH. Wounds that time won't heal: the neurobiology of child abuse. *Cerebrum.* 2000; 2(4):50–67

26. Teicher MH, Andersen SL, Polcari A, Anderson CM, Navalta CP. Developmental neurobiology of childhood stress and trauma. *Psychiatr Clin North Am.* 2002;25:397–426, vii–viii

27. Liu D, Diorio J, Tannenbaum B, et al. Maternal care, hippocampal glucocorticoid receptors, and hypothalamic-pituitary-adrenal responses to stress. *Science.* 1997;277:1659–1662

28. Lauder JM. Hormonal and humoral influences on brain development. *Psychoneuroendocrinology.* 1983;8:121–155

29. Dunlop SA, Archer MA, Quinlivan JA, Beazley LD, Newnham JP. Repeated prenatal corticosteroids delay myelination in the ovine central nervous system. *J Matern Fetal Med.* 1997;6:309–313

30. Sapolsky RM, Uno H, Rebert CS, Finch CE. Hippocampal damage associated with prolonged glucocorticoid exposure in primates. *J Neurosci.* 1990;10:2897–2902

31. Ardeleanu A, Sterescu N. RNA and DNA synthesis in developing rat brain: hormonal influences. *Psychoneuroendocrinology.* 1978;3:93–101

32. Sapolsky RM. Glucocorticoids and hippocampal atrophy in neuropsychiatric disorders. *Arch Gen Psychiatry.* 2000;57:925–935

33. Teicher MH, Andersen SL, Polcari A, Anderson CM, Navalta CP, Kim DM. The neurobiological consequences of early stress and childhood maltreatment. *Neurosci Biobehav Rev.* 2003;27:33–44

34. Carrion VG, Weems CF, Reiss AL. Stress predicts brain changes in children: a pilot longitudinal study on youth stress, posttraumatic stress disorder, and the hippocampus. *Pediatrics.* 2007;119:509–516

35. Gross C, Hen R. The developmental origins of anxiety. *Nat Rev Neurosci.* 2004;5(7):545–552

36. De Bellis MD, Keshavan MS, Clark DB, et al. AE Bennett research award. Developmental traumatology. Part II: brain development. *Biol Psychiatry*. 1999;45:1271–1284
37. Teicher MH, Dumont NL, Ito Y, Vaituzis C, Giedd JN, Andersen SL. Childhood neglect is associated with reduced corpus callosum area. *Biol Psychiatry*. 2004;56:80–85
38. De Bellis MD, Kuchibhatla M. Cerebellar volumes in pediatric maltreatment-related posttraumatic stress disorder. *Biol Psychiatry*. 2006;60:697–703
39. Limperopoulos C, Bassan H, Gauvreau K, et al. Does cerebellar injury in premature infants contribute to the high prevalence of long-term cognitive, learning, and behavioral disability in survivors? *Pediatrics*. 2007;120:584–593
40. Diorio D, Viau V, Meaney MJ. The role of the medial prefrontal cortex (cingulate gyrus) in the regulation of hypothalamic-pituitary-adrenal responses to stress. *J Neurosci*. 1993;13:3839–3847
41. De Bellis MD. The psychobiology of neglect. *Child Maltreat*. 2005;10:150–172
42. De Bellis MD, Keshavan MS, Spencer S, Hall J. N-acetyl-aspartate concentration in the anterior cingulate of maltreated children and adolescents with PTSD. *Am J Psychiatry*. 2000;157:1175–1177
43. Krawczyk DC. Contributions of the prefrontal cortex to the neural basis of human decision making. *Neurosci Biobehav Rev*. 2002;26:631–664
44. Bechara A, Tranel D, Damasio H. Characterization of the decision-making deficit of patients with ventromedial prefrontal cortex lesions. *Brain*. 2000;123(Pt 11):2189–2202
45. Teicher MH. Scars that won't heal: the neurobiology of child abuse. *Sci Am*. 2002;286:68–75
46. McEwen BS. Physiology and neurobiology of stress and adaptation: Central role of the brain. *Physiol Rev*. 2007;87:873–904
47. Cook A, Blaustein M, Spinazzola J, van der Kolk B, eds. *Complex Trauma in Children and Adolescents: White Paper from the National Child Traumatic Stress Network Complex Trauma Task Force*. Los Angeles, CA and Durham, NC: National Child Traumatic Stress Network; 2003
48. Bretherton I. The origins of attachment theory: John Bowlby and Mary Ainsworth. *Dev Psychol*. 1992;28:759–775
49. Cicchetti D, Toth SL. A developmental psychopathology perspective on child abuse and neglect. *J Am Acad Child Adolesc Psychiatry*. 1995;34(5):541–565
50. Ainsworth MS, Bleher MC, Waters E. *Patterns of Attachment: A Psychological Study of the Strange Situation*. Hillsdale, NJ: Lawrence Erlbaum Associates; 1978
51. Cassidy J, Berlin LJ. The insecure/ambivalent pattern of attachment: theory and research. *Child Dev*. 1994;65:971–991
52. Crittenden PM, DiLalla DL. Compulsive compliance: the development of an inhibitory coping strategy in infancy. *J Abnorm Child Psychol*. 1988;16:585–599
53. Schore AN. The effects of early relational trauma on right brain development, affect regulation, and infant mental health. *Infant Ment Health J*. 2001;22:201–269
54. Dube SR, Felitti VJ, Dong M, Chapman DP, Giles WH, Anda RF. Childhood abuse, neglect, and household dysfunction and the risk of illicit drug use: the adverse childhood experiences study. *Pediatrics*. 2003;111:564–572
55. Dube SR, Miller JW, Brown DW, et al. Adverse childhood experiences and the association with ever using alcohol and initiating alcohol use during adolescence. *J Adolesc Health*. 2006; 38(4):444.e1–444.e10
56. Anda RF, Whitfield CL, Felitti VJ, et al. Adverse childhood experiences, alcoholic parents, and later risk of alcoholism and depression. *Psychiatr Serv*. 2002;53:1001–1009
57. Rayworth BB, Wise LA, Harlow BL. Childhood abuse and risk of eating disorders in women. *Epidemiology*. 2004;15:271–278
58. Fang X, Corso PS. Child maltreatment, youth violence, and intimate partner violence: developmental relationships. *Am J Prev Med*. 2007;33(4):281–290

59. Chapman DP, Whitfield CL, Felitti VJ, Dube SR, Edwards VJ, Anda RF. Adverse childhood experiences and the risk of depressive disorders in adulthood. *J Affect Disord*. 2004;82:217–225

60. Wise LA, Zierler S, Krieger N, Harlow BL. Adult onset of major depressive disorder in relation to early life violent victimisation: a case-control study. *Lancet*. 2001;358:881–887

61. Molnar BE, Berkman LF, Buka SL. Psychopathology, childhood sexual abuse and other childhood adversities: relative links to subsequent suicidal behaviour in the US. *Psychol Med*. 2001;31:965–977

62. Giese AA, Thomas MR, Dubovsky SL, Hilty S. The impact of a history of childhood abuse on hospital outcome of affective episodes. *Psychiatr Serv*. 1998;49:77–81

63. Zlotnick C, Ryan C, Miller I, Keitner G. Childhood abuse and recovery from major depression. *Child Abuse Negl*. 1995;19:1513–1516

64. American Psychiatric Association. *Diagnostic and Statistical Manual of Mental Disorders, Fifth Edition (DSM-5)*. Washington, DC: American Psychiatric Press; 2013

65. Terr LC. Childhood traumas: an outline and overview. *Am J Psychiatry*. 1991;148:10–20

66. Macfie J, Cicchetti D, Toth SL. The development of dissociation in maltreated preschool-aged children. *Dev Psychopathol*. 2001;13:233–254

67. Putnam FW, Helmers K, Trickett PK. Development, reliability, and validity of a child dissociation scale. *Child Abuse Negl*. 1993;17:731–741

68. Pollak SD, Cicchetti D, Hornung K, Reed A. Recognizing emotion in faces: developmental effects of child abuse and neglect. *Dev Psychol*. 2000;36:679–688

69. Ford JD, Racusin R, Ellis CG, et al. Child maltreatment, other trauma exposure, and posttraumatic symptomatology among children with oppositional defiant and attention deficit hyperactivity disorders. *Child Maltreat*. 2000;5:205–217

70. Dennis W. *Children of the Creche*. New York, NY: Appleton-Century-Crofts; 1973

71. Lyons-Ruth K, Zoll D, Connell D, Grunebaum HU. The depressed mother and her one-year-old infant: environment, interaction, attachment, and infant development. *New Dir Child Dev*. 1986;(34):61–82

72. Egeland B, Sroufe LA, Erickson M. The developmental consequence of different patterns of maltreatment. *Child Abuse Negl*. 1983;7:459–469

73. Allen R, Oliver JM. The effects of child maltreatment on language development. *Child Abuse Negl*. 1982;6:299–305

74. Culp R, Watkins R, Lawrence H, et al. Maltreated children's language and speech development: abused, neglected, and abused and neglected. *First Lang*. 1991;11:377–389

75. Burke AE, Crenshaw DA, Green J, Schlosser MA, Strocchia-Rivera L. Influence of verbal ability on the expression of aggression in physically abused children. *J Am Acad Child Adolesc Psychiatry*. 1989;28:215–218

76. Perry BD. Neurodevelopmental adaptions to violence: how children survive the intragenerational vortex of violence. http://www.healing-arts.org/tir/perry_neurodevelopmental_adaptations_to_violence.pdf. Accessed February 13, 2014

77. Kendall-Tackett K, Eckenrode J. The effects of neglect on academic achievement and disciplinary problems: a developmental perspective. *Child Abuse Negl*. 1996;20:161–169

78. Perez C, Widom CS. Childhood victimization and long-term intellectual and academic outcomes. *Child Abuse Negl*. 1994;18:617–633

79. Wodarski JS, Kurtz PD, Gaudin JM Jr, Howing PT. Maltreatment and the school-age child: major academic, socioemotional, and adaptive outcomes. *Soc Work*. 1990;35:506–513

80. Eckenrode J, Laird M, Doris J. School performance and disciplinary problems among abused and neglected children. *Dev Psychol*. 1993;29:53–62

81. Kurtz PD, Gaudin JM Jr, Wodarski JS, Howing PT. Maltreatment and the school-aged child: school performance consequences. *Child Abuse Negl*. 1993;17:581–589

82. Shonk S, Cicchetti D. Maltreatment, competency deficits, and risk for academic and behavioral maladjustment. *Dev Psychol.* 2001;37:3–17

83. Loader P. Such a shame—a consideration of shame and shaming mechanisms in families. *Child Abuse Rev.* 1998;7:44–57

84. Schneider-Rosen K, Cicchetti D. Early self-knowledge and emotional development: visual self-recognition and affective reactions to mirror self-images in maltreated and nonmaltreated toddlers. *Dev Psychopathol.* 1991;27:471–478

85. Vondra J, Barnett D, Cicchetti D. Self-concept, motivation, and competence among preschoolers from maltreating and comparison families. *Child Abuse Negl.* 1990;14:525–540

86. Briere J, Runtz M. Differential adult symptomatology associated with three types of child abuse histories. *Child Abuse Negl.* 1990;14:357–364

87. Anda RF, Croft JB, Felitti VJ, et al. Adverse childhood experiences and smoking during adolescence and adulthood. *JAMA.* 1999;282:1652–1658

88. Anda RF, Brown DW, Dube SR, et al. Adverse childhood experiences and chronic obstructive pulmonary disease in adults. *Am J Prev Med.* 2008;34:396–403

89. Kalivas PW, Volkow ND. The neural basis of addiction: a pathology of motivation and choice. *Am J Psychiatry.* 2005;162:1403–1413

90. Volkow ND, Fowler JS, Wang GJ, Swanson JM, Telang F. Dopamine in drug abuse and addiction: results of imaging studies and treatment implications. *Arch Neurol.* 2007;64:1575–1579

91. Chao J, Nestler EJ. Molecular neurobiology of drug addiction. *Annu Rev Med.* 2004;55:113–132

92. Roberto M, Madamba SG, Moore SD, Tallent MK, Siggins GR. Ethanol increases GABAergic transmission at both pre- and postsynaptic sites in rat central amygdala neurons. *Proc Natl Acad Sci U S A.* 2003;100:2053–2058

93. Hillis SD, Anda RF, Felitti VJ, Nordenberg D, Marchbanks PA. Adverse childhood experiences and sexually transmitted diseases in men and women: a retrospective study. *Pediatrics.* 2000;106:E11

94. Hillis SD, Anda RF, Dube SR, Felitti VJ, Marchbanks PA, Marks JS. The association between adverse childhood experiences and adolescent pregnancy, long-term psychosocial consequences, and fetal death. *Pediatrics.* 2004;113:320–327

95. Hillis SD, Anda RF, Felitti VJ, Marchbanks PA. Adverse childhood experiences and sexual risk behaviors in women: a retrospective cohort study. *Fam Plann Perspect.* 2001;33:206–211

96. Anda RF, Felitti VJ, Bremner JD, et al. The enduring effects of abuse and related adverse experiences in childhood. A convergence of evidence from neurobiology and epidemiology. *Eur Arch Psychiatry Clin Neurosci.* 2006;256:174–186

97. Carter CS, Altemus M. Integrative functions of lactational hormones in social behavior and stress management. *Ann N Y Acad Sci.* 1997;807:164–174

98. Felitti VJ, Anda RF, Nordenberg D, et al. Relationship of childhood abuse and household dysfunction to many of the leading causes of death in adults. the adverse childhood experiences (ACE) study [see comment]. *Am J Prev Med.* 1998;14:245–258

99. Dong M, Giles WH, Felitti VJ, et al. Insights into causal pathways for ischemic heart disease: adverse childhood experiences study. *Circulation.* 2004;110:1761–1766

100. Miniño AM, Heron MP, Murphy SL, Kochanek KD. Deaths: Final data for 2004. *National vital statistics reports* [serial online]. 2007;55:October 8, 2007

101. Flaherty EG, Thompson R, Litrownik AJ, et al. Effect of early childhood adversity on child health. *Arch Pediatr Adolesc Med.* 2006;160:1232–1238

102. Masten AS. Ordinary magic: resilience processes in development. *Am Psychol.* 2001;56:227–238

103. Jaffee SR, Caspi A, Moffitt TE, Polo-Tomas M, Taylor A. Individual, family, and neighborhood factors distinguish resilient from non-resilient maltreated children: a cumulative stressors model. *Child Abuse Negl.* 2007;31:231–253

104. Bonanno GA, Mancini AD. The human capacity to thrive in the face of potential trauma. *Pediatrics*. 2008;121:369–375

105. Kim-Cohen J, Caspi A, Taylor A, et al. MAOA, maltreatment, and gene-environment interaction predicting children's mental health: new evidence and a meta-analysis. *Mol Psychiatry*. 2006;11:903–913

106. Breslau N, Lucia VC, Alvarado GF. Intelligence and other predisposing factors in exposure to trauma and posttraumatic stress disorder: a follow-up study at age 17 years. *Arch Gen Psychiatry*. 2006;63:1238–1245

107. Collishaw S, Pickles A, Messer J, Rutter M, Shearer C, Maughan B. Resilience to adult psychopathology following childhood maltreatment: evidence from a community sample. *Child Abuse Negl*. 2007;31:211–229

108. van IJzendoorn MH, Bakermans-Kranenburg MJ, Juffer F. Plasticity of growth in height, weight, and head circumference: meta-analytic evidence of massive catch-up after international adoption. *J Dev Behav Pediatr*. 2007;28:334–343

109. van IJzendoorn MH, Juffer F, Poelhuis CWK. Adoption and cognitive development: a meta-analytic comparison of adopted and nonadopted children's IQ and school performance. *Psychol Bull*. 2005;131:301–316

110. Juffer F, van IJzendoorn MH. Behavior problems and mental health referrals of international adoptees: a meta-analysis. *JAMA*. 2005;293:2501–2515

CHAPTER 11

Long-term Developmental and Behavioral Issues Following Adoption

Lisa Albers Prock, MD, MPH, FAAP

Introduction

Predicting expected developmental or behavioral outcomes for children within the context of adoption is quite a challenge for a variety of reasons. Children with a history of adoption may experience a wide range of life circumstances before joining their adoptive families that may have an effect on their post-adoptive health, development, and long-term potential and outcomes. As a result, heterogeneity and variability of outcomes are to be expected following adoption. Importantly, when considering long-term outcomes, it is critical to acknowledge that the long-term outcomes most relevant for any child are in fact those exhibited in adulthood. However, adult outcome studies describing experiences following adoption in childhood are quite limited in the literature, and those available reflect the experiences of populations of children who joined their families decades before children currently being adopted. As a result, even outcomes currently available and described for adopted individuals in adulthood may be not be entirely reflective of pre- and post-adoptive experiences of current children and adolescents with a contemporary history of adoption. In addition, it is critical to acknowledge that the landscape of domestic and international adoption, including pre-adoptive and post-adoptive experiences and preparation of children and families, has changed dramatically over the past several generations, most notably with an increase in open adoptions and changes in intercountry adoption (see Chapter 1, History of Adoption, on page 1). Finally, it must be acknowledged that evidence about the outcomes of children with a history of adoption are typically based on the population level, whereas individual outcomes are harder to discuss and predict for any given child.

Despite these inherent challenges, adoptive families and professionals working with them are interested in long-term outcomes for children and families following adoption. Adoptive parents may have questions about the long-term effect of their child's history prior to the child's adoption (given reported pre-adoptive experiences, birth family history, or a child's previous presentation or diagnosis) or much later in a child's life, especially if developmental or behavioral concerns emerge. From an adoptive family's perspective, understanding the potential long-term risks for the adoptive child, based on information provided about his or her pre-adoptive experiences and expected post-adoptive environment, is one important factor in supporting the child's optimal development. For children presenting with developmental, behavioral, or emotional concerns following adoption, understanding the etiology of these challenges may assist in identifying appropriate interventions.

Alternatively, clinicians and researchers typically use specific diagnostic categories that describe a child's or adolescent's developmental and behavioral challenges (eg, *Diagnostic and Statistical Manual of Mental Disorders, 5th Edition [DSM-5]; International Classification of Diseases, 9th Edition, Clinical Modification; International Classification of Diseases, 10th Edition, Clinical Modification)* to communicate about aspects of an individual's developmental, behavioral, or emotional presentation and related service needs; determine eligibility to enroll in research studies to ensure participants meet specific consensus-driven criteria; and bill appropriately in medical, mental health, and educational settings. However, rarely does any specific diagnosis used in such clinical or research settings sensitively, specifically, and comprehensively describe an individual adopted (or non-adopted) child's profile. Ideally, studies of long-term outcomes following adoption of a child would consider child-, family-, and geographic-specific variables as they may affect developmental, behavioral, and emotional outcomes for children from infancy through adulthood (see tables 11-1 and 11-2). Relevant post-adoptive outcomes may include those measurable in childhood (eg, cognitive and learning abilities) and later functional outcomes (eg, employment status, emotional health in adulthood) as well as issues that may affect identity development (eg, adoption, transracial adoption) well into adulthood.

Unfortunately, no single study examining pre-adoptive genetics and experiences, post-adoptive experiences, and individual, family, or community variables affecting long-term developmental, academic, or emotional outcome in adults with a history of adoption has been conducted. However, many investigators have examined aspects of pre- and post-adoptive experiences and environments as they have affected adopted children and their families. For many children with a history of adoption, limited information is typically available on many pre-adoptive and genetic factors. As a result, understanding implications of specific risk factors (whether known or unknown) and the limitations of existing literature on adoptive children when considering expected outcomes for any specific child is complex and imprecise. This chapter will consider currently available evidence within the context of supporting children with a history of adoption and their families.

Developmental and Behavioral Outcomes: Challenges Within the Context of Adoption

Developmental and behavioral outcomes are expected to be dynamic and complex for any child in any situation. For example, any child with developmental and behavioral challenges may present with a range of symptoms that may be described to meet specific diagnostic criteria, which hopefully may lead to appropriate treatment strategies. Any child's presentation can be positively or negatively influenced by genetic, environmental, or epigenetic factors. In addition, all children and adolescents may present with a fluctuating combination of symptoms based on their age and ability at presentation, previous interventions provided, and expectations of observers describing clinical symptoms. In other words, descriptions of any given child's behavior and development at any point in childhood or adolescence reflects subjective observations at one point along their developmental or behavioral trajectory.

For children with a history of adoption, pre-adoptive and post-adoptive risk factors (Table 11-1) as well as the child's trajectory in the adoption process may affect a child's presentation (Table 11-2) prior to and following a child's adoption. As a result, each adoptive child's circumstances are likely to be quite unique. Although adoption is a fact of a child's history, the specific reasons for and individual factors related to one's pre- and post-adoptive experiences are more relevant to predicting long-term outcomes than purely a history of adoption alone.

From an evidence-based clinical and research perspective, factors contributing to developmental and/or behavioral concerns may be studied on a population level and may be described as contributing to a relative risk for any specific outcome, albeit not necessarily conferring absolute risk to any specific child. As many variables are often unknown at the time of a child's adoption, caution is warranted in predicting post-adoptive outcomes without being able to factor in the unique aspects of each adoptee's genetics, pre- and post-adoptive history, and environmental factors contributing to potential. In addition, it must be acknowledged that details about many pre-adoptive risk and protective factors are often unknown to families, researchers, clinicians, and educators working with children.

Clearly, positive and negative pre- and post-adoptive factors, as well as the timing of exposures and transitions, dynamically influence developmental trajectories for children with a history of adoption. The theory of risk and protective mechanisms suggests that an accumulation of risk factors contributes to less optimal developmental outcomes while protective factors may buffer negative effects of the risks.[1] With respect to adoption, ideally transitioning to an adoptive family reflects a significant protective mechanism and often changes a child's trajectory by decreasing

Table 11-1. Risk and Protective Factors That May Affect Developmental and Behavioral Outcomes for Adopted Children

Pre-adoptive Factors
Genetic potential Cognitive abilities; learning disabilities; mental health concerns
Prenatal health Maternal nutrition; prenatal exposure to substances of abuse; prescription medications
Pre-adoptive living situation Orphanage; foster care; birth family; presence or absence of at least one nurturing caregiver/role model/protector
Pre-adoptive medical concerns Non-remediated hearing loss or vision loss
Post-adoptive Factors
Family Parental emotional attunement capacity; fiscal and time capacity; number of caregivers/children in the home
Developmental supports Access to typical play; remedial speech and language supports (early invention programs); special education system (Individualized Education Plan, 504) and remedial supports (speech-language therapy, occupational therapy, physical therapy)
Mental health treatment available Trauma-focused cognitive behavioral therapy; behavioral supports for autistic symptoms; psycho-education for child/family on post-adoptive grief/loss and identity development
Relationship support for family Adoption-competent therapists understanding and supporting families by suggesting "when to worry and when to not"
Community supports Routine family/friends for family, especially friends/families who look like adoptee/adoptive family; friends with a history of adoption

exposure to some risk factors over time. Alternatively, transitioning to an adoptive family may add stress if there is a mismatch between parental expectations and a child's capacity. Brodzinsky has also proposed a psychosocial model of adoption adjustment, which includes an additional set of factors in identity development, including coping with the loss of birth parents/family.[2]

While genetic predispositions and prenatal exposures are not modifiable, access to nutrition, health care, emotional support, and appropriate developmental stimulation clearly can be modified in an adoptive family. In addition, critical or sensitive periods may or may not exist for recovery or development of specific skills such as language development. *Resilience* can be defined as reduced vulnerability to environmental risk experiences, the overcoming of a stress or adversity, or a relatively

Table 11-2. Examples of Post-adoptive Developmental/Behavioral Trajectory Contextual Considerations

Factor	Examples of Implications
Age at adoption	Younger children have fewer challenging experiences prior to joining families; older children have more pre-adoptive life experiences, which may be positive or negative.
Number of placements prior to joining permanent family	Transitioning immediately to an adoptive family (norm with private domestic infant adoption) versus time with birth family or multiple foster placements or orphanage life
Time since joining a family	One year after joining a family as a newborn versus one year after joining a family at 6 years of age — different implications for child's likelihood of continued developmental/behavioral change
Trajectory since joining a family	"Honeymoon periods" for older children may be followed by increased behavioral concerns, but 10 years after adoption of a toddler, development and behavioral trajectory more likely reflects child's potential.
Current or previous relationship with birth or foster families	Intermittent interactions with birth family members may contribute to behavioral exacerbations; loss of meaningful birth/foster family members has different meaning for children based on their developmental age.
Stage of adoptive identity development	Transracial adoption may trigger identity concerns as early as preschool; identity development includes integration and making sense of one's history, which may be in opposition to the expectations and desires of joining a family for older adoptees.

good outcome despite risk experiences.[3] In other words, it is an interactive concept in which the presence of resilience has to be inferred from individual variations in outcome among individuals who have experienced significant stress or adversity. Resilience may also encompass resistance to adverse environmental influences, as well as steeling following brief intermittent stressors.[4] Despite the challenges in examining long-term developmental and behavioral outcomes of children and young adults with a history of adoption, this chapter will examine evidence from the literature on implications of specific risk factors while emphasizing the unique aspects of each child's experience.

Cognitive and Educational Outcomes Following Adoption

Cognitive abilities for all humans are thought to be largely influenced by genetic factors with substantial contributions from environmental supports or detractors and epigenetic factors through childhood and adolescence.[5] Largely positive outcomes have been described for domestically adopted infants with respect to development and attachment security; yet relatively fewer healthy infants are currently available for adoption worldwide than ever before. However, the preponderance of research suggests that even the majority of children with special needs adopted at older ages have positive outcomes with their adoptive families. Joining a caring and nurturing family, whether via birth or adoption, is expected to be a protective factor for all children, but for some children with challenging experiences, even the most optimal family environment will not completely ameliorate pre-adoptive experiences.

Studies examining the heritability of cognitive abilities often use adoption status as a predictor variable rather than potentially a mediator of cognitive outcome. However, one meta-analysis reviewing 62 studies and including 77,767 adopted children[6] considered the potential positive or negative effect of adoption at various ages on cognitive (IQ) and academic outcomes for children and adults. The study suggested that adoption alone was not a predictor of IQ. Specifically, it was found that overall IQ of adopted children did not vary significantly from their non-adopted environmental siblings or peers. However, others have described significant differences between adoptive parents' IQ and their adopted children's IQ.[7]

The same meta-analysis[6] found that despite no statistically significant change in mean IQ score for adopted versus population cognitive abilities, adoptive status doubled a child's chance of having learning disabilities requiring special education or other services (12.8% for children with a history of adoption vs 5.5% for non-adopted children). In addition, adoption after the age of 1 year predicted less optimal school achievement when compared with non-adopted peers. Clearly there are many potential factors known to increase the likelihood of learning disabilities (eg, genetic predisposition to learning disabilities, limited language or educational exposure) that were not examined. The authors also suggest that social-emotional demands may exacerbate learning challenges for children with a history of adoption. In addition, especially for older adoptees with a history of international adoption, it may take 4 to 6 years or more before children have achieved a communicative language level in their new primary language that will allow them to learn as fluently in their new language and demonstrate their cognitive abilities.[8]

Mental Health Issues and Seeking Support Following Adoption

Regardless of the reasons, children with a history of adoption are overrepresented in inpatient and outpatient mental health facilities. Five percent to 12% of adopted children are seen in outpatient mental health settings, representing 2.5 to 6 times the population rate for children in general.[9] It has been suggested that perhaps adoptive families, who have been described as typically high-functioning, with a desire to provide a stable home for a child, and generally from higher-than-average socioeconomic background,[10] may have a lower threshold and greater resources for engaging with mental health professionals to access support. However, the specifics of each adopted child's circumstances (eg, time spent in challenging pre-adoptive living arrangements, birth family history of mental health concerns, exposure to domestic violence, loss of meaningful relationships in life to date) are not often reported or known to families prior to or following adoption. In some cases, access to mental health services may be transient or required. For example, for children with a history of domestic public adoption, ongoing counseling after they join a new family may be an expected part of the transition process. Similarly, children with known significant trauma history or anxiety/mood issues often benefit from long-term therapy, but this access to supports may not represent long-term mental health needs.

Although questions are frequently asked about mental health outcomes given a child's history of adoption in childhood, many factors may be far more predictive of behavioral outcomes than a child's adoptive status. For example, certain risk factors (eg, prenatal substance exposure, pre-placement deprivation, older age at adoptive placement) increase a child's likelihood of social and emotional concerns in childhood and beyond.[11-13] Increasing age (especially adoption beyond 24 months of age) and history of multiple adversities[14] at the time of adoption have been associated with an increased risk of internalizing and externalizing symptoms.[15] Analysis of data provided for the National Longitudinal Study of Adolescent Health suggests that background characteristics, early maltreatment, and peer and family relations were associated with antisocial behavior, but adoption status alone contributed little or no additional predictive power.[16] Although overall, epidemiologic studies suggest that adoptees are at increased risk of behavioral and mental health concerns, the type of adoption may also affect the relative degree of risk. One meta-analysis[17] considered behavioral challenges and mental health referrals for children with a history of international or domestic adoption in contrast with non-adopted controls in a range of developed countries (Europe, North America, Asia) and reviewed 64 articles about behavioral problems and 34 articles about mental health referrals published between 1961 and 2004. The authors concluded that adoptees (n=25,281 cases; 80,260 controls) were more likely to present with behavioral problems than non-adoptees, although effect sizes were small (D, 0.16–0.24); adoptees were over-represented in mental health settings; international adoptees demonstrated more behavioral concerns than non-adopted controls, but effect sizes were small (D, 0.07–0.11); and international adoptees showed fewer total, externalizing, and internalizing behavior problems than domestic adoptees and were less often referred to mental health services (international adoptees D, 0.37; domestic adoptees D, 0.81).

One systematic review of existing studies suggested that at least a subpopulation of children with a history of intercountry adoption are at greater risk of long-term developmental, behavioral, and emotional concerns when compared with population risk.[18] This review, commissioned by the Swedish government, suggested that children with a history of international adoption have a 2- to 3-times greater chance of later psychiatric problems and relationship difficulties when compared with their non-adopted peers. In general, the older a child was at the time of adoption, the greater the risk that he or she would later have identified psychiatric or social adjustment challenges. Although several studies do not support a significantly greater risk for major developmental and psychiatric concerns after intercountry adoption, sampling bias and validity of outcome measurements may have influenced the conclusions. Irhammar and Cederblad[18] concluded that a small proportion of adoptees may show severe symptoms and may be overrepresented in clinical samples, whereas many children who are healthy and develop well are only documented in larger cohort studies.

Perception of mental health challenges can vary depending on the reporter. For example, one study examining the mental health of US adolescents adopted when younger than 2 years[19] studied parent, teacher, and child self-reports and used a structured diagnostic interview (Diagnostic Interview for Children and Adolescents [DICA]) to compare adolescent's profiles with *DSM* criteria for behavioral and emotional concerns. Strengths of this study include the use of DICA for a more in-depth assessment of potential concerns than typically obtained from questionnaires alone and the inclusion of domestic (n=178) and international (n=514) adoptees as well as non-adoptees (n=540). Importantly, the demographics of the domestic adoptees were not described (eg, public vs private placement), and the international adoptee demographics (eg, 60.3% female; 89.7% adopted from South Korea) are not typical of most international adoptees. However, researchers found that most individuals adopted as infants did not meet diagnostic criteria for any disorder, but a subset of adoptees appeared to be at risk for externalizing disorders (effect size 0.18 to 0.46). For example, the odds of meeting criteria for oppositional defiant disorder (ODD) or attention-deficit/hyperactivity disorder (ADHD) were approximately twice as high in this study's adoptees compared with non-adoptees. In contrast, the prevalence of conduct disorder, major depressive disorder, and separation anxiety disorder was not associated with adoption status. Interestingly, even though children adopted internationally joined their families at significantly later ages, they were at statistically less risk of externalizing concerns compared with domestic adoptees after controlling for other variables, including family socioeconomic status and gender. It is also noteworthy that teachers rated international adoptees as more anxious than non-adoptees, although parents and children did not report anxiety symptoms. Overall, adolescents with a history of adoption (whether domestic or international) in this study were approximately twice as likely to have had contact with a mental health professional.

Developmentally, it is interesting to note that international adoptees have been described as presenting with fewer[20] and more[14,21-23] behavioral concerns in adolescence compared with early and middle childhood. As a typical part of the identity development process, adolescents naturally are expected to consider who they are in the world, including how they came to be part of an adoptive family and making sense of their adoptive history, which may affect the degree of testing and acting-out behaviors. Some investigators have described children who had been residing with their family for more than 12 years demonstrating fewer externalizing behaviors. For transracial adoptees, it has been hypothesized that given obvious differences in physical appearance when compared with their adoptive parents, greater awareness of their adoptive status may contribute to increased behavioral concerns prior to adolescence.[20] Again, it is critical to note that the nature of international adoption and acceptability of transracial adoption has changed dramatically over the past several decades (see Chapter 1); therefore, the generalizability of existing studies is limited.

Similar to other mental health concerns, risk of substance use for any child or young adult may be affected by a range of factors, including genetic and environmental risk and protective. Importantly, alcoholism and other forms of substance use are often multifactorial and multigenerational and associated with preexisting mental health concerns such as ADHD or anxiety disorders, which users may be attempting to self-medicate with illicit substances. One study examining the complex relationship among birth family history, adoptive family history, and substance abuse suggests that a birth parent history of substance use approximately doubles an adopted person's history of substance use (OR 2.09 for drug abuse if birth parent history of drug abuse). Interestingly, birth sibling history of drug use and adoptive sibling history of drug use were nearly identical in affecting an adoptee's risk of substance use (OR 1.84 for birth siblings; OR 1.95 for adoptive siblings).[24] In other words, birth and adoptive family factors significantly affect one's use of substances.

Effect of Pre-adoptive Deprivations: Implications of Studies of Previously Institutionalized Children

Studies of children who were previously institutionalized (PI) provide a unique opportunity to examine the resilience and vulnerability of children. For all children who join their families beyond the newborn period, inherent cognitive potential as well as a range of pre-adoptive experiences may affect long-term outcomes for children, adolescents, and adults. Although pre-adoptive potential and birth family experiences are less easy to study as they are often unknown, experiences of children transitioning to families from institutions have been widely described. Resilience and vulnerability to severe deprivation have been described by researchers examining the post-adoptive trajectory of internationally adopted children with a history of institutionalization.

Deprivation may occur on a range of levels and to various degrees. Gunnar and colleagues[25] have suggested that when considering outcomes for PI children, 3 different planes of privation may have an effect on a child's health and well-being: basic nutritional, hygienic, and medical needs; stimulation and opportunity to engage with the environment in a way that supports motor, cognitive, language, and social development; and stable interpersonal relationships allowing children to develop an attachment relationship with a consistent caregiver. Similar planes of deprivation may occur for children experiencing deprivation in a birth or foster family. Importantly, although these levels of privation may be theoretically described and separated, they are not independent factors in a child's real-life experience. However, an appreciation of these different planes of support or privation informs our understanding of factors that may affect children residing with families or in institutions. Some aspects of a child's pre-adoptive history are easier to ascertain than others. For example, while access to nutrition can be crudely observed by examining a child's growth chart, access to a stable interpersonal relationship is much harder to quantify. Although it is likely that access to adequate nutrition increases the likelihood of interpersonal relationships with those providing the nutrition, the degree of privation suffered before adoption is essentially impossible to determine for any child and may be significant.

Although all families and child welfare institutions are unique, the overwhelmingly negative long-term effect of institutional life on a child's growth and development has been well described for more than a century in many different countries. Fortunately, PI children transitioning from living in orphanages to living with foster or adoptive families have demonstrated an immense human capacity for developmental plasticity and recovery of many functions. Although a number of investigators have examined the outcomes of children adopted internationally in the past several decades, the results of 2 key longitudinal adoption studies and one ongoing foster care study are notable and continue to shed insight on pre-adoptive experiences and post-placement resilience. All 3 are longitudinal epidemiologic studies examining children adopted from Romania to the United Kingdom and to Canada or transitioning from institutional care to foster care in Romania (Bucharest Early Intervention Project [BEIP]). (See Table 11-3.)

Taken together, longitudinal studies examining the developmental and behavioral outcomes for these children have demonstrated significant cognitive, behavioral, and emotional improvement for PI children throughout childhood and adolescence, albeit with recovery not always complete.[12,29,46–49] In general, PI children have been reported to have relatively higher rates of poor attention, hyperactivity, difficulty with emotional regulation, and elevated levels of anxiety as well as difficulties later in life with intimate social attachments, emotional regulation, and interpretation of facial expression.[20,36,45,50–57] In general, PI children are expected to demonstrate healthy attachments with their adoptive parents, although the classification of their

Table 11-3. Romanian Longitudinal Studies

	English and Romanian Adoptees Study[26-36]	Canadian Study[37,38]	Bucharest Early Intervention Project[39-45]
Type of study	Stratified random sample	Cohort follow-up	Randomized foster care intervention
Study population	Romanian adoptees (N=155, including 144 children residing exclusively in institutions before adoption) adopted from Romania into families in the United Kingdom at younger than 42 months divided into 3 groups based on months of institutionalization prior to adoption <6 mo (n=58) 6–24 mo (n=59) 24–42 mo (n=48) Control group (n=52) with domestic adoption <5 mo	Romanian adoptees (N=75) adopted by families in British Columbia divided into 2 groups based on age at adoption Early adoptees: <4 mo at adoption (n=29) Romanian orphanage: >8 mo at age of adoption (n=46) Control: Canadian born, not adopted (n=46)	Romanian children aged 6 to 30 months (N=136); institutionalized children in Romania randomized to foster care or care as usual 68 to foster care 68 care as usual (of whom only 20 remain institutionalized in 2011, but analyses as per intent to treat) n=72 (never institutionalized, raised in families)
Analysis compares	Domestic UK adoption controls Romanian adoption <6 mo 6–24 mo 24–42 mo	Canadian-born, non-adopted controls Romanian adoption <4 mo >8 mo	Community controls Randomized groups: Foster care vs care as usual

attachment relationship with their adoptive parents is more likely to be insecure.[50-54] Indiscriminate friendliness is common (more than two-thirds of PI preschool children) and may persist for years following adoption.[36,50] Despite an increased risk of long-term concerns on a population level, cognitive and emotional improvement following transition to adoptive families is still expected for the majority of children. Similarly, it is expected that children without a history of institutionalization but with some deprivation may also experience some degree of post-adoptive recovery of functioning.

Delays in or variations from the normal progression of a child's development prior to adoption have been attributed to multiple factors common for children residing in institutions or depriving environments, including, but not limited to, malnutrition, emotional neglect via lack of a consistent emotional connection with caregivers, and lack of developmentally stimulating opportunities or experiences. Additional factors such as prenatal exposure to alcohol, environmental exposures including lead, and genetic or neurologic disorders may also cause or contribute to children's developmental outcomes, although these factors may not be identified prior to adoption, if ever. In general, post-adoptive improvements of children's developmental skills and behaviors are routinely expected when children join their families following institutionalization. Eventually, after years of residing with adoptive parents, children's ongoing developmental or behavioral challenges may represent innate disorders, irreversible consequences of early life experiences, or a combination.

Certain factors, such as quality of care and length of institutionalization, are especially predictive of outcomes. Historical and contemporary studies confirm a relationship between length of time and quality of care received while a child resides in an institution and that child's long-term health and development following adoption. Length of time residing in an institution is positively correlated with a child's risk of presenting with developmental, behavioral, and emotional concerns after international adoption.[26–36,39–45] In the BEIP, the timing of placement with foster families correlated with improvements in cognitive, language, behavioral, emotional, and attachment outcomes that were most significant for children with the least time in an orphanage.[39,40,44,58] Longitudinal studies of children adopted from Romanian orphanages into adoptive families in the United Kingdom suggested no measureable differences between children adopted prior to 6 months of age and age-matched peers without a history of institutionalization.[26,27,36] Other investigators have found that with less depriving environments, children adopted at younger than 12 or 24 months were indistinguishable from non-institutionalized peers.[6,17,39] Quality of care provided in an institution is also correlated with children's post-adoptive outcomes, as orphanages associated with improved child health and development outcomes typically provide children with adequate nutrition and health care, a lower child-to-caregiver ratio (3:1 vs 10:1), a lower total number of caregivers over the life of the child, and caregivers who recognize and respond to the distress and vocalizations of children.[39–41,59] Unfortunately, despite this well-documented fact, economic and political conditions typically prevent most children residing in an institution from experiencing optimal conditions.[60]

Although concerns with self-regulation have been widely described for PI children,[17] there is a fair amount of variability with respect to outcomes described in various populations. Zeanah et al have estimated that approximately 20% of PI children (compared with approximately 6% of US children[61]) will reach a clinical threshold for an anxiety disorder, while 19% of PI children (compared with approximately 9% of US children[62]) meet criteria for ADHD.[44] Internalizing concerns (eg, anxiety, depression) have been described in some samples of PI children,[63] while others have not described an increase in internalizing concerns for PI children.[15] Some studies have suggested that internalizing symptoms (versus externalizing symptoms) are much more likely to improve after joining a stable family,[39,41,42–45] but follow-up into adolescence has not yet been described.

Epidemiologic studies examining the outcomes of children adopted from institutions have generally been limited in their implications and generalizability by lack of pre-adoptive information (positive or negative); nonrandom adoption of children from institutions; and lack of an appropriate comparison group. However, findings from the BEIP randomized foster care intervention study (Table 11-3) have provided important information about early indications of mental health and the capacity of recovery in nurturing foster care settings. Relative to children remaining in orphanage care, PI children demonstrated dramatic improvements in developmental domains over time despite well-described growth and developmental delays at the time of joining families.[39,64] Long-lasting developmental challenges for PI children have specifically been described for children adopted after 6 months of age.[65] Despite overall cognitive competence, specific vulnerabilities have been described for PI children, including relative weaknesses with executive functioning, language, and memory.[50]

Mental health concerns remained for children transitioning out of BEIP foster care despite developmental and cognitive improvements. Even in preschool years, a substantial number of children with a history of institutionalization presented with diagnosable psychiatric disorders (53% of children ever institutionalized vs 22% of children never institutionalized). However, relatively shortly after transitioning to foster care homes, children demonstrated greater attention to tasks and greater positive affect in comparison with their still institutionalized peers.[41,66] Children transitioned to caring and committed foster families from institutions (at a mean age of 22 months) were comparable to peers who were never institutionalized with resolution of internalizing symptoms (eg, anxiety, mood symptoms). The effect on improvement of internalizing symptoms was especially notable for girls. Unfortunately, a similar effect of foster care was not noted for externalizing behavioral symptoms for children of either gender, suggesting that these symptoms are less amenable to recovery by transitioning to new living circumstances.[41,44]

Neural Underpinnings of Post-adoptive Behavioral, Emotional, Cognitive, and Mental Health Issues

Behavioral or emotional concerns reported by parents, teachers, and children or youth themselves reflect observable symptoms that may contribute to mental health diagnoses and inform treatment approaches. However, a large range of risk and protective factors may contribute to these symptoms. For example, substantial evidence in animals and humans suggests that a history of previous institutionalization may contribute to a range of neural structure and functional outcomes, although specific brain structure and region effects have not been entirely consistent across studies (Table 11-4).[67-70] There are also a range of genetic variables known to affect mental health outcomes that are not routinely evaluated in clinical settings.

While the reasons for persistent behavioral challenges in the setting of cognitive and emotional improvement are not certain, it is likely because of ongoing adversity or risk factors during periods of neurodevelopment.[71] It is critical to acknowledge that exposure to adversity is not expected to affect developing brains of children uniformly, but rather that certain periods of brain development and certain brain regions may be exquisitely vulnerable to insults at various points in time. While human evidence is still emerging, there is already strong evidence in adult animals that exposure to stress increases the growth and activity of the amygdala, with perhaps even greater effect of stress on the amygdala of developing animals.[68] The

Table 11-4. Neuroimaging and Children Who Were Previously Institutionalized

Imaging Study/ Citation	Population and Findings	Comments
English Romanian adoptee Romanian adoptees to United Kingdom and UK control adolescents[67]	n=14 adolescents adopted from Romania to United Kingdom n=11 adolescents never institutionalized Mean age at magnetic resonance imaging (MRI): ~16 years Structural MRI findings: significantly smaller total white and gray matter; smaller left hippocampus; larger right amygdala for adolescents with history of institutionalization (HI) compared with controls	Suggestion of global (total white and gray matter) and specific (smaller left hippocampus; larger right amygdala) effects with HI *Note:* size of hippocampus and amygdala not corrected for total brain size
Previously institutionalized, then adopted to United States; and non-adopted US controls[68]	n=34 previously institutionalized children adopted to United States (average age = 8.4 y) n=28 non-adopted children (average age = 9.4 y) Structural MRI findings suggest amygdala was increased in size relative to total brain volume for children if adopted at older than 15 months	Amygdala increased in size if adopted at older than 15 months; did not replicate ERA findings of smaller hippocampus/ larger amygdala. *Note:* younger age than Mehta's study of English Romanian adoptee population

Table 11-4. Neuroimaging and Children Who Were Previously Institutionalized, continued

Imaging Study/ Citation	Population and Findings	Comments
Previously institutionalized, then adopted to United States; and non-adopted US controls[69]	n=7 Romanian adoptees; n=7 US non-adoptees Structural MRI findings suggest smaller whole brain white and gray matter for adoptees with HI compared with peers. Diffusion tensor imaging suggested reduced apparent diffusion coefficients/fractional anisotropy across all white matter tracts for those with HI, most significantly in left uncinate fasciculus	While all white matter tracts appeared to have decreased diffusion, particularly the left uncinate fasciculus, findings suggest a general decrease in white matter integration.
Bucharest Early Intervention Project: Romanian institutionalized, randomized to foster care and community controls[70]	n=20 typically developing Romanian children n=29 children exposed to institutional rearing n=25 children with HI and exposed to foster care Exposure to institutionalization decreased cortical gray matter. Foster care remediates white matter deficits compared with care as usual group. Electroencephalographic alpha power partially mediated by white matter growth.	White (but not gray matter) growth in response to foster care Controlling for total brain volume eliminates amygdala-specific findings.

long-lasting effect of environmental stressors has been hypothesized to correlate with the relative resistance of amygdala cells to show recovery once a stressor is removed, unlike many other brain regions.[72] Similar to animal studies and relevant to increased behavioral regulation challenges, PI children have been described as having a relationship between amygdala structure and function and emotion and behaviors, including an exaggerated amygdala response to emotional faces,[71] increased anxiety and reduced social competence related to amygdala development, and increased amygdala volumes and decreased neural connections between the amygdala and the cortex years after joining adoptive families.[67,69]

Indiscriminate behavior directed at unfamiliar adults has been one specific area of interest for a number of researchers. The exact neurobiological mechanism for developing and maintaining indiscriminate and intimate behaviors directed at unfamiliar adults, including willingness to walk off with a stranger, is not clear, but deficits in face processing found in PI children have been suggested to contribute to these behaviors.[73,74]

Face processing is described as an environmentally shaped skill that assists in guiding social interactions. Relative to age-matched peers without a history of institutional care, PI children are less likely to correctly identify the emotional expressions of faces[75] and tend to show neural hypo-activation on electroencephalographic measures.[54] It has been suggested that social deprivation in institutional settings may not provide for experiences necessary to hone these skills.[76] In addition, emotional facial expressions can be highly arousing for PI children and may contribute to behavioral regulation challenges, including increased impulsivity.[74,76]

Summary

Consistent with many of the specific examples cited previously, a recent monograph[60] summarized current research as well as implications for practice and policy for children raised without permanent parents, including those with a history of institutionalization or foster care. After an extensive review of the worldwide literature, the editors summarized their findings by concluding that infants and young children being reared in most child welfare institutions are substantially delayed in their physical, neurobiological, cognitive, and social-emotional development. For children fortunate enough to transition to family environments (eg, adoptive or foster families), immediate and substantial improvement is observed in all domains. However, it is noteworthy that challenges and deficiencies in all developmental domains can persist at higher than expected rates even after transitioning to families. Developmental implications were particularly noteworthy after 6 to 24 months of institutionalization, depending on the severity of the depriving institutional conditions, the particular developmental outcome measure, and other factors.

As reviewed previously, evidence from a range of longitudinal studies suggests that transition to a caring and supportive family, whether adoptive or foster, promotes significant improvements, albeit not complete recovery, with respect to cognitive and emotional deficiencies for PI children.[77] Although a history of institutional care clearly carries risks for emotional, behavioral, and developmental challenges, this is based on increased risk for a population of children with significant variability among individuals within this population. While absolute risk and protective or ameliorative factors are not known, increased time in a challenging environment and therefore age at placement with a foster or adoptive family are some of the most influential predictors of outcomes. It is important to note that while increased time in an orphanage may carry increased risk for later outcomes, children in any institution may experience differential risk, protective factors, or individual resilience that contributes to post-adoptive variability with respect to cognitive, emotional, and behavioral outcomes.

In conclusion, most individuals with a history of adoption in infancy are well adjusted and psychologically healthy in childhood, adolescence, and adulthood. With multiple adverse risk factors prior to adoption and increased age at adoption, children are at greater risk for a range of developmental and behavioral concerns. One subset of adoptees appears to be at greater risk for meeting criteria for externalizing disorders such as ADHD and ODD. However, further research to understand pre-adoptive factors, identify children at greater risk of later developmental and behavioral concerns, identify mediating factors, and communicate effective post-adoptive interventions is required to improve the capacity of families and health care professionals to address challenges that may occur for any child and family following adoption.

References

1. Rutter M. Psychosocial resilience and protective mechanisms. In: Folf J, Masten AS, Cicchetti D, Nuechterlein KH, Weintraub S, eds. *Risk and Protective Factors in the Development of Psychopathology.* Cambridge, England: Cambridge University Press; 1990:181–214

2. Brodzinsky DM. Adjustment to adoption: a psychosocial perspective. *Clin Psychol Rev.* 1987;7(1):25–47

3. Rutter M. Implications of resilience concepts for scientific understanding. *Ann N Y Acad Sci.* 2006;1094:1–12

4. Castle J, Groothues C, Beckett C, et al. Parents' evaluation of adoption success: a follow-up study of intercountry and domestic adoptions. *Am J Orthopsychiatry.* 2009;79(4):522–531

5. Bouchard TJ Jr. Genetic and environmental influences on adult intelligence and special mental abilities. *Hum Biol.* 1998;70(2):257–279

6. van IJzendoorn MH, Juffer F, Poelhuis CW. Adoption and cognitive development: a meta-analytic comparison of adopted and nonadopted children's IQ and school performance. *Psychol Bull.* 2005;131(2):301–316

7. Capron C, Duyme M. Assessment of effects of socio-economic status on IQ in a full cross-fostering study. *Nature.* 1989;340:552–554

8. Gindis B. Cognitive, language, and educational issues of children adopted from overseas orphanages. *J Cogn Educ Psychol.* 2005;4(3):291–315

9. Haugaard JJ. Is adoption a risk factor for the development of adjustment problems? *Clin Psychol Rev.* 1998;18(1):47–69

10. Hellerstedt WL, Madsen NJ, Gunnar MR, Grotevant HD, Lee RM, Johnson DE. The International Adoption Project: population-based surveillance of Minnesota parents who adopted children internationally. *Matern Child Health J.* 2008;12(2):162–171

11. Nulman I, Rovet J, Greenbaum R, et al. Neurodevelopment of adopted children exposed in utero to cocaine: the Toronto Adoption Study. *Clin Invest Med.* 2001;24(3):129–137

12. Beckett C, Maughan B, Rutter M, et al. Do the effects of early severe deprivation on cognition persist into early adolescence? Findings from the English and Romanian adoptees study. *Child Dev.* 2006;77(3):696–711

13. Sharma AR, McGue M, Benson P. The emotional and behavioral adjustment of United States adopted adolescents, part II: age at placement. *Child Youth Serv Rev.* 1996;18(1–2):101–114

14. van der Vegt EJ, van der Ende J, Ferdinand RF, Verhulst FC, Tiemeier H. Early childhood adversities and trajectories of psychiatric problems in adoptees: evidence for long lasting effects. *J Abnorm Child Psychol.* 2009;37(2):239–249

15. Gunnar MR, van Dulmen MH; International Adoption Project Team. Behavior problems in post-institutionalized internationally adopted children. *Dev Psychopathol.* 2007;19(1):129–148

16. Grotevant HD, van Dulmen MH, Dunbar N, et al. Antisocial behavior of adoptees and nonadoptees: prediction from early history and adolescent relationships. *J Res Adolesc.* 2006;16(1):105–131

17. Juffer F, van IJzendoorn MH. Behavior problems and mental health referrals of international adoptees: a meta-analysis. *JAMA.* 2005;293(20):2501–2515

18. Irhammar M, Cederblad M. Outcomes of intercountry adoption in Sweden. In: Selman P, ed. *Intercountry Adoption: Developments, Trends and Perspectives.* London, United Kingdom: British Agencies for Adoption and Fostering; 2000:143–163

19. Keyes MA, Sharma A, Elkins IJ, Iacono WG, McGue M. The mental health of US adolescents adopted in infancy. *Arch Pediatr Adolesc Med.* 2008;162(5):419–425

20. van IJzendoorn MH, Juffer F. The Emanuel Miller Memorial Lecture 2006: adoption as intervention. Meta-analytic evidence for massive catch-up and plasticity in physical, socio-emotional, and cognitive development. *J Child Psychol Psychiatry.* 2006;47(12):1228–1245

21. Colvert E, Rutter M, Beckett C, et al. Emotional difficulties in early adolescence following severe early deprivation: findings from the English and Romanian adoptees study. *Dev Psychopathol.* 2008;20(2):547–567

22. Verhulst FC, Althaus M, Versluis-den Bieman HJ. Problem behavior in international adoptees. I. An epidemiological study. *J Am Acad Child Adolesc Psychiatry.* 1990;29(1):94–103

23. Tieman W, van der Ende J, Verhulst FC. Psychiatric disorders in young adult intercountry adoptees: an epidemiological study. *Am J Psychiatry.* 2005;162(3):592–598

24. Kendler KS, Sundquist K, Ohlsson H, et al. Genetic and familial environmental influences on the risk for drug abuse: a national Swedish adoption study. *Arch Gen Psychiatry.* 2012;69(7):690–697

25. Gunnar MR, Bruce J, Grotevant HD. International adoption of institutional reared children: research and policy. *Dev Psychopathol.* 2000;12(4):677–693

26. Rutter M. Developmental catch-up, and deficit, following adoption after severe global early privation. English and Romanian Adoptees (ERA) Study Team. *J Child Psychol Psychiatry.* 1998;39(4):465–476

27. Rutter M, Andersen-Wood L, Beckett C, et al. Quasi-autistic patterns following severe early global privation. English and Romanian Adoptees (ERA) Study Team. *J Child Psychol Psychiatry.* 1999;40(4):537–549

28. Rutter ML, Kreppner JM, O'Connor TG. Specificity and heterogeneity in children's responses to profound institutional privation. *Br J Psychiatry.* 2001;179(2):97–103

29. Rutter M, O'Connor TG; English and Romanian Adoptees Study Team. Are there biological programming effects for psychological development? Findings from a study of Romanian adoptees. *Dev Psychol.* 2004;40(1):81–94

30. Rutter M, Sonuga-Barke EJ. X. Conclusions: overview of findings from the era study, inferences, and research implications. *Monogr Soc Res Child Dev.* 2010;75(1):212–229

31. Rutter M, Kumsta R, Schlotz W, Sonuga-Barke E. Longitudinal studies using a "natural experiment" design: the case of adoptees from Romanian institutions. *J Am Acad Child Adolesc Psychiatry.* 2012;51(8):762–770

32. Rutter M. Resilience as a dynamic concept. *Dev Psychopathol.* 2012;24(2):335–344

33. O'Connor TG, Bredenkamp D, Rutter M; English and Romanian Adoptees Study Team. Attachment disturbances and disorders in children exposed to early severe deprivation. *Infant Ment Health J.* 1999;20(1):10–29

34. O'Connor TG, Rutter M. Attachment disorder behavior following early severe deprivation: extension and longitudinal follow-up. English and Romanian Adoptees Study Team. *J Am Acad Child Adolesc Psychiatry.* 2000;39(6):703–712

35. O'Connor TG, Rutter M, Beckett C, Keaveney L, Kreppner JM. The effects of global severe privation on cognitive competence: extension and longitudinal follow-up. English and Romanian Study Team. *Child Dev.* 2000;71(2):376–390

36. O'Connor TG, Marvin RS, Rutter M, et al. Child-parent attachment following early institutional deprivation. *Dev Psychopathol.* 2003;15(1):19–38

37. Fisher L, Ames EW, Chisholm K, Savoie L. Problems reported by parents of Romanian orphans adopted to British Columbia. *Int J Behav Dev.* 1997;20(1):67–82

38. LeMare L. Follow-up on the Romanian Adoptee study. Presented at Joint Council on International Children's Services, Washington, DC, April 10, 2002

39. Nelson CA, Zeanah CH, Fox NA, Marshall PJ, Smyke AT, Guthrie D. Cognitive recovery in socially deprived young children: the Bucharest Early Intervention Project. *Science.* 2007;318(5858):1937–1940

40. Nelson CA, Furtado EA, Fox NA, Zeanah CH. The deprived human brain: developmental deficits among institutionalized Romanian children—and later improvements—strengthen the case for individualized care. *Am Sci.* 2009;97(3):222–224

41. Bos K, Zeanah CH, Fox NA, Drury SS, McLaughlin KA, Nelson CA. Psychiatric outcomes in young children with a history of institutionalization. *Harv Rev Psychiatry.* 2011;19(1):15–24

42. Zeanah CH, Smyke AT, Koga SF, Carlson E; Bucharest Early Intervention Project Core Group. Attachment in institutionalized and community children in Romania. *Child Dev.* 2005;76(5):1015–1028

43. Zeanah CH, Smyke AT, Dumitrescu A. Attachment disturbances in young children. II: indiscriminate behavior and institutional care. *J Am Acad Child Adolesc Psychiatry.* 2002;41(8):983–989

44. Zeanah CH, Egger HL, Smyke AT, et al. Institutional rearing and psychiatric disorders in Romanian preschool children. *Am J Psychiatry.* 2009;166(7):777–785

45. Zeanah CH, Gunnar MR, McCall RB, Kreppner JM, Fox NA. Sensitive periods. *Monogr Soc Res Child Dev.* 2011;76(4):147–162

46. Snedeker J, Geren J, Shafto CL. Starting over: international adoption as a natural experiment in language development. *Psychol Sci.* 2007;18(1):79–87

47. Roberts JA, Pollock KE, Krakow R. Continued catch-up and language delay in children adopted from China. *Semin Speech Lang.* 2005;26(1):76–85

48. Johnson DE, Guthrie D, Smyke AT, et al. Growth and associations between auxology, caregiving environment, and cognition in socially deprived Romanian children randomized to foster vs ongoing institutional care. *Arch Pediatr Adolesc Med.* 2010;164(6):507–516

49. van IJzendoorn MH, Bakermans-Kranenburg MJ, Juffer F. Plasticity of growth in height, weight, and head circumference: meta-analytic evidence of massive catch-up after international adoption. *J Dev Behav Pediatr.* 2007;28(4):334–343

50. Fox NA, Almas AN, Degnan KA, Nelson CA, Zeanah CH. The effects of severe psychosocial deprivation and foster care intervention on cognitive development at 8 years of age: findings from the Bucharest Early Intervention Project. *J Child Psychol Psychiatry.* 2011;52:919–928

51. van den Dries L, Juffer F, van IJzendoorn MH, Bakermans-Kranenburg MJ. Infants' physical and cognitive development after international adoption from foster care or institutions in China. *J Dev Behav Pediatr.* 2010;31(2):144–150

52. Behen ME, Helder E, Rothermel R, Solomon K, Chugani HT. Incidence of specific absolute neurocognitive impairment in globally intact children with histories of early severe deprivation. *Child Neuropsychol.* 2008;14(5):453–469

53. Hodges J, Tizard B. Social and family relationships of ex-institutional adolescents. *J Child Psychol Psychiatry*. 1989;30(1):77–97

54. Moulson MC, Fox NA, Zeanah CH, Nelson CA. Early adverse experiences and the neurobiology of facial emotion processing. *Dev Psychol*. 2009;45(1):17–30

55. Loman MM, Johnson AE, Westerlund A, Pollak SD, Nelson CA, Gunnar MR. The effect of early deprivation on executive attention in middle childhood. *J Child Psychol Psychiatry*. 2013;54(1):37–45

56. MacLean K. The impact of institutionalization on child development. *Dev Psychopathol*. 2003;15(4):853–884

57. McDermott J, Westerlund A, Zeanah CH, Nelson CA, Fox NA. Early adversity and neural correlates of executive function: implications for academic adjustment. *Dev Cogn Neurosci*. 2012;2(Suppl 1):S59–S66

58. Smyke AT, Zeanah CH, Fox NA, Nelson CA, Guthrie D. Placement in foster care enhances quality of attachment among young institutionalized children. *Child Dev*. 2010;81(1):212–223

59. Dennis W. *Children of the Crèche*. New York, NY: Appleton-Century-Crofts; 1973

60. McCall R, van IJzendoorn MH, Juffer F, Groark C, Groza V. *Children Without Permanent Parents: Research, Practice and Policy*. Hoboken, NJ: Wiley-Blackwell; 2012

61. National Institute of Mental Health. Any anxiety disorder among children. http://www.nimh.nih.gov/statistics/1ANYANX_child.shtml. Accessed February 13, 2014

62. National Institute of Mental Health. Attention deficit hyperactivity disorder among children. http://www.nimh.nih.gov/statistics/1ADHD_CHILD.shtml. Accessed February 13, 2014

63. Casey BJ, Glatt CE, Tottenham N, et al. Brain-derived neurotrophic factor as a model system for examining gene by environment interactions across development. *Neuroscience*. 2009;164(1):108–120

64. Groark CJ, McCall RB, Fish L; the Whole Child International Evaluation Team. Characteristics of environments, caregivers, and children in three Central American orphanages. *Infant Ment Health J*. 2011;32(2):232–250

65. McLaughlin KA, Fox NA, Zeanah CH, Nelson CA. Adverse rearing environments and neural development in children: the development of frontal electroencephalogram asymmetry. *Biol Psychiatry*. 2011;70(11):1008–1015

66. Ghera MM, Marshall PJ, Fox NA, et al. The effects of foster care intervention on socially deprived institutionalized children's attention and positive affect: results from the BEIP study. *J Child Psychol Psychiatry*. 2009;50(3):246–253

67. Mehta MA, Golembo NI, Nosarti C, et al. Amygdala, hippocampal and corpus callosum size following severe early institutional deprivation: the English and Romanian Adoptees study pilot. *J Child Psychol Psychiatry*. 2009;50(8):943–951

68. Tottenham N, Hare TA, Quinn BT, et al. Prolonged institutional rearing is associated with atypically larger amygdala volume and emotion regulation difficulties. *Dev Sci*. 2010;13(1):46–61

69. Eluvathingal TJ, Chugani HT, Behen ME, et al. Abnormal brain connectivity in children after early severe socioemotional deprivation: a diffusion tensor imaging study. *Pediatrics*. 2006;117(6):2093–2100

70. Sheridan MA, Fox NA, Zeanah CH, McLaughlin KA, Nelson CA. Variation in neural development as a result of exposure to institutionalization early in childhood. *Proc Natl Acad Sci U S A*. 2012;109(32):12927–12932

71. Tottenham N, Hare TA, Millner A, Gilhooly T, Zevin JD, Casey BJ. Elevated amygdala response to faces following early deprivation. *Dev Sci*. 2011;14(2):190–204

72. Vyas A, Pillai AG, Chattarji S. Recovery after chronic stress fails to reverse amygdaloid neuronal hypertrophy and enhanced anxiety-like behavior. *Neuroscience*. 2004;128(4):667–673

73. Chisholm K. A three year follow-up of attachment and indiscriminate friendliness in children adopted from Romanian orphanages. *Child Dev.* 1998;69(4):1092–1106

74. Tottenham N, Sheridan MA. A review of adversity, the amygdala and the hippocampus: a consideration of developmental timing. *Front Hum Neurosci.* 2010;3(68):1–18

75. Fries AB, Pollak SD. Emotion understanding in postinstitutionalized Eastern European children. *Dev Psychpathol.* 2004;16(2):355–369

76. Tottenham N. Risk and developmental heterogeneity in previously institutionalized children. *J Adolescent Health.* 2012;51(2 Suppl):S29–S33

77. Smyke AT, Zeanah CH, Gleason MM, et al. A randomized controlled trial comparing foster care and institutional care for children with signs of reactive attachment disorder. *Am J Psychiatry.* 2012;169(5):508–514

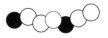

CHAPTER 12

Long-term Growth and Puberty Concerns for Adopted Children

Patrick W. Mason, MD, PhD, FAAP

You look at your schedule and see a new patient listed at 9:15 am. The schedule only says, "New patient from Russia." As you enter the room you meet Sasha, an active 23-month-old little blond-haired boy. After your thorough history, you know little more. Sasha has been home for 2 weeks and has been very healthy. He has a good appetite, sleeps well, and seems to be adjusting well to his new family. His past history reveals little information about his birth family. The medical information provided to his new family was brief and confusing. He reportedly had perinatal encephalopathy and vegito-visceral syndrome. Little else was known before he was adopted. Your physical examination was fairly routine, and you think you are going to stay on schedule because there is little here to do. Lastly you look at the growth chart that your nurse has plotted. Clearly this must be wrong. This healthy looking child can't be this far below the growth curve. You ask to remeasure him yourself and get the same points. The family asks about his size and wonders if he will be able to grow and catch up. What do you tell them?

Growth in Adoption: Experience With International Adoption

Growth is one of the most fundamental things that differentiates children from adults. This chapter will examine what is known about the effect that early life environment may have on a child's ability to grow and how adoption can influence this. It will also examine the implications of the often rapid catch-up that many will experience following their adoption.

As children are followed after their adoption, their health care professionals begin to comprehend the multitude of issues they present with as they join their new family. Studies continue to implicate early pre-adoption environments as one of the major causes of adoptees' impairments. On arrival to their new family, children appear to be at risk for a wide variety of medical and developmental abnormalities that are clearly outlined in this manual. Problems such as infections, untreated medical conditions, malnutrition, and speech and motor delays are far more common in children available for adoption than many health care professionals may be used to seeing in their practice. In addition, one of the most common and consistent abnormalities seen on arrival to a new family is poor growth. The etiology of growth failure is likely varied. The child's health care team must be aware of the potential causes and be prepared to work with the family to ensure adequate catch-up in the adopted child's growth.

Environmental Influences of Growth

A child's ability to grow to his or her full potential appears related to many issues, including genetics, nutrition, medical conditions, pre- and postnatal exposures, and the hormonal milieu, to name a few. The environment in which a child lives is well known to influence growth rate and ultimately growth outcome. Much has been written about how poverty, war, and malnutrition can influence growth.[1-3] Children who are adopted, especially those adopted internationally, are often coming from less than ideal settings, including situations of profound neglect and deprivation. The influence of deprivation and neglect on growth has received significant attention recently, although the effect of adverse living conditions on growth has been described for centuries. In the 1200s, King Frederick II of Sicily performed the first studies of deprivation by isolating infants to see if they developed an "innate" language. These infants not only failed to develop language but also failed to grow, and they died quickly because of lack of attention.[4] More recent reports have continued to document that children living in less than ideal settings generally have poor growth and high mortality rates.[4-6] Spitz[7,8] noted that without consistent attention, children living in foundling homes exhibited poor growth and development as well as a high mortality rate despite evidence of adequate nutrition. Talbot et al[9] noted a strong correlation between poor growth and a high incidence of abandonment, neglect, and maternal psychopathology, which improved in a subset of children after a psychologic intervention program was initiated for the family.

Widdowson[10] reported on the growth of children in 2 German orphanages run by 2 very different women. One was a caring woman who was very attentive to the needs of the children, while the second was a domineering and unpleasant woman. Despite similar food rations, children under the care of the loving woman grew better than did those cared for by the unpleasant matron. In an example of a crossover study, the directors were reassigned after 6 months to the other's orphanage. In addition, the strict woman was given increased rations. Despite this, the children under her care who had previously been growing well had a decreased growth rate. The children who were then under the care of the loving woman grew better despite their past poor growth and with fewer caloric rations.

Growth Following Adoption

Reports such as that of Widdowson[10] are very compelling and suggest a significant effect of institutional care and deprivation on subsequent growth. Although an estimated 226 million children younger than 5 years worldwide suffer growth stunting,[1] in the past a typical pediatric practitioner would evaluate such children only rarely. This changed, however, over the last 20 years with the dramatic expansion of international adoption. Following the Christmas day execution of Nicolae and Elena Ceaușescu in 1989 and the subsequent publicity surrounding the children housed under deplorable conditions in orphanages, large number of Western families went to Romania to adopt children. The subsequent breakup of the former Soviet Union and the relaxation of adoption rules in China had led to a large number of institutionalized children coming to the United States and Europe. Since the arrival of the first Romanian children in 1990, more than 200,000 children have been adopted internationally and brought into the United States. Now physicians and practitioners in almost every specialty have likely cared for a growing number of children who were adopted internationally. As our experience grows, we are beginning to recognize the effect that early environmental neglect has on children's health, development, and growth.

Johnson et al[11] first reported on growth impairment in children adopted from Eastern European orphanages. They found that one-third of the children adopted from Romania had evidence of growth failure on arrival. They also noted that the orphanage environment had an ongoing effect on the physical growth of the child, with height z scores decreasing as the length of institutionalization increased. They estimated that a child lost roughly 1 month of growth in height for every 2.6 months that he or she lived in an orphanage ($r = -0.79$). Miller and Hendrie[12] noted a similar correlation between growth failure and the duration of institutionalization in girls adopted from China, with a deviation of 1 month of height from mean age levels for each 2.86 months spent in the orphanage ($r = 0.90$, $P = 0.001$). Although the validity of such measurements in predicting the extent of growth stunting is debated, these studies do point out the cumulative influence that these environments may exert on the growing young child.

The ongoing negative effect on growth of a child's early life was further studied by Miller et al,[13] who reviewed changes in growth of children in a Russian orphanage. They found that 25% of the children had a height z score less than -2 at entry into the orphanage and that this number increased almost 40% while the children were in the orphanage.

Multiple studies have all continued to demonstrate the negative influence on growth of institutionalization.[14–17] Miller et al[18] found that this negative influence was not noted only in children from Eastern Europe; they found that children adopted from Guatemala had a mean height z score of -1.04. Moreover, growth stunting was significantly greater in children adopted from an orphanage compared with those adopted from a foster care family. Children adopted from Ethiopia[19] were found to have less stunting in growth (mean height z score -0.64 at arrival), likely related to the fact that they spent more time with their birth family than children adopted from other countries.

A growing number of studies show the extent of growth stunting seen in children adopted internationally (Table 12-1). Van Ijzendoorn et al[28] performed a meta-analysis of 33 papers in which growth of adopted children was reported. They noted that adopted children were on average more than 8 cm smaller than their peers at the time of their adoption. Adoption at a younger age had less of an effect on height

Table 12-1. Review of Anthropometric Measurements for Children Adopted Internationally

Studies	Weight z Score	Height z Score	Head Circumference z Score
Johnson et al, 1992[11] Romania, N=65	-1.10	-1.68	-1.06
Proos et al, 1992[20] India, N=114	-0.94	-2.25	-1.98
Miller et al, 1995[16] 22 countries, N=129	-0.76	-1.36	-1.03
Johnson et al, 1996[21] Russia, N=210	-1.71	-2.09	-1.15
Albers et al, 1997[22] Eastern Europe, N=56	-1.05	-1.41	-1.25
Rutter, 1998[15] Romania, N=111	-2.2 ±2.4	-2.3 ±1.7	- 2.2 ±1.3
Johnson et al, 1999[23] Romania, N=59	-3.56 ±2.0	-2.47 ±1.29	-2.08 ±1.53
Johnson, 2000[24]	-1.62 ±1.49	-1.25 ±1.15	-1.36 ±1.3
Miller and Hendrie, 2000[12] China, N=192	-1.17	-1.51	-1.43
Mason et al, 2000[25] Eastern Europe, N=339	-1.67	-2.03	N/A
Miller et al, 2005[18] Guatemala, N=50	-1.00	-1.04	-1.08
Miller et al, 2009[26] Eastern Europe, N=138	-1.41	-1.23	-0.63
Palacios et al, 2010[27] Mixed, N=289	-1.48	-1.46	-0.71

but no difference on changes in weight and head circumference when compared with children adopted at an older age.

What about growth in children adopted from the US foster care system? The effect of a poor environment does not seem to honor geopolitical borders. Although fewer studies have been reported, children adopted from the US foster care system also exhibit growth stunting and catch-up following permanent placement.[29,30] It is also a growing trend that children adopted domestically may have the opposite growth issue, with more adoptees showing obesity.

Psychosocial Short Stature: A Possible Mechanism?

Clearly, growth failure is a common feature seen in children adopted from international and domestic foster care settings. The etiology of poor growth is likely multifactorial and includes issues such as prematurity, intrauterine growth failure, genetics, prenatal and postnatal exposures, nutritional deficiencies, and medical illnesses. The nomenclature for this phenomenon of poor growth in children living under neglectful and deprived conditions has varied throughout the years but is now commonly termed *psychosocial short stature* (PSS).[2] By understanding the multiple presentations and possible mechanisms behind PSS, we may better understand the root causes of the institutional short stature seen in our adopted population and can tailor treatments to ensure catch-up growth.

Psychosocial short stature is a failure in growth that occurs in association with emotional deprivation or psychologic harassment for which there is no other explanation.[31] Several distinct subtypes have been described that pertain to children residing in institutional care settings. The first pattern (type 1) occurs in infants under stress or deprivation. Babies characteristically demonstrate poor growth and decreased appetite but show normal growth hormone (GH) response.[31] This growth failure may be related to the absence of touch and use of calories for growth.[32]

The second pattern (type 2A) is seen in older children living in stressful or deprived environments. These children do not experience weight loss but demonstrate bizarre behaviors including abnormal food rituals and hyperphagia.[33,34] This form of growth failure appears to be caused by reversible GH deficiency.[33,34] After removing children from these situations and placing them in a caring, nurturing environment, there is a return to normal GH secretion and evidence of catch-up growth. Miller et al[35] showed the reversible nature of GH insufficiency in a child who had normalization of his GH profile following removal from his stressful environment. Improvement in GH release appears to occur through an increase in GH pulse amplitude with no change in pulse frequency.[36,37] A subset of older children (type 3) has been found to present with anorexia, symmetric growth failure (height and weight), and more normal GH response to provocative testing.[38,39] Children adopted from international orphanages have been shown to demonstrate each of these growth patterns on arrival, suggesting that the stunting seen in many adopted children may be consistent with PSS.

One of the hallmarks of PSS is the reversible nature of growth failure when a child is removed from the environment. King and Taitz[40] reported on the catch-up growth of children following abuse and found that 55% of the children showed catch-up growth (an increase of >1 z score) compared with an increase in only 11% for children remaining in their original homes. Wyatt et al[29] examined 45 preschool children after placement into foster care and found an above average increase in height velocity and an increase in mean height standard deviation (SD) of 0.61. Colombo et al[41] noted a greater increase in growth of previously malnourished children who were placed in adoptive homes than those who remained in their original home or were institutionalized. Gohlke et al[42] demonstrated that children with PSS who were removed from their adverse environment had a marked improvement in height velocity as well as an increase in GH release.

To make the argument that the observed growth failure in children adopted from international orphanages is similar to children from Western societies with PSS, significant catch-up growth needs to be observed. Two studies[43,44] examined the growth of 240 female Korean orphans adopted into the United States and showed that all of the girls had evidence of growth improvement, with a correlation between the extent of catch-up and the age of the children at adoption. Johnson et al[45] reported a mean growth velocity of +5.5 SD for children adopted from Romania. Benoit et al[14] reported in their study that all children adopted at younger than 6 months and 87% of those adopted at older than 6 months had caught up within 1 year post-adoption. Despite significant growth stunting on arrival, Rutter[15] found catch-up in weight and height for most children in a cohort of Romanian adoptees, with only 1% of the children with height below the third percentile at follow-up. Loman et al[46] found that after a mean of 8 years in their newly adopted family, post-institutionalized children had a significant catch-up in height (-1.99 SD at adoption vs -0.08 SD at follow-up). This catch-up was similar regardless of whether the adoptees were from Eastern Europe, Asia, or South America. Miller et al[47] reported that for children adopted from Eastern Europe, there was an increase in mean height SD score from -1.22 at 2 weeks post-adoption to -0.59 after 6 months following their adoption. In their meta-analysis of adoption publications, van IJzendoorn et al[28] found that most studies reported an overall catch-up in height and weight that was similar to age-matched peers before puberty. Head circumference also improved but lagged behind non-adopted peers even 4 years after the adoption.

The ability to return to age norms may be related to several factors, including the age at placement and the extent of stunting on arrival. Johnson[24] reported that catch-up to age norms had been achieved by 78% of Romanian children who had been adopted before 18 months of age. Older children at adoption demonstrated a similar height velocity but, because of the greater deficit at arrival, failed to fully catch up.[43] Miller et al[47] also found that improvement in height was associated with a younger age and greater extent of growth failure at the time of adoption and higher caloric intake in the first 6 months after adoption. Mason et al[25] demonstrated a similar correlation with greater height catch-up and age, height at the time of adoption, and body mass index following adoption, with these 3 variables accounting for 57% of the variance ($r^2 = 0.57$, $P = 0.001$). Palacios et al[27] tried to determine if there was a rate of catch-up following adoption similar to the 1 month of height loss for every 3 months spent in an orphanage prior to the adoption as reported by Johnson et al[11] and Miller et al.[12] They noted a recovery rate of 2.76 months of height each year following adoption for the first 2 years. This rate of recovery decreased, however, to 1.32 months per year after the third year post-adoption.

As noted, many children adopted from institutional settings around the world have evidence of growth failure that appears to be directly related to the duration of time spent in the orphanage setting. It is likely that many factors contribute to this institutional short stature. Although there is compelling evidence to suggest that adopted children are likely PSS, this has yet to be fully demonstrated. Furthermore, the exact mechanisms in which the environment is able to influence the child's growth have not been determined. Numerous theories, however, have been proposed to understand the cause of PSS. Green et al[48] suggested that nutritional factors are unlikely to have a role because of the rapidity of hormonal changes. Changes in sleep patterns have been proposed to be a cause of other forms of GH abnormalities.[49,50] Children with PSS have been shown to have unusual sleep patterns that may lead to abnormal GH secretion,[51] as maximal GH release occurs during sleep.[52] Children who remain in a stressful environment not only fail to show the expected improvement in spontaneous GH production but also to grow in response to administration of GH,[53,54] suggesting that growth failure may also be related to GH insensitivity.

Stress as an Influence on Growth?

One potential mechanism in which the external environment could affect growth might be mediated through the hypothalamic-pituitary-adrenal (HPA) "stress" axis. The HPA axis has clearly been shown to have a significant effect on the body's growth response. By understanding this system, we may be able to ultimately understand the causes and prevent underlying abnormalities.

Animal studies have shown that lifelong changes in the responsiveness to stress can be controlled through early life experiences. Using animal handling models[55,56] as well as animal models of prenatal maternal stress, alcohol consumption, and malnutrition,[57,58] investigators have demonstrated that one can influence permanent development of the HPA axis, creating abnormal levels of stress hormones, which have been shown to correlate with poor cognitive[59] and emotional functioning[60,61] as well as poor growth. Numerous experiments with rodents have demonstrated the ability of acute stressors to increase HPA axis hormone levels and a concomitant decrease in GH levels.[62–71]

Similar to findings in animals, children who have experienced early life adverse events appear to be at risk of developing an abnormal stress response later in life.[72–76] Carlson and Earls[77] demonstrated that children living in an orphanage with poor quality of care have lower baseline morning cortisol levels and abnormally elevated noon and evening values compared with children living in an enriched environment. Similarly, a blunted morning response with a lower drop in evening cortisol was noted in children in foster care settings.[78–80] Bruce et al[81] found that for children in foster care, a low level of morning cortisol correlated with more severe neglect.

When a child is removed from an adverse environment, we know that growth catch-up is a fundamental component of recovery. Less is known as to whether observed growth changes following adoption correlate with a change in the HPA axis of the child after living in a nurturing family or whether these adverse changes are lifelong, as is the case for animals. Gunnar et al[82] reevaluated children from Romania 6½ years after their adoption and found that a subset of children at an older age still had significantly higher cortisol values then did children adopted after less time in an orphanage. Studies are currently ongoing to examine whether responsiveness of the HPA axis occurs following adoption and if these changes correlate with the child's ability to grow.

Long-term Effect of Growth: Precocious Puberty?

Growth delay appears to be a consistent finding in children being raised under adverse conditions in orphanages or many US foster care settings. There appears to be a strong correlation between the extent of growth failure and the time a child spent in an adverse environment. Although the mechanisms for growth loss have yet to be fully explained, they may share components with psychosocial growth failure. As pediatric practitioners begin to care for these children, they can confidently counsel new families on the likelihood of catch-up growth. While not inevitable, growth improvements occur, but they occur so commonly that it is appropriate to delay an evaluation for poor growth for at least 3 to 6 months post-arrival in anticipation of this expected improvement. If an increase in growth velocity has not occurred by 6 months post-adoption, a referral to a pediatric endocrinologist is likely warranted.

These rapid growth changes may, however, come at a price, especially for girls. Several studies and anecdotal accounts from parents have suggested that girls who were internationally adopted may be at risk for early puberty, which may ultimately affect final adult height. Initially, studies described girls adopted from India and Bangladesh who had evidence of early puberty.[83] All of the girls were small on arrival (-2.1 SD) into their new families and exhibited pronounced catch-up growth following their adoption (an improvement of 3.2 SD). Each of these girls was noted to have early puberty, with 4 having periods by age 7.6 years. This led to the suggestion that early puberty was related to the increased metabolic activity exhibited during catch-up growth.

Proos et al[84] later reported that girls from India who were adopted by Swedish families also experienced puberty significantly earlier than Swedish and Indian control groups. The majority of girls were malnourished on arrival, but following adoption, most had significant improvement in growth. Several other investigators have since reported a relationship between the timing of puberty and catch-up growth.[85,86] In contrast to these reports, Job and Quelquejay[87] studied 4 children adopted by a single family and showed no relationship between catch-up growth and precocious puberty.

Virdis et al[88] described 19 girls adopted from developing countries who demonstrated signs of puberty by age 6.9 years. Girls who were older at the time of adoption showed evidence of greater malnutrition and had the greatest delay in bone age. One year post-adoption, these differences were no longer observed. Several girls had their puberty medically delayed using gonadotropin-releasing hormone (GnRH) agonist and demonstrated a slowing in their bone age advancement and ultimately a greater predicted final height. Non-treated girls had a rapid advancement through puberty with a corresponding rapid change in bone age, resulting in heights lower than predicted and suggesting an overall negative effect on final adult height. When examining the phases of growth throughout development, Proos et al[89] found that the childhood phase of growth was shorted by 1.5 years because of early pubertal development.

Soriano-Guillén et al[90] recently reported on 44 children adopted in Spain (37 internationally and 7 domestic) who presented with central precocious puberty. They found an increased relative risk of central precocious puberty in adopted children compared with non-adopted children of 27.82 (18.28 for domestically adopted; 30.33 for internationally adopted).

The concerns of early puberty and its effect on ultimate adult height in adopted children led Mul et al[91] to examine the benefits of GH therapy for girls undergoing pharmacologic delay of puberty. They reported that the addition of GH in adopted girls undergoing hormonal delay with GnRH agonist resulted in a greater height velocity and increased predicted adult height than those receiving GnRH agonist alone. This finding differs from that of Tuvemo et al,[92] who found little benefit in final height with GnRH agonist, GH, or both. Several fundamental differences existed between the studies, including duration of treatment and method of predicting height prior to treatment, which would affect interpretation of the results. Further studies are needed to determine normal course and ultimate final adult heights of international adoptees. In addition, the use of GH to augment height gain following delay of puberty needs further evaluation.

A growing number of studies have now reported on the development of puberty for young adopted children. One of the controversies that exist is whether these children are truly precocious. Soriano-Guillén et al[90] found that the average age of diagnosis for the children in their study was 7.04 years. Studies in the United States have found a similar trend, with an earlier onset of pubertal changes as first reported by Herman-Giddens et al[93] with a mean age of Tanner 2 breast development being 10 ±1.8. By most accounts, the ages of pubertal onset for many adopted girls based on these more contemporary standards would not likely meet criteria of early puberty. The concerning finding, however, is that unlike the findings of Herman-Giddens et al,[93] who found an increase in the time between breast budding and menarche, Virdis et al[88] reported a more rapid development. This trend of rapidly progressing puberty may be of greater concern for the young girl and her family than the actual age of onset for breast budding. Our own review of the expected age of menarche in countries from which most children had been adopted (Figure 12-1) revealed that the girls who are demonstrating early puberty are doing so not only by US standards but also standards in their birth countries. Therefore, a

Figure 12-1.
Mean Age of Menarche in Countries of Adoption

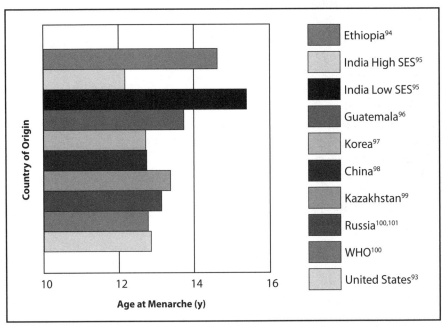

The mean age of menarche is reported for several countries from which most children are adopted and is compared to US mean values. Abbreviations: SES, socioeconomic status; WHO, World Health Organization.

genetic norm for this early puberty is unlikely. Clearly, there are some limitations in interpreting data to date. Sampling and recall bias as well as cross-sectional research and small sample size limits conclusions that can be made for any specific child. Further studies examining this trend are still needed for confirmation; however, the clinician should be aware of this potential acceleration of puberty.

While much is known about the risk of early puberty for girls adopted from abroad, little has been reported about possible risks for boys. Bourguignon et al[85] noted early puberty in one boy. Baron et al[86] reported that of 99 French families surveyed, early puberty was reported in 44.9% of the girls (49) compared with only 8.6% of the boys (3 out of 35 boys surveyed). Soriano-Guillén et al[90] noted early puberty in 5 boys for an incidence rate of 34.08 per million-person years (MPYs) at risk, compared with 265.8 MPYs for girls and 0.96 MPYs for non-adopted boys living in Spain. Etiology of this female predominance for early puberty is not fully understood. It may be an extension of the significantly higher rates of idiopathic central precocious puberty seen in girls in general. Other causes of early puberty specific to the population of adopted girls cannot be excluded. As further studies examine the basis of early puberty in girls, the differential expression of puberty between boys and girls in this population may become apparent.

What Is the Etiology of Early Puberty for Adopted Children?

What, then, is the etiology of early puberty for adopted girls, and how common is early puberty in this group of children? The relative risk for girls adopted internationally is unknown, and data to determine this are limited. The risk of early puberty does appear higher in general than for children residing in their new countries. In Belgium, girls who were adopted appeared to be at an 80-times increased risk of early puberty than girls born in Belgium.[102] Teilmann et al[103] estimated the rate of early puberty to be 20-times higher in adopted girls than native Danish girls, and Soriano-Guillén et al[90] found a relative risk of 27.82 for adopted girls compared with non-adopted Spanish girls.

The rate for this increased risk has yet to be calculated for children adopted into the United States. Mason et al's survey of 193 girls found that 30% (57 of 193) had early breast development and 12% (23 of 193) had menarche by mean age of 10.5 ±2.6 years[25]; this is the only survey to date reporting early puberty in adopted children. The low number of reports from the United States may reflect a negative referral bias given ongoing controversy surrounding the definition of normal and thus early age of puberty in the country. Table 12-2 reviews several studies on pubertal timing in girls following international adoption.

The question remains, however, as to the etiology of the observed early rates of puberty for the adopted girl. Multiple factors are likely to play a role. Improved nutrition and rapid growth changes have been implicated.[83–86] Teilmann et al[105]

Table 12-2. Review of Pubertal Timing in Girls Following International Adoption

Study	Marshall and Tanner[104]	Herman-Giddens et al[93]	Proos et al[84]	Baron et al[86]	Mason et al[25]
Subjects	192	15,439 (Caucasian)	107	30	193
Breast	11.2 ±1	10 ±1.8			8.8 ±2.5
Menarche	13.5 ±1	12.9 ±1.2	11.6	11.3	10.5 ±2.6

found that adopted girls had an earlier activation of their pituitary and gonadal activity than did non-adopted girls. Other influences are also likely to play a role. The effect of early deprivation and stress may be influencing this risk of early puberty. The HPA stress axis has been shown to have an effect on the timing of puberty in animal models as well as clinical cases.[106–109] Reports have demonstrated the effect of early life in an orphanage setting on the HPA axis of adopted children,[77,82] so this may be playing a role. The report of Krstevska-Konstantinova et al[102] may call the relationship between early puberty and deprivation in question because it found that children who migrated into Belgium with their families also had an increased rate of early puberty. It did not, however, measure cortisol values or the response of the HPA axis to stress, so there may still be a role for this axis affecting early puberty. Other factors such as environmental toxins and endocrine disrupters could perhaps explain the relationship between a child's environment and risk of early and rapid puberty changes.[110] Further multicenter studies will be needed to clarify not only the relative risk of early puberty but also the possible etiology of these changes.

Conclusion

We are beginning to appreciate the consequences of an adopted child's early environment on subsequent growth and puberty. Children who are adopted are frequently much smaller than their aged-matched peers on arrival to their new family. The influences and mechanisms responsible for institutional short stature have yet to be fully explained but are likely multiple. The majority of children show significant and rapid catch-up in their growth, which makes evaluation by a physician unnecessary for most of them. The hormonal mechanisms that govern these changes are unknown at present but may be similar to those previously reported for PSS. Growth acceleration may come at the price of early puberty for girls. Precocious puberty may be associated with acceleration of the pubertal process, leading to early menarche and premature cessation of bone elongation. These physical changes of puberty may cause further stress for the affected child and her adopted family. At the present time, there is insufficient evidence to support pharmacologic intervention to delay puberty or enhance growth. Further studies are needed to determine if this approach offers any advantages for the child. As Western families adopt more children from outside the United States, these children will seek medical services at increased frequencies. Many adopted children quickly overcome the effect of their early environment and demonstrate rapid improvement in growth and development. Health care professionals need to be aware of these potential problems to address these issues following adoption and anticipate problems that may develop. Only with future research will we be able to understand the etiology of the issues and help alleviate the difficulties that new parents and children must overcome as they become a family.

References

1. United Nations Children's Fund. *The State of the World's Children 1998*. New York, NY: Oxford University Press; 1998
2. Waterlow JC. Post-neonatal mortality in the Third World. *Lancet*. 1988;2(8623):1303
3. Martorell R, Mendoza F, Castillo R. *Poverty and Stature in Children*. Vol 14. New York, NY: Raven Press; 1988
4. Gardner L. Deprivation dwarfism. *Sci Am*. 1972;227:76–82
5. Chapin H. A plan of dealing with atrophic infants and children. *Arch Pediatr*. 1908;25:491–496
6. Chapin H. Are institutions for infants necessary? *JAMA*. 1915;64:1–3
7. Spitz R. Hospitalism, an inquiry into the genesis of psychiatric conditions in early childhood. *Psychoanal Study Child*. 1945;1:53–74
8. Spitz R. Hospitalism, a follow-up report. *Psychoanal Study Child*. 1946;2:113–117
9. Talbot NB, Sobel EH, Burke BS, Lindemann E, Kaufman SB. Dwarfism in healthy children: its possible relation to emotional, nutritional and endocrine disturbances. *N Engl J Med*. 1947;236:783–793
10. Widdowson E. Mental contentment and physical growth. *Lancet*. 1951;1:1316–1318
11. Johnson DE, Miller LC, Iverson S, et al. The health of children adopted from Romania. *JAMA*. 1992;268(24):3446–3451
12. Miller LC, Hendrie NW. Health of children adopted from China. *Pediatrics*. 2000;105(6):E76
13. Miller LC, Chan W, Litvinova A, Rubin A, Tirella L, Cermak S. Medical diagnoses and growth of children residing in Russian orphanages. *Acta Paediatr*. 2007;96(12):1765–1769
14. Benoit TC, Jocelyn LJ, Moddemann DM, Embree JE. Romanian adoption. The Manitoba experience. *Arch Pediatr Adolesc Med*. 1996;150(12):1278–1282
15. Rutter M. Developmental catch-up, and deficit, following adoption after severe global early privation. English and Romanian Adoptees Study Team. *J Child Psychol Psychiatry*. 1998;39(4):465–476
16. Miller LC, Kiernan MT, Mathers MI, Klein-Gitelman M. Developmental and nutritional status of internationally adopted children. *Arch Pediatr Adolesc Med*. 1995;149:40–44
17. Groze V, Ileana D. A follow-up study of adopted children from Romania. *Child and Adolescent Social Work Journal*. 1996;13(6):541–565
18. Miller L, Chan W, Comfort K, Tirella L. Health of children adopted from Guatemala: comparison of orphanage and foster care. *Pediatrics*. 2005;115(6):e710–e717
19. Miller L, Tseng B, Tirella L, Chan W, Feig E. Health of children adopted from Ethiopia. *Matern Child Health J*. 2008;12(5):599–605
20. Proos LA, Hofvander Y, Wennqvist K, Tuvemo T. A longitudinal study on anthropometric and clinical development of Indian children adopted in Sweden. I. Clinical and anthropometric conditions at arrival. *Ups J Med Sci*. 1992;97(1):79–92
21. Johnson D, Albers L, Iverson S, et al. Health status of Eastern European orphans referred for adopton. *Pediatr Res*. 1996;39:134A

22. Albers LH, Johnson DE, Hostetter MK, Iverson S, Miller LC. Health of children adopted from the former Soviet Union and Eastern Europe. Comparison with preadoptive medical records. *JAMA.* 1997;278(11):922–924

23. Johnson D, Aronson J, Federici R, et al. Profound, global growth failure afflicts residents of pediatric neuropsychiatric institutes in Romania. *Pediatr Res.* 1999;45:126A

24. Johnson DE. Long-term medical issues in international adoptees. *Pediatr Ann.* 2000;29(4):234–241

25. Mason P, Narad C, Jester T, Parks J. A survey of growth and development in the internationally adopted child. *Pediatr Res.* 2000;47:209A

26. Miller BS, Kroupina MG, Iverson SL, et al. Auxological evaluation and determinants of growth failure at the time of adoption in Eastern European adoptees. *J Pediatr Endocrinol Metab.* 2009;22(1):31–39

27. Palacios J, Roman M, Camacho C. Growth and development in internationally adopted children: extent and timing of recovery after early adversity. *Child Care Health Dev.* 2010;37(2):282–288

28. van IJzendoorn M, Bakermans-Kranenburg M, Juffer F. Plasticity of growth in height, weight and head circumference: meta-analytic evidence of massive catch-up after international adoption. *J Dev Behav Pediatr.* 2007;28(4):334–343

29. Wyatt D, Simms M, Horwitz S. Widespread growth retardation and variable growth recovery in foster children in the first year after initial placement. *Arch Pediatr Adolesc Med.* 1997;151:813–816

30. Pears K, Fisher P. Development, cognitive, and neuropsychological functioning in preschool-aged foster children: associations with prior maltreatment and placement history. *J Dev Behav Pediatr.* 2005;26:112–122

31. Blizzard RM, Bulatovic A. Syndromes of psychosocial short stature. In: Lifshitz F, ed. *Pediatric Endocrinology.* 3rd ed. New York, NY: Marcel Dekker, Inc; 1996

32. Field T. Massage therapy for infants. *J Dev Behav Pediatr.* 1995;16:105–111

33. Powell GF, Brasel JA, Blizzard RM. Emotional deprivation and growth retardation simulating idiopathic hypopituitarism. I. Clinical evaluation of the syndrome. *N Engl J Med.* 1967;276(23):1271–1278

34. Powell GF, Brasel JA, Raiti S, Blizzard RM. Emotional deprivation and growth retardation simulating idiopathic hypopituitarism. II. Endocrinologic evaluation of the syndrome. *N Engl J Med.* 1967;276(23):1279–1283

35. Miller JD, Tannenbaum GS, Colle E, Guyda HJ. Daytime pulsatile growth hormone secretion during childhood and adolescence. *J Clin Endocrinol Metab.* 1982;55(5):989–994

36. Albanese A, Hamill G, Jones J, Skuse D, Matthews DR, Stanhope R. Reversibility of physiological growth hormone secretion in children with psychosocial dwarfism. *Clin Endocrinol (Oxf).* 1994;40(5):687–692

37. Stanhope R, Adlard P, Hamill G, Jones J, Skuse D, Preece MA. Physiological growth hormone (GH) secretion during the recovery from psychosocial dwarfism: a case report. *Clin Endocrinol (Oxf).* 1988;28(4):335–339

38. Skuse D, Albanese A, Stanhope R, Gilmour J, Voss L. A new stress-related syndrome of growth failure and hyperphagia in children, associated with reversibility of growth-hormone insufficiency. *Lancet.* 1996;348(9024):353–358

39. Gohlke BC, Frazer FL, Stanhope R. Body mass index and segmental proportion in children with different subtypes of psychosocial short stature. *Eur J Pediatr.* 2002;161(5):250–254

40. King JM, Taitz LS. Catch up growth following abuse. *Arch Dis Child.* 1985;60(12):1152–1154

41. Colombo M, de la Parra A, Lopez I. Intellectual and physical outcome of children undernourished in early life is influenced by later environmental conditions. *Dev Med Child Neurol.* 1992;34(7):611–622

42. Gohlke BC, Frazer FL, Stanhope R. Growth hormone secretion and long-term growth data in children with psychosocial short stature treated by different changes in environment. *J Pediatr Endocrinol Metab.* 2004;17(4):637–643

43. Winick M, Meyer KK, Harris RC. Malnutrition and environmental enrichment by early adoption. *Science.* 1975;190(4220):1173–1175

44. Lien NM, Meyer KK, Winick M. Early malnutrition and "late" adoption: a study of their effects on the development of Korean orphans adopted into American families. *Am J Clin Nutr.* 1977;30(10):1734–1739

45. Johnson D, Miller L, Iverson S, et al. Post-placement catch-up growth in Romanian orphans with psychosocial short stature. *Pediatr Res.* 1993;33:89A

46. Loman MM, Wiik KL, Frenn KA, Pollak SD, Gunnar MR. Postinstitutionalized children's development: growth, cognitive, and language outcomes. *J Dev Behav Pediatr.* 2009;30(5):426–434

47. Miller BS, Kroupina MG, Mason P, et al. Determinants of catch-up growth in international adoptees from Eastern Europe. *Int J Pediatr Endocrinol.* 2010;107252:1–8

48. Green WH, Campbell M, David R. Psychosocial dwarfism: a critical review of the evidence. *J Am Acad Child Psychiatry.* 1984;23(1):39–48

49. Guilhaume A, Benoit O, Gourmelen M, et al. Relationship between sleep stage IV deficit and reversible HGH deficiency in psychosocial dwarfism. *Pediatr Res.* 1982;16:299–303

50. Wolff G, Money J. Relationship between sleep and growth in patients with reversible somatotropin deficiency (psychosocial dwarfism). *Psychol Med.* 1973;3:18–27

51. Mouridsen SE, Nielsen S. Reversible somatotropin deficiency (psychosocial dwarfism) presenting as conduct disorder and growth hormone deficiency. *Dev Med Child Neurol.* 1990;32(12):1093–1098

52. Sassin JF, Parker DC, Mace JW, Gotlin RW, Johnson LC, Rossman LG. Human growth hormone release: relation to slow-wave sleep and sleep-walking cycles. *Science.* 1969;165(3892):513–515

53. Frasier SD, Rallison ML. Growth retardation and emotional deprivation: relative resistance to treatment with human growth hormone. *J Pediatr.* 1972;80(4):603–609

54. Tanner JM. Resistance to exogenous human growth hormone in psychosocial short stature (emotional deprivation). *J Pediatr.* 1973;82(1):171–172

55. Levin S. Infantile experience and resistance to physiological stress. *Science.* 1957;126(3270):405

56. Meaney MJ, Aitken DH, van Berkel C, Bhatnagar S, Sapolsky RM. Effect of neonatal handling on age-related impairments associated with the hippocampus. *Science.* 1988;239(4841 Pt 1):766–768

57. Ogilvie KM, Rivier C. Prenatal alcohol exposure results in hyperactivity of the hypothalamic-pituitary-adrenal axis of the offspring: modulation by fostering at birth and postnatal handling. *Alcohol Clin Exp Res.* 1997;21(3):424–429

58. Clarke AS, Wittwer DJ, Abbott DH, Schneider ML. Long-term effects of prenatal stress on HPA axis activity in juvenile rhesus monkeys. *Dev Psychobiol.* 1994;27(5):257–269

59. Lupien SJ, McEwen BS. The acute effects of corticosteroids on cognition: integration of animal and human model studies. *Brain Res Rev.* 1997;24(1):1–27

60. de Haan M, Gunnar MR, Tout K, Hart J, Stansbury K. Familiar and novel contexts yield different associations between cortisol and behavior among 2-year-old children. *Dev Psychobiol.* 1998;33(1):93–101

61. Schmidt LA, Fox NA, Rubin KH, et al. Behavioral and neuroendocrine responses in shy children. *Dev Psychobiol.* 1997;30(2):127–140

62. Armario A, Lopez-Calderon A, Jolin T, Castellanos JM. Sensitivity of anterior pituitary hormones to graded levels of psychological stress. *Life Sci.* 1986;39(5):471–475

63. Kokka N, Garcia JF, George R, Elliot HW. Growth hormone and ACTH secretion: evidence for an inverse relationship in rats. *Endocrinology.* 1972;90(3):735–743

64. Brown GM, Martin JB. Corticosterone, prolactin, and growth hormone responses to handling and new environment in the rat. *Psychosom Med.* 1974;36(3):241–247

65. Armario A, Castellanos JM, Balasch J. Adaptation of anterior pituitary hormones to chronic noise stress in male rats. *Behav Neural Biol.* 1984;41(1):71–76

66. Schalch DS, Reichlin S. Plasma growth hormone concentration in the rat determined by radioimmunoassay: influence of sex, pregnancy, lactation, anesthesia, hypophysectomy and extracellular pituitary transplants. *Endocrinology.* 1966;79(2):275–280

67. Kuhn CM, Pauk J, Schanberg SM. Endocrine responses to mother-infant separation in developing rats. *Dev Psychobiol.* 1990;23(5):395–410

68. Rivier C, Vale W. Involvement of corticotropin-releasing factor and somatostatin in stress-induced inhibition of growth hormone secretion in the rat. *Endocrinology.* 1985;117(6):2478–2482

69. Smith EL, Coplan JD, Trost RC, Scharf BA, Rosenblum LA. Neurobiological alterations in adult nonhuman primates exposed to unpredictable early rearing. Relevance to posttraumatic stress disorder. *Ann N Y Acad Sci.* 1997;821:545–548

70. Barbarino A, Corsello SM, Della Casa S, et al. Corticotropin-releasing hormone inhibition of growth hormone-releasing hormone-induced growth hormone release in man. *J Clin Endocrinol Metab.* 1990;71(5):1368–1374

71. Barinaga M, Bilezikjian LM, Vale WW, Rosenfeld MG, Evans RM. Independent effects of growth hormone releasing factor on growth hormone release and gene transcription. *Nature.* 1985;314(6008):279–281

72. Elizinga BM, Schmahl CG, Vermetten E, van Dyck R, Bremner JD. Higher cortisol levels following exposure to traumatic reminders in abuse related PTSD. *Neuropsychopharmocology.* 2003;28(9):1656–1665

73. Gunnar MR, Brodersen L, Nachmias M, Buss K, Rigatuso J. Stress reactivity and attachment security. *Dev Psychobiol.* 1996;29(3):191–204

74. Nachmias M, Gunnar M, Mangelsdorf S, Parritz RH, Buss K. Behavioral inhibition and stress reactivity: the moderating role of attachment security. *Child Dev.* 1996;67(2):508–522

75. Halligan SL, Herbert J, Goodyer IM, Murray L. Exposure to postnatal depression predicts elevated cortisol in adolescent offspring. *Biol Psychiatry.* 2004;55(4):376–381

76. Brown ES, Varghese FP, McEwen BS. Association of depression with medical illness: does cortisol play a role? *Biol Psychiatry.* 2004;55(1):1–9

77. Carlson M, Earls F. Psychological and neuroendocrinological sequelae of early social deprivation in institutionalized children in Romania. *Ann N Y Acad Sci.* 1997;807:419–428

78. Fisher P, Gunnar M, Dozier M, Bruce J, Pears K. Effects of a therapeutic intervention for foster children on behavior problems, caregiver attachment and stress regulatory neural systems. *Ann N Y Acad Sci.* 2006;1094:215–225

79. Fisher P, Van Ryzin M, Gunnar M. Mitigating HPA axis dysregulation associated with placement changes in foster care. *Psychoneuroendocrinology.* 2011;36(4):531–539

80. Dozier M, Manni M, Gordon M, et al. Foster children's diurinal production of cortisol: an exploratory study. *Child Maltreat.* 2006;11(2):189–197

81. Bruce J, Pears K, Levine S, Fisher P. Morning cortisol levels in preschool-aged foster children: differential effects of maltreatment type. *Dev Psychbiol.* 2009;51(1):14–23

82. Gunnar MR, Morison SJ, Chisholm K, Schuder M. Salivary cortisol levels in children adopted from Romanian orphanages. *Dev Psychopathol.* 2001;13(3):611–628

83. Adolfsson S, Westphal O. Early pubertal development in girls adopted from Far-Eastern countries. *Pediatr Res.* 1981;15:82

84. Proos LA, Hofvander Y, Tuvemo T. Menarcheal age and growth pattern of Indian girls adopted in Sweden. I. Menarcheal age. *Acta Paediatr Scand.* 1991;80(8–9):852–858

85. Bourguignon JP, Gerard A, Alvarez Gonzalez ML, Fawe L, Franchimont P. Effects of changes in nutritional conditions on timing of puberty: clinical evidence from adopted children and experimental studies in the male rat. *Horm Res.* 1992;38(Suppl 1):97–105

86. Baron S, Battin J, David A, Limal JM. [Precocious puberty in children adopted from foreign countries]. *Arch Pediatr.* 2000;7(8):809–816

87. Job JC, Quelquejay C. Growth and puberty in a fostered kindred. *Eur J Pediatr.* 1994;153(9): 642–645

88. Virdis R, Street ME, Zampolli M, et al. Precocious puberty in girls adopted from developing countries. *Arch Dis Child.* 1998;78(2):152–154

89. Proos L, Karlberg J, Hofvander Y, Tuvemo T. Pubertal linear growth of Indian girls adopted in Sweden. *Act Paediatr Scand.* 1993;82:641–644

90. Soriano-Guillén L, Corripio R, Labarta J, et al. Central precocious puberty in children living in Spain: incidence, prevalence and influence of adoption and immigration. *J Clin Endocrinol Metab.* 2010;95(9):4305–4313

91. Mul D, Oostdijk W, Waelkens JJ, Schulpen TW, Drop SL. Gonadotrophin releasing hormone agonist treatment with or without recombinant human GH in adopted children with early puberty. *Clin Endocrinol (Oxf).* 2001;55(1):121–129

92. Tuvemo T, Gustafsson J, Proos LA. Growth hormone treatment during suppression of early puberty in adopted girls. Swedish Growth Hormone Advisory Group. *Acta Paediatr.* 1999;88(9):928–932

93. Herman-Giddens ME, Slora EJ, Wasserman RC, et al. Secondary sexual characteristics and menses in young girls seen in office practice: a study from the Pediatric Research in Office Settings network. *Pediatrics.* 1997;99(4):505–512

94. Zegeye DT, Magabiaw B, Mulu A. Age at menarche and the menstrual pattern of secondary school adolescents in northwest Ethiopia. *BMC Womens Health.* 2009;9:29

95. Rao S, Joshi S, Kanade A. Height velocity, body fat and menarcheal age of Indian girls. *Indian Pediatr.* 1998;35(7):619–628

96. Kahn A, Schroeder D, Martorell R, Rivera J. Age at menarche and nutritional supplementation. *J Nutrition.* 1995;125(Suppl 4):1090–1096

97. Cho G, Park H, Shin J, et al. Age at menarche in a Korean population: secular trends and influencing factors. *Eur J Pediatr.* 2010;169(1):89–94

98. Song Y, Ma J, Hu P, Zhang B. [Geographic distribution and secular trend of menarche in 9-18 year-old Chinese Han girls]. *Beijing Da Xue Xue Bao.* 2011;43(3):360–364

99. Facchini F, Fiori G, Bedogni G, et al. Puberty in modernizing Kazakhstan: a comparison of rural and urban children. *Ann Hum Biol.* 2008;35(1):50–64

100. Wang Y, Adair L. How does maturity adjustment influence the estimates of overweight prevalence in adolescents from different countries using an international reference? *Int J Obes Relat Metab Disord.* 2001;25(4):550–558

101. Iampol'skaia Iu A. [Dynamics of puberty levels in girls of Moscow]. *Gig Sanit.* 1997;May-June(3):29–30

102. Krstevska-Konstantinova M, Charlier C, Craen M, et al. Sexual precocity after immigration from developing countries to Belgium: evidence of previous exposure to organochlorine pesticides. *Hum Reprod.* 2001;16(5):1020–1026

103. Teilmann G, Main K, Skakkebaek N, Juul A. High frequency of central precocious puberty in adopted and immigrant children in Denmark. *Horm Res.* 2002;58:135

104. Marshall WA, Tanner JM. Variations in pattern of pubertal changes in girls. *Arch Dis Child.* 1969;44(235):291–303

105. Teilmann G, Boas M, Petersen J, et al. Early pituitary-gonadal activation before clinical signs of puberty in 5- to 8-year old adopted girls: a study of 99 foreign adopted girls and 93 controls. *J Clin Endocrinol Metab.* 2007;92(7):2538–2544

106. Rabin D, Gold PW, Margioris AN, Chrousos GP. Stress and reproduction: physiologic and pathophysiologic interactions between the stress and reproductive axes. *Adv Exp Med Biol.* 1988;245:377–387

107. Rivier C, Rivier J, Vale W. Stress-induced inhibition of reproductive functions: role of endogenous corticotropin-releasing factor. *Science.* 1986;231(4738):607–609

108. Magiakou MA, Mastorakos G, Webster E, Chrousos GP. The hypothalamic-pituitary-adrenal axis and the female reproductive system. *Ann N Y Acad Sci.* 1997;816:42–56

109. Compagnucci CV, Compagnucci GE, Lomniczi A, et al. Effect of nutritional stress on the hypothalamo-pituitary-gonadal axis in the growing male rat. *Neuroimmunomodulation.* 2002;10(3):153–162

110. Parent AS, Teilmann G, Juul A, Skakkebaek NE, Toppari J, Bourguignon JP. The timing of normal puberty and the age limits of sexual precocity: variations around the world, secular trends, and changes after migration. *Endocr Rev.* 2003;24(5):668–693

CHAPTER 13

Attachment and the Adopted Child

Christine Narad Mason, DNP, C-PNP; Susan Branco Alvarado, MAEd, LPC; and Patrick W. Mason, MD, PhD, FAAP

Introduction

Jack is a 15-month-old boy adopted from Kazakhstan 2 weeks ago. His mother, father, and grandmother are present at today's initial evaluation visit. When you enter the room and sit down, Jack promptly climbs into your lap, and his mother says, "Jack is always going over to strangers and trying to go home with the neighbors when they visit. I'm in a chat group online with other parents from the orphanage we adopted from and one of the mothers said that this sounded like reactive attachment disorder. Is it, and what do we do about it?"

Having an understanding of attachment theory and the current literature, you know this is a complex question that may not be answered in the first evaluation visit with a newly adopted child.

Attachment as an infant to a primary caregiver is one of the cornerstones of child development and paramount for the development of a lifetime of healthy relationships. Attachment, as initially defined by John Bowlby, is a persisting attribute for a person to seek close proximity to another person regardless of the situation but especially in times of distress.[1] This relationship is characterized by affinity and reciprocity between the child and caregiver. Decreased or adverse attachment can lead to a poor parenting cycle and interference with normal growth and developmental milestone achievement. Although Bowlby's attachment theory was initially met with some resistance 30 years ago, it is now generally accepted.[2] It is important to note that attachment is only one aspect of relationship development and should not be considered in a vacuum.[2] Temperament, match between child and adult, environment, and issues outside the parental relationship can also play a significant role in the parent-child relationship. The majority of children who are internationally adopted and many children adopted out of foster care lack the opportunity to attach to a primary caregiver because of a lack of caregiving or inconsistency in caregivers.[3] This is particularly true among children raised within institutional settings. Within an Iranian orphanage, researchers found that although the physical environment and medical care were satisfactory, the psychosocial environment was severely impaired.[4] The caregiver ratio ranged between one caregiver to 10 children on the day shift to one caregiver to 50 children on the evening and night shifts. Aside from meeting basic needs, the children were without companionship for much of the day because of the caregiver's multitude of additional responsibilities. Most of the children were found to have significant delays in physical, emotional, and behavioral development.

A prospective study looking at the amount of time caregivers spent with children in a Russian orphanage also found human contact lacking.[5] The researchers followed 138 children without special needs ranging in age from 1 month to 4 years. The children were evaluated every 10 minutes for 5 hours. During this period, 65% of infants, 43% of toddlers, and 46% of preschoolers were alone. In general, the children spent 50% of their time alone and only 27% with a caregiver. This information is vital and verifies that the children have had very limited time to form a securely attached relationship with a caregiver.

Cultural and language differences, if present, are other variables that may interfere with the development of an attached relationship with a new parent following an international adoption.[6]

When considering the minimal amount of human interaction many children experience prior to their placement, it's not surprising that many international and domestic adoptees come to their new families with attachment "issues." Within the adoption community, there is a plethora of misinformation widely shared about attachment difficulties. At this time, there is limited information available on long-term outcomes of attached relationships in internationally adopted children, and most of this literature focuses on children raised in orphanages and not foster care situations. This chapter will focus on the tenants of attachment theory and attachment research as they relate to adopted children and their parents throughout the adopted child's life.

Basic Theory of Attachment

There are 30 infants, 2 to a bed, in a Chinese orphanage with 3 caregivers during the day and 2 at night. Caregiver Xu has been taking care of the same 10 infants for the past year. She has found a better paying job in the city and is leaving the orphanage. What might the effect of this departure be on the children?

In this case, a lot will depend on the amount of neglect that a child experienced at the hands of the caregiver. The institutional environment is characterized by deprivation and neglect in which caregivers are unable or unwilling to meet basic needs for nurturing, safety, and protection.[7] Caregiver-child ratios in child care centers, which can be used as a proxy indicator for institutional care, predict infant attachment.[8] Researchers have found that children experiencing lower caregiver-to-infant ratios (one caregiver to 3 or fewer children) are more likely to have secure attachment (72%) compared with children experiencing higher caregiver-to-child ratios (one caregiver to 3 or more children), who were more likely to have insecure attachments (57%).[8]

Information on attachment was virtually nonexistent until John Bowlby began working with the World Health Organization reviewing the world's literature on the effects of long-term institutionalization on personality development of children.[9] In 1951, *Maternal Care and Mental Health* was published, detailing findings that children became acutely distressed when they were "separated from those they know and love" and including recommendations of how best to avoid, or at least mitigate, short- and long-term ill effects.[10]

Two films, *Grief: A Peril in Infancy* (1947) by René Spitz[11] and *A Two-Year-Old Goes to the Hospital* (1952) by John Robertson,[12] visually portrayed, for the first time, the detrimental effect of children being separated from their mothers and the impact this had on the child's ability to trust the parent. These classic films brought attention to attachment in children and were instrumental in further developing Bowlby's work.[9] During the 1950s and 1960s, attachment theory permeated the fields of child psychiatry, psychology, pediatrics, and nursing, leading to the more liberal parental visitation policies present in hospitals today.[9]

Prior to Bowlby's work, there was a widely held belief, which persists today, that children attached to their mother primarily because of food, and dependency on the mother for a personal relationship was actually secondary.[9,13] In 1951, Bowlby described a link between ethology (the study of animal behavior) and human infants based on the work of Konrad Lorenz (Nobel Prize winner credited with founding the discipline).[9,14] Ethology provided the foundation for the argument that children were not attached to their mothers primarily for food but also for attention and protection. Bowlby's theory was in part based on the behavior of newly hatched birds. Baby birds feed themselves, yet they still have an affinity for the mother bird. Bowlby believed that infants have a genetic predisposition to facilitate bonding between themselves and their caregiver because infants are completely dependent on the primary caregiver for meeting all their needs, not just feeding.

Experiments of Harry Harlow[9,15] further defined our understanding of attachment. In these studies, infant monkeys were separated from their mothers and given an option of a cloth monkey or a wire monkey who dispensed food. The rhesus monkey babies consistently preferred the soft cloth-covered monkey over the wire monkey, even when they were fed solely by the wire monkey. When stressed, the baby monkey consistently went to the cloth monkey for comfort. Furthermore, when infant monkeys were kept in total isolation and deprived of contact with other infant monkeys or mother monkeys over an 8-month period, they had permanent mental health problems similar to the characteristics of a child with an autism spectrum disorder today. After several different experimental models, it was found that if the baby monkey was reunited with the mother before 90 days of deprivation (the equivalent of 6 months of age in a human baby), the infant monkey returned to normal behavior.[15] This research was important because it stressed the need to prevent isolation and provide a nurturing environment early in life. Because many of the early studies of attachment theory were conducted in a prospective manner, researchers were able to understand the trauma of childhood separation and prospectively trace the features of separation behaviors. By building a theory based on observations of the child's behavior in defined situations and recording the child's behavior, feelings, and thoughts, patterns could be identified. These patterns shed light on how the child's personality developed in relation to the parent-child relationship.

Bowlby's initial observations on abnormal attachment behavior in institutionalized children remain relevant today. Canadian researchers investigating long-term attachment behavior in children adopted from Romanian orphanages stratified the time the children spent within the orphanage before their adoption.[16,17] Using a parent report questionnaire, attachment behavior was assessed. The results indicated that the Romanian children adopted after 8 months of age were more likely than Romanian children adopted before 4 months of age and non-adopted, Canadian-born children to exhibit lower attachment scores and greater indiscriminately friendly behavior. A follow-up study was performed 3 years later on the same group of children using an attachment security questionnaire and parental report to see if these differences were maintained.[18] The children adopted after 8 months of age continued to show indiscriminate friendly behavior but no longer exhibited any difference in the rate of insecure attachment when compared with the other control groups. Those children who originally had more insecure attachment did, however, exhibit significantly more behavioral problems than the control group.

O'Connor, Rutter, and the English and Romanian Adoptees Study Team found that children adopted prior to 4 months of age had fewer issues of disrupted attachment[19,20]; their data also suggested that a close association existed between the duration of time in the orphanage and resulting deprivation and the degree of attachment disorder behaviors in children who were adopted after 8 months of age.[18] These studies are congruent with Harlow's research with infant rhesus monkeys discussed earlier.[14]

Process of Attachment

Attachment behavior is aimed at keeping the caregiver close for protection during infancy.[9] There are 4 phases recognized in infancy: pre-attachment, attachment in the making, clear-cut attachment, and goal-corrected attachment.[9] These phases are influenced by the infant's need to keep the object of preferred attachment close for nurturing, safety, and protection. While the chronologic timing may be different for children who are internationally adopted, the chronologic order of the phases is applicable.

The first phase is pre-attachment. During the first month of life, a newborn exhibits behaviors to bring the primary caregiver closer, including crying, smiling, rooting, clinging, sucking, looking at people, synchronizing movements with adult speech, and distinguishing the primary caregiver's voice.[9] The feeding gaze is one example of behavior used to entice the primary caregiver in this phase.

Jade is a 22-month-old female adopted from Korea one month ago. She started child care 2 weeks ago. When dropped off at child care by her mother, she will scream, cry, and cling to her mother's leg. Once her mother leaves, she continues to cry and cling to the door of the child care. While at child care, she is cranky and does not want to participate with her peers. When her mother comes to pick her up, she hides under a table.

Jade's screaming, crying, and clinging to her mother's leg may have nothing to do with attachment and more to do with the tremendous amount of change she has experienced in the past weeks. Not all behaviors children exhibit are related to an attachment issue. From an attachment perspective, in this case, it is more likely that Jade has not yet developed an attachment to her mother and therefore is not able to go to her mother for protection during this stressful time. It will be important for Jade's mother to recognize that Jade is cueing distress, not defiance, and to provide a nurturing environment for her at this time of crisis. This may include delaying child care until Jade is more adjusted to her new home.

The second phase is attachment in the making. This phase extends into the second half of the first year of life. During this phase, the infant singles out and selectively smiles at the primary caregiver.[9] An example of this phase is the selective social smile a young infant gives on purpose to the primary caregiver to promote attachment.

Mia is a 3-year-old girl who was adopted from Ethiopia at 2 years of age and has been cared for in the home by her mother while her father works during the week. The family comes into the office for a visit. Dad is upset because Mia cries whenever she is left with her father for the first 30 minutes and then will settle down and play. As soon as Mia's mother returns, she will insist on spending time with her. How will you counsel this family?

Mia is showing signs of secure attachment to her mother. Her behavior also indicates the concept of hierarchy of attachment relationships. Mia has placed her mother in the first hierarchy position, as would be expected given that she has spent more time at home interacting and getting to know her mother. She also demonstrates signs of distress when her mother leaves; however, she is able to settle down after a short amount of time and appears to be able to depend on her father to meet her needs when her mother is not around. This indicates that her father is in the secondary hierarchy position, but Mia upgrades him into the primary position when mother is unavailable and downgrades him again when her mother returns. This is a normal process that securely attached children participate in regardless of adoptive status. It is important for her father to spend time alone with Mia without her mother around to help develop their relationship. In some cases, alone time with her father may be too stressful for Mia. Another alternative to supporting the development of healthy attachment with both parents includes playfully engaging with her father while reading, rolling a ball among all 3 with Mia seated with her mother but facing her father, or playing hide-and-seek, with Mia and her father seeking her mother and vice versa.

In typically developing infants, phase 3, clear-cut attachment, begins during the second half of the first year. Behaviors of this phase are designed to draw the primary caregiver closer emotionally and physically by crying, squirming, smiling, and using newly developed locomotive skills to move closer to the primary caregiver.[9]

Zoe is an 18-month-old girl who has begun to run up and down the steps at home. She enjoys running up the steps away from her father, calling out, "Daddy, find me!" while hiding around the corner of the stairs. Her father joins in this game by acting as if he cannot see Zoe in her hiding place and calling out, "Where is Zoe? Where did my Zoe go?" while running up and down the steps.

This is an example of using gross motor skills to bring the caregiver closer to the child while exploring the environment in a safe manner. Being in control of the game and having her father as an active participant is helping Zoe master her separation response.

Peekaboo and hide-and-seek are games that the child will use to practice controlled engagement and disengagement with the primary caregiver.

The second year encompasses the fourth phase, goal-corrected attachment, in which the child begins to anticipate and influences the primary caregiver's behavior. The child also develops recognition of the cause-and-effect components of the parent-child relationship.[9] For example, the child can purposefully cry to bring the caregiver closer. The primary goal of each of these phases is for the child's needs to be met. If this occurs, positive attachment and security and protection have developed. However, if the child's needs are not met, negative attachment and lack of security can occur.

Alex is a 2-year-old boy adopted from Guatemala who has been home for one year. The family has a new puppy. Alex has never had a pet and is very scared of the new dog. When the dog barks, Alex will cry and call out, "Mama, help!" What can his mother do to help Alex with his fear?

Alex is making his needs known very clearly—he is scared of the new puppy and has identified his mother as a source of protection from his fear of the dog. His mother can help him to overcome this fear by facilitating supervised interactions with the puppy to help Alex feel more confident and less scared. By providing support or scaffolding during the interaction, his mother can demonstrate how to pet the puppy or throw the ball to the puppy, and Alex can learn how to explore a new situation with his mother's nurturing support and protection.

Separation Response

Robertson, in association with Bowlby, initially identified protest, despair, and denial/detachment as the 3 phases in the separation response of a child from the mother.[21] Bowlby further put forth the concept that grief and mourning were present in children.[22] This concept was pivotal in advancing the 4 phases of grief in adulthood (ie, numbness, yearning and protest, disorganization and despair, and finally reorganization), which in turn is an important component in parental attachment behaviors (see Types of Attachment on page 267).[23,24]

Mary Salt Ainsworth, a student of Bowlby, further advanced knowledge about the separation response and is credited with having performed the first ethologically based infant-mother attachment study in Uganda.[25,26] Through this research, Ainsworth was able to identify patterns of attachment from observations within a select group of mothers and children. She separated these patterns of behavior into 3 distinct categories: securely attached, insecurely attached, and not yet attached. When in the presence of their mothers, securely attached infants cried less and more freely explored their surroundings. Their mothers showed high levels of maternal sensitivity to the needs of their infants. In contrast, insecurely attached infants cried more, even when held by their mother, and were more tentative in their exploration. The mothers of the insecurely attached infants were found to be less sensitive and less attuned to their infant's needs. The infants not yet attached showed no distinction between the mother and other caregivers. These patterns were consistent with Ainsworth's later work with mother-child dyads in Baltimore.[27] A key finding from this research is that most of the attachment interaction patterns were established within the first 3 months of the child's life.[27–29] It is unknown if the first 3 months following adoption are as critical a period.

Circle of Security

To help assess how securely attached a child and parent relationship might be, Ainsworth developed the Strange Anxiety Scale.[27] The Strange Situation is a 20-minute controlled situation in which the child is placed under distress and the interaction between the child and caregiver is observed and recorded on video through a one-way mirror. One parent and the child of interest are brought to the playroom for a set amount of time before the parent gets up and leaves the child. How the child and parent handle the departure is observed as well as what the child does while the parent is gone. After a set amount of time, the parent returns to the room and the reunion between the parent and child is observed. In the second phase, after a set amount of time, a stranger comes into the room, sits quietly, and does not interact with the child. The parent leaves the room, then after a specific time, returns to the room and the stranger leaves. The behaviors of the parent and child are observed and categorized into a specific pattern of attachment.[25]

The Circle of Security is a helpful tool to assess the effect of the Strange Situation on the parent and child.[30,31] Observations that occur during the Strange Situation are categorized in terms of the attachment behavior system, and interactions are assessed to evaluate how well the parent and child work together and how effective the parent is at reading the child's cues to promote nurturing, closeness, and security from the parent. The Circle of Security provides a visual illustration of what Marvin and Whelan describe as the "dynamic dance" that takes place between the primary caregiver and child (Figure 13-1).[30,31]

Throughout the dynamic dance, the child is presenting the parent with signals for what he or she needs and the parent responds accordingly. The type of interaction present can be classified as ordered or non-ordered attachment. The goal of attachment behaviors is to keep the primary caregiver close, thereby providing protection and comfort to the child. How close the child wants to be to the primary caregiver will depend on the situation that is occurring. Children will use a variety of behaviors to bring the primary caregiver closer or to bring themselves closer to the primary caregiver (eg, creeping, crawling). The mechanism chosen depends on the perceived stress of the stimulus.

Figure 13-1.
Circle of Security

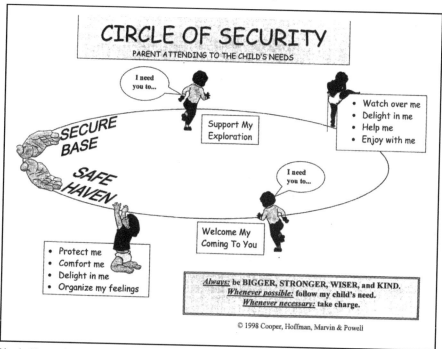

Used with permission.

Katie is a 36-month-old girl adopted from Vietnam at 9 months of age. She is learning to climb a slide at the playground. Katie climbs the first few steps and gets scared and starts to cry. Her father pats her back and offers encouraging words. He helps Katie up the last step and holds her hand while she goes down the slide. At the bottom of the slide, he gives her a big hug and tells her what a good job she did. Katie gets very excited and goes around, climbing up the steps again. At the top of the slide she gets scared and says, "Daddy, hold hand," which her father does. Katie goes around, climbing up the steps again; this time she tells her father, "Me do." At the top, her father notices that she is getting teary; from the bottom of the slide, he holds out his arms and says, "Daddy's here to catch you, Katie." Giggling, Katie slides down into her father's arms for a big hug.

This is an example of a parent and child who are freely moving around the Circle of Security. When Katie is scared and working on the Safe Haven side of the circle, her father offers comfort and protection while helping to move her to the Secure Base side of the circle so she can master the task of sliding. Her father is not speeding up the process but taking his cues from Katie and helping to support her in her new experience.

Children and parents should be able to move freely around the Circle of Security and go from a safe haven, where the child is able to obtain comfort and nurturing, to the secure base, where the child is able to explore the environment with relative ease and minimal anxiety. An attachment problem can become apparent for multiple reasons beyond the scope of this chapter when the parent or child has become stuck in one area of the circle or is unable to ask for or provide the necessary comfort or exploration needed. When this occurs, treatment would be important so the caregiver can learn to provide a secure base from which the infant or child is able to obtain nurturing or protection or explore the environment around him or her. It is important for the parent to understand the dynamic dance that takes place. For some parents this is intuitive, while others may need assistance.[30]

Sasha is a 5-year-old boy adopted from Russia. His mother has enrolled him into T-ball for the summer. Sasha becomes very shy around the other team players and will cling to his mother and hide behind her legs as soon as they get to the baseball field. He will not sit with the other children on the bench and becomes frantic, trying to climb into his mother's arms, when it is his turn to bat. His mother will carry him to the plate and hand him the bat, saying, "Sasha be a big boy and stop crying; it's your turn to bat," while walking away. When this happens, Sasha will just stand still holding the bat until he is out.

Sasha is clearly cueing his need for comfort and protection and is on the Safe Haven side of the circle. His mother is focused on having Sasha explore the Secure Base portion of the circle and is not responding to his need to make the environment safe so he feels he is able to seek out new adventures. Sasha and his mother are not functioning on the same portion of the circle; this will make it hard for them to form a securely attached relationship.

Parents and children must be able to move around the Circle of Security in a free-flowing manner depending on the needs of the child, and parents must readjust to the developmental level of the child. During infancy and early childhood, children learn to participate in various activities such as play to explore their surroundings. As a child gains more confidence, he or she is able to increase the distance and time spent away from the caregiver. By 3½ years of age, a child who has had the opportunity to form a secure attached relationship will be able to spend half a day to an entire day away from the primary caregiver.[9] Adolescents are able to spend weeks or months away from home but still need to return to home base.[9,31] More research is needed to understand if these parameters are applicable for children who were adopted internationally and their parents.

Kyle is a 9-year-old boy adopted from Ethiopia at 2 years of age. He is going to sleepaway camp for the first time. In preparation for the weeklong trip, his parents have been arranging sleepovers with friends for the past few months. The night before camp, Kyle and his parents are talking. Kyle says, "I think you are going to miss me while I'm gone, so I'm going to put this picture of me beside your bed so you can see me before you go to sleep."

"That is a very good idea, Kyle," says his mother.

"It's such a good idea," says his father, taking a picture of Kyle and his parents off the wall, "that I think you should take this with you."

"This is great! I'm so excited to go camping for a whole week! It will be like one long sleepover, and then I'll come home and tell you all about what I did."

"We will have a celebration when you come home," says his mother.

This is an example of a family working together to make a new experience less stressful for the child. Kyle is miscuing about his true concern of missing his parents, but his parents are able to see through the miscue and to address the real concern of Kyle missing his parents. They also had a plan in place that helped Kyle to become more familiar with the sleepover process before the long camp trip. Kyle is excited about the camp and already making plans for a reunion with his parents.

Types of Attachment

Through Ainsworth's Strange Anxiety Scale, 4 general patterns of attachment were found to be present: secure, autonomous; insecure, avoidant-dismissing; insecure, ambivalent-preoccupied; and insecure, disordered (disorganized or insecure or other pattern).[27] The Circle of Security is a helpful tool for understanding how the child and parent interact to create these patterns of attachment.[31]

Secure, Autonomous Attachment

Secure attachment occurs when the child has a responsible caregiver who is able to recognize cues for protection and comfort. Additionally, the primary caregiver responds to the cues in a manner that is prompt and appropriate to the situation. The parent also has the skill to anticipate when the child perceives he or she is in an adverse or frightening situation.[32] In the secure child, autonomous parent pattern, the parent and child have the ability to interact with each other effortlessly between the nurturing and exploration components of the Circle of Security.[30,31] The child is able to give appropriate cues for what he or she needs at any given point in time, and the parent is able to read these cues and respond appropriately. If, for some reason, a mistake or a disruption in the relationship occurs, it is easily repaired, and the dyad can return to its normal pattern of interaction.[31]

Josie is a 3-year-old girl adopted from China. Last week, her mother fell and broke her leg. Neighbors cared for Josie overnight. When her mother returns home, Josie will not go and see her mother immediately. Josie's mother sits in the same room as Josie and talks to her, saying, "Josie, Mommy missed you so much last night, and she didn't want to be in the hospital without you. All I could think about was how we missed reading our bedtime story. Do you think we could read one now that I am home and you could come and sit on the couch next to me?" Josie runs to the bookcase to find a very long storybook and sits by her mother.

Josie's mother has addressed the fact that she was not available to Josie last night and offered a repair in the relationship by making up for the missed story time last night. Because they are securely attached, this action is able to repair the disruption in the relationship, and they are able to move forward.

Insecure, Avoidant-Dismissing Attachment

In the insecure, avoidant-dismissing pattern, the child and parent tend to stay in the exploration portion of the Circle of Security and minimize nurturing needs.[31] Anxious, avoidant attachment occurs when the child has no confidence that needs will be responded to in a helpful manner. Often the child is rebuffed for the behavior that is requesting protection and security. The child tries to become emotionally self-sufficient and with time becomes more narcissistic. In this pattern, the child

Travis is a 4-year-old boy who was adopted from Russia. He is learning to ride a bike without training wheels. His mother made sure he put on his bike helmet and elbow pads prior to the lesson. His mother starts the lesson by giving Travis a push forward on his bike. As Travis begins to roll forward, he starts to teeter and falls off his bike into a tree. Travis gets angry and starts to kick the bike. His mother responds by picking up the bike and telling Travis it is time for a second try. On the next try, the same thing happens. This time he scrapes his knee. His mother again responds by picking up the bike and telling Travis it is time for another try. This time Travis kicks the tree for getting in his way. What is going on here?

Travis is sending a miscue to his mother, and she is reading the miscue instead of the covered-up feelings. Travis was most likely upset and scared from riding his bike for the first time without training wheels. When he fell off the bike and started to kick the tree in anger, which may have been covering up fear, his mother ignored the emotions (Safe Haven portion of the circle) associated with the new task of riding the bike and focused instead on the task at hand (Secure Base portion of the circle). His mother did provide protection for Travis' physical being, but she is neglecting his emotional need for comfort. In addition, Travis is sending a miscue to his mother by not talking about how scared he is doing this for the first time. Travis is working on the Safe Haven portion of the circle and giving miscues to look as if he is on the Secure Base side of the circle where his mother is functioning.

often miscues the parent and the parent reads the miscue rather than the true need of the child. Basic protection needs are often met, but the child's underlying emotional needs are often neglected. If a disruption in the relationship occurs, the dyad has a complex and anxious pattern of recovery. Children who have undergone repeated rejections exhibit this type of attachment behavior.[31,32]

Insecure, Ambivalent-Preoccupied Attachment

In the insecure, ambivalent-preoccupied pattern, the parent overly focuses on nurturing and limits the child's ability to explore the environment. The child often appears to be overly dependent on the parent and unable to seek out adventure. Caregiver inconsistency in early life contributes to this pattern of attachment behavior and is often exhibited as enmeshment of those in the dyad. When disruption in the relationship occurs, there is a very complex, intimate, and anxious

Loannie is a 14-year-old girl adopted from Romania at 3 years of age. Her father, Mr Daran, reports that he is concerned about the interaction between his daughter Loannie and her mother on a recent school field trip they chaperoned. Loannie did not want to leave her mother's side, was hesitant to walk with her peer group to view the exhibits, and depended on her mother to choose her lunch items, although her father was standing next to her in line. At one point on the trip, Loannie became very frantic when her mother went to the bathroom without telling her; when her mother returned, Loannie demanded that she hold her hand for the rest of the trip. In the gift shop, Loannie told her father that she wanted to get a pencil set like her friend Meg, but when her mother came over, she let her mother choose a stuffed animal for her. Mr Daran reports that when he chaperoned a previous field trip earlier in the year without Mrs Daran, Loannie did not behave this way; however, he has noticed that Loannie no longer goes on playdates with friends. As you gather more information, you notice that Loannie looks to her mother to answer the questions that you are asking, even one as benign as, "What color do you like?" You also notice that as Mr Daran discusses his concerns, Loannie's mother waves her over to the chair next to her, and she eventually sits in her mother's lap.

This is a complicated situation; you will likely need the help of a pediatric mental health care professional familiar with identifying and treating attachment issues. In this interaction, you have observed

1. Loannie and her mother have a close relationship with each other.
2. Loannie and her father have a different relationship with each other (which you know is possible because children do not attach to all adults in the same manner).
3. Loannie's mother enticed Loannie to sit with her when she felt she was being criticized by the father.
4. Loannie is not acting like a "typical" teenager.

   This leads you to believe that Loannie and her mother may be having some problems in the way they are attached to each other. You must also consider that her parents may have other issues going on and that Loannie is getting caught in the middle.

recovery that takes place.[31,33] Children often exhibit behavior closer to one type of attachment pattern than another; however, some children develop unpredictable attachment patterns.

Insecure, Disordered Attachment

The disordered pattern of attachment is characterized by disorganization or insecure or other patterns in which the parent is fearful of or angry at the child. Often the underlying cause is the parent's own history with abuse, childhood trauma, or current trauma that makes it difficult for the parent to look beyond his or her circumstances to the needs of the child.[31] These patterns often result when the primary caregiver exhibits bipolar illness or has been physically or sexually abused.[32] Dyads who are working in these areas of attachment patterns are often not on the Circle of Security completely and have no set pattern for recovering from a disruption in the relationship. For the parent and child, this is a high-risk attachment pattern.[31]

Daniel is a 4-year-old boy adopted from Russia at 18 months of age. You initially followed him for a year after his adoption. His parents have returned for your counseling because they are having trouble with Daniel's temper tantrums. Daniel will shout, scream, bite, pinch, and hit when he is told "No." He has become so violent that he broke his mother's nose when he was kicking to get away from her to run into the street. His parents tell you that they are concerned about their ability to keep Daniel safe and that they are becoming scared of him. His mother has been placed on antidepressants because the adoption has not turned out the way she planned and she is overwhelmed with Daniel's behaviors. In the examination room, Daniel's mother tells him to leave the blood pressure cuff alone. Daniel charges at his mother and you notice that she flinches. What are your assessment and next steps?

Your assessment is that Daniel has disorganized attachment. You are concerned about his show of violent behavior toward his caregivers. You are also concerned that Daniel's mother may be being abused or have been abused in the past based on her guarded behavior when Daniel charges after her. You know this is a family that needs counseling immediately because things will not get better without professional help.

Disrupted Attachment

When a child experiences separation, it is seen "as a fundamental threat to their well-being" and therefore a disruption of the attachment bond with the parent.[34] The degree of distress will be based on the child's age, length of separation, and experience. The child undergoes 3 phases of separation from a primary caregiver. The first phase during initial separation is called *protest*. The child experiences extreme anger and fear. Depending on the child's age, a search is commenced to find the missing object of attachment. This phase can last from a few hours to longer than a week. When the primary caregiver cannot be found, the child moves into the second phase, *despair*. Sadness and a decrease in emotional expression are apparent. Lastly, the final phase is *detachment*. The child will play with less energy, there is an absence of joy, and the child can appear listless.[34] Hostile behavior increases over time. On return of the caregiver, the child will often ignore him or her. Older children who have experienced successful attached relationships are able to discuss an upcoming separation from the primary caregiver and plan for the return of that caregiver. It was proposed by Bowlby that separation from the mother was as serious as withholding food from an infant.[34]

Angelina is a 3-year-old girl adopted from China. Angelina was abandoned at a police station, and her history prior to entering the orphanage is unknown. A single mother initially adopted Angelina at 18 months of age. At 21 months of age, it became clear that Angelina had an underlying medical condition that would require frequent hospitalizations and long-term speech, physical, and occupational therapy. For various reasons, her mother decided she could not continue to parent Angelina, and she was placed in foster care for re-adoption. At 28 months of age, Angelina was adopted by a 2-parent family in another state who felt better able to handle her medical and developmental needs. Since the time of her second adoption, Angelina has been non-expressive verbally and physically. If she perceives that she has done something wrong, she will stand in a catatonic solider position looking down at the floor for longer than an hour. If her mother or father leaves her sight, she becomes angry and will rip books or throw pillows. When the missing parent returns, she will ignore the parent and hit him or her if the parent comes close to her. In the middle of the night, her father has found her crying while hiding under a table. As the new pediatrician for this family, what will you do?

There are many issues at play in this case. Most important is the history of multiple disrupted attachments that occurred between Angelina and her birth family, her orphanage caregivers, her first adoptive mother, and her foster family prior to her placement with 2 new parents in a new environment. It is easy to see that this child is confused and has not had the consistency needed to transition from one situation to another. It will be very important for her new parents to be consistent and responsive to Angelina's needs to begin to build trust and start to form an attached relationship.

Pilowsky and Kates[35] discuss the disruption of an attached relationship and how this affected children in the foster care system. The researchers found that permanency was a key stabilizing component for children previously shifted from one foster care home to another. This information can be applied to a child adopted internationally who routinely had multiple caregivers and then enters a new home environment where all the rules and norms are unknown and new.

The ability to anticipate separation events is a necessary component for children to master. Anticipation provides the foundation for formation of relationships throughout the life span. The child and adult must have experienced responsiveness and security to make the transition from primary caregiver to other significant relationships. The child's expectations, as well as the primary caregiver's responsiveness, are an important component of this process. Open communication and the ability to discuss fears, anger, and sadness must occur for positive attachment to be present. For children with a history of multiple challenges to a healthy attachment relationship, routine strategies to support attachment between parent and child are critical, but the support of a good attachment-knowledgeable therapist can be helpful in facilitating a healthy attachment pattern.

Persistence of Patterns

Once a pattern of attachment is established, it tends to persist throughout life. Each pattern is self-perpetuating. For example, the anxious-ambivalent child is often whiny and clingy, while the anxious-avoidant child is distant and a bully. These behaviors will elicit an unpleasant response from the primary caregiver, resulting in further negative attention for the child. These patterns of behavior internalize into the child's perceptions of how a relationship should function. Children in orphanages around the world have not had the opportunity to form a secure attachment bond and are therefore at greater risk for anxious-ambivalent or anxious-avoidant behavior.

Vorria et al[36] examined Greek children in long-term institutionalized care and were interested in the concept set forth by Bowlby that children would fare better in homes than institutions. Children 9 to 11 years of age living in an orphanage were matched with children in a control group of the same age, gender, and school living in 2-parent families. Caregivers and teachers participated by answering a questionnaire that elicited information about each child's behavior. This information was augmented by classroom observation. The institutionalized children were found to be more passive, inattentive, and involved in nonproductive activities compared with the control group. Parent and teacher questionnaires indicated more conduct and emotional difficulties in the institutionalized group of children. The institutionalized children also exhibited an increased tendency to seek affection from their teacher and engaged in more superficial relationships with peers. Institutionalized girls showed significant emotional problems and poor school performance compared with controls, while institutionalized boys exhibited more conduct, hyperactivity, and decreased task involvement than the control group.

Smyke et al[37] also studied 3 groups of children: those living in Romanian orphanages, a "pilot" unit in which caregiver-child ratios were low, and noninstitutionalized peers. They found that children in the orphanage group had indiscriminant friendliness and were more emotionally labile when compared with the pilot unit and noninstitutionalized peer group. These findings illustrate the importance of the child-caregiver relationship in the overall well-being of children in detrimental situations such as orphanages.

Other Variables

Underlying medical, genetic, developmental, or environmental problems can influence attachment behaviors. Although there is limited research available about adopted children and attachment, there is a fair amount of literature available on children with other underlying issues and their ability to form attachments to their caregivers.

Underlying Medical Issues

Children who are premature do not have a significantly increased risk of having attachment problems when compared with full-term infants; however, they do have an increased risk of the anxious-resistant pattern of attachment if they experienced a prolonged hospital stay.[38] Children with failure to thrive have been found to have significantly higher rates of anxious attachment and may be influenced by caregivers' past traumatic events or current experiences.[38]

Children with underlying neurologic disorders such as cerebral palsy have slightly higher rates of insecure attachment (40%), which is most likely related to the challenges parents face when caring for a child with special needs.[38] On the other hand, children with other cognitive abnormalities, such as Down syndrome and autism spectrum disorder, have been found to form secure attachments with a primary caregiver.[38]

Caregiver Influences on Attachment

Several studies have looked at maternal-fetal attachment (MFA) and may be helpful in understanding maternal attachment in adoption. Windridge and Berryman[39] reported that women 35 years or older had lower MFA scores than those in their mid-20s. This is an interesting finding because the majority of adoptive mothers are older, with an age range of 40 to 50 years.[40] First-time mothers had higher MFA scores than experienced mothers, and the MFA had an inverse correlation to the number of children in low-risk but not high-risk women.[39] In other words, MFA scores lowered with an increased number of children. This would support Ames' recommendation for the adoption of one child at a time.[16] This information would suggest that a mother age 43 adopting 2 children from Russia would be at risk for having lower MFA than a mother in her 20s adopting one child. Clearly, further study is needed in this area. In addition, very little is known about the effect of the father on the attachment of the newly adopted child.

The effects of early deprivation can and do affect relationships into adulthood. Long-term follow-up studies of women raised in institutions for part or all of their lives reveal problems with relationships.[41-43] Each of these studies revealed that formerly institutionalized women were more likely than the control group to have poor psychosocial functioning and severe parenting problems. The degree of these problems could be tempered by positive relationship experiences. For instance, women who experienced positive school relationships were more likely to have a successful marriage.[42,43] The ex-institutionalized care group and the control group of mothers showed the same degree of play and conversational interaction with their children.[41] However, the children of ex-institutionalized women were more likely to have their cues for attention ignored.

Child Care or School

Following adoption, many parents find that they need to go back to work and place children within child care settings. This reality often raises many concerns and anxiety for the newly adoptive parents as they consider attachment issues for their child. Unfortunately, little research has been done to help guide the parents or their health care team in making these decisions. Some professionals recommend that, if possible, the parents should stay home with their new child for as long as possible to help facilitate attachment. The concern is that spending prolonged time with a nanny or child care staff will help facilitate attachment with the nonfamilial caregiver and not the parents. While this advice makes sense, there is little research currently available that helps confirm or refute this opinion. The parents should work with their health care team to discuss available child care options and determine which make the most sense.

Prior to placement, the parents should spend as much time as possible with the child, providing an opportunity for the child to understand the role of the parents. Several professionals suggest that only the parents should care for the child in this transition period. They should be the only ones who feed, dress, bathe, and put the child down for sleep. In this way, the child begins to understand and seeks the parents as the new primary caregiver. Transition to the child care setting should proceed slowly, if possible, perhaps a couple of hours a day or with the parents present at first. This may allow the child to feel more comfortable in the new setting. The parents, child care staff, and health care team should remain diligent in monitoring how the child is doing with this transition.

Sleep

An additional factor that may influence the adopted child's attachment to a primary caregiver is sleep disturbances, which are common in many adopted children. Research indicates that the developmental of sleep-wake organization in the first 3 years of life may be related to regulatory function emerging through child-caregiver relationships.[38] Mothers with underlying sleep disorders have been recognized to have a more distorted or disengaged relationship with their infants, putting the dyad at risk for attachment problems.[38]

Reactive Attachment Disorder

Frustrated parents enter your office reporting that their 4-year-old, adopted at age 2, has reactive attachment disorder (RAD). They offer proof of this diagnosis by showing you a checklist of symptoms they downloaded from a Web site advertising treatment of children with RAD. How can this family best be aided?

Having a clear understanding of the incidence of RAD will help you to provide appropriate referrals to help this family transition and assist them in building a securely attached relationship with their child.

As mentioned previously, the Internet offers seemingly endless information on attachment disorders for adoptive parents, and the topic of attachment and specifically reactive attachment disorder (RAD) is much discussed. Some sites offer checklists with RAD symptoms for parents to diagnose their adoptive children should problematic behaviors exist. In reality, there are no current studies that show the actual percentages of adopted children who have been diagnosed with RAD or the accuracy of parental checklists. Chaffin et al[44] state that "there is very little systematically gathered epidemiologic information on RAD. In its absence, much of what is believed about RAD is based on theory, clinical anecdotes, case studies, and extrapolated from laboratory research on humans and animals."

Reactive attachment disorder is now grouped in the trauma- and stressor-related disorders category of the fifth edition of the *Diagnostic and Statistical Manual of Mental Disorders (DSM-5)*. The *DSM-5* breaks RAD into 2 distinct disorders. The emotionally withdrawn or inhibited pattern is now referred to as RAD, and the indiscriminately social or disinhibited pattern is called *disinhibited social engagement disorder.*[45]

The broad definition in the preceding edition of the *DSM* had previously led to what some would consider an overdiagnosis of RAD, particularly within individuals with a history of adoption. Furthermore, there is no one standard, reliable, and empirically validated screening tool to definitively diagnose RAD. Zeanah[46] found that disinhibited/indiscriminant RAD can be present in adopted children despite an attached relationship with the parent. This implies that there is still much for us to learn despite promising measures that can more helpfully identify a child's attachment category and patterns, ie, the Child Attachment Interview[47] and Circle of Security evaluation protocol.

Jake, an 11-year-old boy adopted at age 6, spent his formative years in his birth mother's care. His pre-adoption records describe him as having been left alone; tied to his crib for extended periods, possibly days; and severely neglected. He was removed from his birth mother's care at age 2 and was taken to an orphanage housing hundreds of children ranging in age from infants to teenagers. During this period, he received little individual attention of any sort and often competed for food and resources. When his parents adopted him, he was malnourished and presented with global developmental delays. He demonstrated persistent displays of emotional flatness and was unresponsive to his parents' overtures of comfort or soothing. He showed no parental preference and rarely, if ever, expressed joy in his interactions with them.

Jake's experience with neglect and abuse by his mother has a direct effect on how he is viewing the world and his new family. A key component to helping Jake and his parents is the ability of the family members to develop trust. His parents need to be attuned, vigilant, and consistent in their daily care of Jake to promote an attached relationship. Because of the multiple traumas Jake has experienced, professional care by an experienced counselor with an understanding of adoption issues is vital.

Parental Barriers to Secure Attachment Relationships

A family arrives for its first post-adoption clinic visit. The adopted 18-month-old appears to be energetic and intermittently clingy and fidgety throughout the visit. The mother reports feeling differently than she had expected about the adoption. She reports experiencing fleeting thoughts of regret about the adoption and an overwhelming sense of anxiety and fear. What would be the best guidance for this family?

Some evidence suggests that parents may experience a post-adoption depression (PAD), described as being similar to postpartum depression. Post-adoption depression should be considered early and addressed immediately by a licensed mental health professional with experience working with adoptive parents. If not treated, PAD can interfere with successful and healthy attachment relationships because it hinders the caregiver's ability to respond in a consistent, nurturing, and protective manner to the child. It can also place the child at high risk for further neglect or the development of additional abuse.

Post-adoption depression is increasingly being discussed in electronic mailing lists and blogs for adoptive parents. Foli and Thompson's *The Post-Adoption Blues: Overcoming the Unforeseen Challenges of Adoption*[48] highlighted PAD for the adoption community and professionals alike. Senecky et al,[49] however, found no cases of depression developing in Israeli women caused by their adoption and that each woman who was depressed after an adoption was also depressed before the adoption. Clearly, this area needs further research to see if women, and perhaps their partners, are at increased risk of depression as a consequence of their adoption.

In addition to possible depression, caregivers may also experience increased stress due to their adoption. Narad and Mason[50] found that 43.4% of adopted parents surveyed experienced increased levels of stress (>85th percentile on the Parenting Stress Index) and that more fathers were highly stressed compared with mothers (50% vs 41%). Although this study was small and additional studies need to be performed, it does point out that all parents may experience significant levels of stress before, during, and after an adoption of a child. Health care professionals need to be aware of these potential issues when evaluating the successful integration of a new child into a family.

Finally, a parent's attachment style has been shown to be predictive of the type of relationship the parent develops with his or her children, as evidenced by Hesse and Main's studies used to develop the Adult Attachment Interview.[51] Parents with ambivalent, avoidant, anxious, or disorganized attachment styles are at greater risk of developing a non-securely patterned relationship with their children. These parents most likely will need professional assistance to build securely attached relationships with their child.

PSYCHOSOCIAL MODIFIERS

Few studies have examined how detrimental early life experiences affect a child's mental disorders. Zeanah et al[52] studied whether removing children from an adverse orphanage environment and transitioning them to foster care would decrease the chance of psychiatric illnesses. One-hundred thirty-six institutionalized children between the ages of 6 and 30 months were randomly assigned to ongoing institutional care or foster care after baseline assessments. Both of these groups were compared with a matched cohort of typical family-raised children recruited from Bucharest pediatric clinics. McLaughlin et al[53] examined attachment in these children at 30 months, 42 months, 54 months, and 8 years of age using the Disturbances of Attachment Interview. They showed that adverse attachment decreased after 30 months in foster care, back to levels equal to those children who were in home care. Children placed in foster care prior to 2 years of age exhibited fewer signs of disorganized attachment. Smyke et al[54] examined attachment disorders in the foster care group and noted that they had less inhibited types of RAD, while disinhibited attachment was effected to a lesser extent. Interestingly, children with lower cognitive functions had higher associations of RAD.[55]

Adverse Therapies

Caring for a child with attachment issues or problems can be very difficult for any family. The negative effects early life experiences may have on a child may be difficult to overcome and often require a tremendous amount of time and energy from everyone involved. Unfortunately, out of desperation, families may seek therapies that are controversial because they have not been shown to be effective or have led to injury or death. These therapies include licking therapy, holding therapy, regression therapy, rebirthing therapy, rage reduction, and heavy metal therapy.[56] These therapies should be avoided, and practitioners who are advising families should caution against their use.

Summary

A growing body of literature has evolved on the effect of early life experiences not only on a child's cognitive development but on how the child and family can form a secure and enduring relationship. We do know that there is a direct correlation between caregiver-child ratios, with the lower ratio in an attentive parent mitigating risk factors in the environment, emotionally and psychologically.[33] More information is being learned through new measures assessing attachment, and we now realize that attachment is a 2-way dance between caregivers and children. By understanding the mechanisms essential in developing healthy attachment relationships, we may better understand how to help children who experience adversity in early life and their new parents develop a positive relationship to successfully integrate an adopted child into a new family. Attachment between a parent and an adopted child requires patience and often guidance from well-trained professionals. As we learn more about the effect of adverse environments on a child as well as mediating factors, treatments can be designed to minimize these effects for the child and parent.

References

1. Bowlby J. *Attachment and Loss*. 2nd ed. Vol 1. New York, NY: Basic Books; 1982
2. Rutter M. Clinical implications of attachment concepts: retrospective and prospective. *J Child Psychol Psychiatry*. 1995;36(4):549–571
3. O'Connor TG, Rutter M. Attachment disorder behavior following early severe deprivation: extension and longitudinal follow-up. English and Romanian Adoptees Study Team. *J Am Acad Child Adolesc Psychiatry*. 2000;39(6):703–712
4. Hakimi-Manesh Y, Mojdehi H, Tashakkori A. Short communication: effects of environmental enrichment on the mental and psychomotor development of orphanage children. *J Child Psychol Psychiatry*. 1984;25(4):643–650
5. Tirella LG, Chan W, Cermak SA, Litvinova A, Salas KC, Miller LC. Time use in Russian baby homes. *Child Care Health Dev*. 2008;34(1):77–86
6. Sherwen LN, Smith DW, Cueman MA. Common concerns of adoptive mothers. *Pediatr Nurs*. 1984;10(2):127–130
7. Dozier M, Rutter M. Challenges to the development of attachment relationships faced by young children in foster and adoptive care. In: Cassidy J, Shaver PR. *Handbook of Attachment: Theory, Research and Clinical Applications*. 2nd ed. New York, NY: Guilford Press; 2008
8. Sagi A, Lamb MF, Lewkowicz KS, Shoham R, Dvir R, Fates D. Security of infant-mother, -father and -metapelet among kibbutz reared Israeli children. In: Bretherton I, Waters E, eds. *Growing Points of Attachment Theory and Research, Monographs of the Society for Research in Child Development*. 1985;50(1–2):257–275

9. Bowlby J. *A Secure Base: Parent-Child Attachment and Healthy Human Development.* London, United Kingdom: Basic Books; 1988

10. Bowlby J. *Marital Care and Mental Health.* Geneva, Switzerland: World Health Organization; 1946

11. Spitz RA. *Grief: A Peril in Infancy* [film]. Akron, OH: University of Akron Psychology Archives; 1947

12. Robertson J. *A Two-Year-Old Goes to the Hospital* [film]. London, United Kingdom: Tavistock Child Development Research Unit; 1952

13. Gribble K. Mental health, attachment and breastfeeding: implications for adopted children and their mothers. *Int Breastfeed J.* 2006;1:5

14. Konrad Lorenz, classical ethology, and imprinting. http://www.psychology.sunysb.edu/ewaters/552/PDF_Files/lorenz.pdf. Accessed February 13, 2014

15. Adoption History Project. Harry F. Harlow, monkey love experiments. http://darkwing.uoregon.edu/~adoption/studies/HarlowMLE.htm. Accessed February 13, 2014

16. Ames EW. *The Development of Romanian Orphanage Children Adopted To Canada.* Burnaby, British Columbia: Simon Fraser University; 1997

17. Morison SJ, Ames EW, Chisholm K. The development of children adopted from Romanian orphanages. *Merrill Palmer Q.* 1995;41(4):411–430

18. Chishom K. A three year follow-up of attachment and indiscriminate friendliness in children adopted from Romanian orphanages. *Child Dev.* 1988;69(4):1092–1106

19. O'Connor TG, Rutter M, Beckett C, Keaveney L, Kreppner JM. The effects of global severe privation on cognitive competence: extension and longitudinal follow-up. English and Romanian Adoptees Study Team. *Child Dev.* 2000;71(2):376–390

20. Rutter M. Developmental catch-up, and deficit, following adoption after severe global early privation. English and Romanian Adoptees Study Team. *J Child Psychol Psychiatry.* 1998;39(4):465–476

21. Robertson J, Bowlby J. A Two-Year-Old Goes to Hospital: a scientific film. *Proc R Soc Med.* 1952;46:425–427

22. Bowlby J. Separation anxiety. *Int J Psychoanal.* 1960;41(2–3):89–113

23. Bowlby J, Parkes CM. Separation and loss within the family. In: Anthony EJ, ed. *The Child in his Family.* New York, NY: J Wiley; 1970

24. Parke RD, Coltrane S, Buriel R, Dennis J, Powers J. Economic stress, parenting, and child adjustment in Mexican-American and European-American families. *Child Dev.* 2004;75(6):1632–1656

25. Ainsworth MDS. The development of infant-mother interactions among the Ganda. In: Foss BM, ed. *Determinants of Infant Behavior.* New York, NY: Wiley; 1963:67–104

26. Ainsworth MDS. *Infancy in Uganda: Infant Care and the Growth of Love.* Baltimore, MD: Johns Hopkins University Press; 1967

27. Ainsworth MDS. Attachment theory and its utility in cross-cultural research. In: Leiderman PH, Tulkin SE, Rosenfeld A, eds. *Culture and Infancy.* New York, NY: Academic Press; 1978:49–67

28. Ainsworth MDS. Attachment: retrospect and prospect. In: Parkes CM, Stevenson-Hinde J, eds. *The Place of Attachment in Human Behavior.* New York, NY: Basic Books; 1982

29. Ainsworth MDS. Mary D. Salter Ainsworth. In: O'Connell AN, Russo NF, eds. *Models of Achievement: Reflections of Prominent Women in Psychology.* New York, NY: Columbia University Press; 1983:201–219

30. Attachment–Caregiving & the Circle of Security: Part I: Child Patterns: Identifying Children's Healthy and High Risk Attachment Behaviors: An Evidence-Based Clinical Training Course. Presented by faculty of the Mary D. Ainsworth Child-Parent Attachment Clinic, University of Virginia School of Medicine, 2006

31. Cooper G, Hoffman K, Marvin R, Powell B. The Circle of Security project: attachment-based intervention with caregiver-pre-school child dyads. *Attach Hum Dev.* 2002;4(1):107–124

32. Boris NW, Zeanah CH. Clinical disturbances of attachment in infancy and early childhood. *Curr Opin Pediatr.* 1998;10(4):365–368

33. Zeanah CH, Boris NW, Larrieu JA. Infant development and developmental risk: a review of the past years. *J Am Acad Child Adolesc Psychiatry.* 1997;36(2):165–178

34. Cassidy JSP. *Handbook of Attachment: Theory, Research and Clinical Applications.* New York, NY: The Guilford Press; 1999:21

35. Pilowsky D, Kates W. Foster children in acute crisis: assessing critical aspects of attachment. *J Am Acad Adolesc Psychiatry.* 1996;35(8):1095–1097

36. Vorria P, Rutter M, Pickles A, Wolkind S, Hobsbaum A. A comparative study of Greek children in long-term residential group care and in two-parent families: I. Social, emotional and behavioural differences. *J Child Psychol Psychiatry.* 1998;39(2):225–236

37. Smyke A, Dumitrescu A, Zeanah C. Attachment disturbances in young children. I. The continuum of caretaking causality. *J Am Acad Child Adolesc Psychiatry.* 2002;41(8):972–982

38. Carlson E, Sampson M, Sroufe L. Implications of attachment theory and research for development-behavioral pediatrics. *J Dev Behav Pediatr.* 2003;24(5):364–379

39. Windridge K, Berryman J. Women's experiences of giving birth after 35. *Birth.* 1999;26(1):16–23

40. Mercer R, Ferketich S. Maternal-infant attachment of experienced and inexperienced mothers during infancy. *Nurs Res.* 1994;43(6):344–351

41. Dowdney L, Skuse D, Rutter M, Quinton D, Mrazek D. The nature and qualities of parenting provided by women raised in institutions. *J Child Psychol Psychiatry.* 1985;26(4):599–625

42. Quinton D, Rutter M, Liddle C. Institutional rearing, parenting difficulties and marital support. *Psychol Med.* 1984;14(1):107–124

43. Rutter M, Quinton D. Long-term follow-up of women institutionalized in childhood: factors promoting good functioning in adult life. *Br J Dev Psychol.* 1984;2(3):191–204

44. Chaffin M, Hanson R, Saunders BE, et al. Report of the APSAC task force on attachment therapy, reactive attachment disorder, and attachment problems. *Child Maltreat.* 2006;11(1):76–89

45. Black C, Zeanah CH. Reactive attachment disorder and disinhibited social engagement disorder. In: Cautin R, Lilienfeld S, eds. *The Encyclopedia of Clinical Psychology.* Hoboken, NJ: Wiley-Blackwell. In press

46. Zeanah CH. Disturbances of attachment in young children adopted from institutions. *J Dev Behav Pediatr.* 2000;21(3):230–236

47. Shmueli-Goetz Y, Target M, Fonagy P, Datta A. The Child Attachment Interview: a psychometric study of reliability and discriminant validity. *Dev Psychol.* 2008;44(4):939–956

48. Foli KJ, Thompson JR. *The Post-Adoption Blues: Overcoming the Unforeseen Challenges of Adoption.* Emmaus, PA: Rodale; 2004

49. Senecky Y, Agassi H, Inbar D, et al. Post-adoption depression among adoptive mothers. *J Affect Disord.* 2009;115(1–2):62–68

50. Narad C, Mason P. Parental Stress with International Adoption. Presented at American Academy of Pediatrics National Conference & Exhibition, Washington DC, October 2009

51. Hesse E, Main M. Disorganized infant, child and adult attachment: collapse in behavioral and attentional strategies. *J Am Psychoanal Assoc.* 2000;48(4):1097–1127

52. Zeanah C, Egger H, Smyke A, et al. Institutional rearing and psychiatric disorders in Romanian preschool children. *Am J Psychiatry.* 2009;166(7):777–785

53. McLaughlin K, Zeanah CH, Fox N, Nelson C. Attachment security as a mechanism linking foster care placement to improved mental health outcomes in previously institutionalized children. *J Child Psychol Psychiatry.* 2012;53(1):46–55

54. Smyke AT, Zeanah CH, Gleason MM, et al. A randomized controlled trial comparing foster care and institutional care for children with signs of reactive attachment disorder. *Am J Psychiatry.* 2012;169(5):508–514

55. McDermott JM, Westerlund A, Zeanah CH, Nelson CA, Fox NA. Early adversity and neural correlates of executive function: implications for academic adjustment. *Dev Cogn Neurosci.* 2012;2 (Suppl 1):S59–S66

56. O'Connor TG, Zeanah CH. Attachment disorders: assessment strategies and treatment approaches. *Attach Hum Dev.* 2003;5(3):223–244

CHAPTER 14

Speech and Language Outcomes After International Adoption

Sharon Glennen, PhD, CCC–SLP

The evidence is clear that early development in deprived environments is detrimental to cognitive and language development.[1-7] Although orphanages vary widely in the quality of care provided to children, almost all have a lack of consistency in caregivers, most do not provide adequate communicative or cognitive stimulation, and many are unable to provide children with proper nutrition or medical care.[2,4,8,9] The result is children with neurologic differences that affect physical growth,[2,4,9] social-emotional abilities,[7,9,10] cognition,[1,5,6] and ultimately language and speech development.[3,11,12] When children are adopted from orphanages, most arrive home with mild delays in cognition and language. This finding is consistent in children adopted from Eastern Europe,[3,6] China,[13,14] and Guatemala.[15] Children adopted from abroad out of foster care typically arrive home with fewer developmental delays[15]; however, foster care in other countries varies widely in quality, especially in terms of environmental stimulation and caregiver interactions.

When children are adopted, their environment changes from language deprived to language enriched. Most families who adopt internationally are better educated and earn higher incomes than the general population.[16,17] Children raised in families with these characteristics consistently score higher than peers on tests of vocabulary and academic ability.[18,19] The question is whether the stimuli and nurturance offered by adoptive families can fully counteract the effects of early deprivation, especially in the area of language development. Information from the Bucharest Early Intervention Project (BEIP) Core Group in Romania indicates that an enriched environment with consistent caregivers is a powerful intervention for children with developmental language delays.[12,20] The BEIP compared children who remained in orphanage care to children who were moved from orphanages into foster care and to children in the community who lived with their families. At age 30 months, children who remained in orphanage care had poor language abilities across all measures.[12] Children who recently moved into foster care did slightly better, and children who lived in foster care for more than 12 months had language abilities equal to non-adopted children in the surrounding community. However, other factors also affected language outcomes in these children. Children who moved into foster care at younger ages had better language outcomes than children who moved into foster care at older ages.[21] Thus, adoption into an enriched home provides a significant boost toward overcoming the effect of early environmental deprivation, but the rebound is less pronounced for children adopted at older ages.

The detrimental effect of orphanage care is not the only factor affecting language and speech development in children who are internationally adopted. Children who are adopted from one country to another must also switch languages. At adoption, most children have mild delays in the birth language, then abruptly start over in the language of their adopted country.[3] The transition from one language to another, coupled with developmental delays in the birth language, puts newly adopted children behind in the language-learning process. This language gap widens with the age of adoption. Children adopted at young ages have a relatively small gap to bridge and make the language transition quickly.[22–24] In contrast, children adopted from abroad as preschoolers or at school age have wider gaps to bridge and thus need more time to achieve proficiency in the adopted language.[25]

The transition from one language to another makes it difficult to assess language and speech development in children who were internationally adopted.[22,26] A common misconception is to categorize internationally adopted children as bilingual and attribute all language and speech delays to bilingual language-learning patterns.[23,25,26] However, internationally adopted children are only bilingual for a brief period after adoption.[26,27] Most adoptive families do not speak the birth language and without consistent input, it quickly disappears. Anecdotal evidence suggests this occurs within 4 to 8 months of adoption for most children.[27] Once the birth language disappears, the child's only remaining language is the new adopted language, which is far from proficient. The result is a period when the internationally adopted child lacks proficiency in any language.[26] Children adopted at younger ages have enough time to work through this period and fully learn their new language before school begins.[22,24] However, children adopted at older ages need more time to bridge the language gap and often begin school before they are proficient.[25,27] Children adopted at older ages are at risk of falling behind in school if they lack language proficiency when they begin.

Thus, parents and professionals need to understand typical patterns of language learning during the transition period to identify children who are not making sufficient progress toward learning the new language. This chapter will review typical patterns of speech and language development in children who are adopted internationally. Because language-learning patterns vary with age of adoption, information has been divided into 3 sections: children adopted before age 2 years, children adopted at preschool ages (3 to 5 years), and children adopted at school ages (5 years and older). Each section includes guidelines for assessing language and speech in newly adopted children, criteria for determining who is at risk, and information about speech-language therapy options.

Children Adopted Before Age 2 Years

The majority of infants and toddlers adopted from abroad rapidly learn their new adopted language.[11,13,22] Typical patterns of language development in children adopted at this age are well documented, leading to clear guidelines for who is developing normally and who needs to be referred for early intervention (EI).[11,22] This section will discuss recommended language and speech assessment practices for newly arrived children and guidelines for referring infants and toddlers for speech and language intervention. Typical patterns of language development through the early school years will be reviewed, along with information about speech and language disorders in children who are internationally adopted.

Infants and Toddlers: The First Few Months Home

Most internationally adopted infants and toddlers raised in orphanage settings arrive home with low-average delays in language and speech. This is true for children adopted from China,[3-14] Eastern Europe,[3] and Guatemala[15] and likely holds true for children adopted from other countries. Children raised in international foster care are also at risk for these delays but not as frequently, nor to the same degree, as those raised in orphanages.[15] Children adopted at younger than 2 years who arrive home with more than mild delays in language or cognition are not typical and should immediately be referred for EI.[3,22]

Newly adopted infants and toddlers can validly be assessed using pre-linguistic measures of language and speech.[22] These include measures of social-communicative abilities (ie, eye contact, frequency of communication, and intent of communication), use of gestures, complexity of expressive vocalizations (ie, frequency of vocalizing, type of vocalizations, number of consonant sounds, and phonetic complexity and variety of vocalizations), and symbolic play (ie, developmental levels of play with everyday objects such as spoons, cups, and dolls) (Box 14-1). The benefit of using pre-linguistic measures is that they develop continuously across languages and are relatively similar across cultures. Infant/toddler assessment measures that evaluate such skills can be used with confidence to determine which children are developing typically and which are at risk.

Several researchers have used the Communication and Symbolic Behavior Scales Developmental Profile (CSBS-DP)[28] to assess newly arrived infants and toddlers.[3,13,22] The CSBS-DP assesses pre-linguistic abilities and has well-developed norms. As a group, newly arrived internationally adopted children from Eastern

Box 14-1. Language and Speech Assessment for Newly Arrived Internationally Adopted Infants and Toddlers

Pre-linguistic Communication Abilities	When to Refer for Speech-Language Intervention
• Social communicative abilities — Eye contact — Frequency of communication — Intent of communication (ie, attention, request, protest, comment)	Social communication should be normal for the child's age. Refer any child with poor eye contact or who infrequently attempts to communicate to others.
• Use of gestures — Variety of gestures — Gestures combined with vocalizations — Gestures combined with gaze shifts (from object to person and back) — Complexity of gestures (single vs combination gestures)	Use of gestures for communication should be low-average to average for the child's age. Refer any child with mild or greater delays in gestural communication.
• Vocalizations — Frequency of vocalizations — Vocalizations used to communicate — Variety of vocalizations (ie, number of syllables, repeating versus non-repeating syllables and sounds) — Sound inventory (consonants heard within vocalizations) — Production of first words (for children adopted after age 16 months)	Some newly adopted children may be unusually quiet. In secure play-based settings, the child should begin to vocalize. With the exception of expressing words, vocalization abilities should be low-average or better for the child's age.
• Symbolic play — Developmental level of play (ie, banging vs true symbolic) — Variety of play (ie, variety of objects used and actions performed) — Use of combinations in play (eg, pouring into a cup, then drinking from it)	Symbolic play should be low-average to average for the child's age. Refer any child with mild or greater delays in symbolic play abilities.

Comprehension Abilities in the Adopted Language	
• Early comprehension after 3 months home — Comprehension of simple commands and first words — Developmental quotient score for word comprehension on the MacArthur-Bates Communicative Development Inventory (CDI): Words and Gestures	Children adopted after age 12 months should quickly show signs of comprehending the new language. Refer any child who is not rapidly developing these skills. CDI developmental quotient for word comprehension should be 47 or higher (see page 287). Refer any child who falls below this threshold.

Europe averaged scores of 88 on the CSBS-DP, which was below the expected average of 100 but still within normal limits.[3] Children adopted from China scored similarly on the same measure.[13] One year later, children with scores of 80 or higher were doing well; those with scores of lower than 80 were not.[22] Note that a standard score of 80 is the recommended CSBS-DP test criteria for referring any child to EI. In summary, newly arrived internationally adopted infants and toddlers tend to score in the low-average range on measures of pre-linguistic language abilities. Those who score in the mildly delayed range or lower (standard scores <80) are at risk and should be referred for speech and language intervention.

Measures of pre-linguistic language and speech are reliable indicators for predicting future language and speech development in newly adopted children.[3,13,22] In addition, for children adopted after age 12 months, early measures of vocabulary comprehension in the new language are highly predictive of future language growth. In contrast, early measures of expressive vocabulary production are not.[22] Because the development of comprehension usually precedes expression, it provides a better measure of the rate of early language learning in the first few months home. Children who acquire the adopted language at a faster rate tend to make the language transition quickly and do well over time. Those who learn at a slower rate lag behind their peers when tested at older ages.[22,23]

Vocabulary comprehension checklists such as the MacArthur-Bates Communicative Development Inventory (CDI): Words and Gestures (CDI-WG)[29] can be given to parents to measure these abilities. However, because newly adopted children are in the process of learning the new language, standard norms for these measures cannot be used. Instead, vocabulary comprehension scores can be converted to developmental quotient (DQ) scores.[22,23] The number of vocabulary words understood is matched to the 50th-percentile age equivalent using test norms. The age-equivalent score is then converted to DQ using the following formula: DQ = developmental age/chronologic age × 100. For example, a 17-month-old child who comprehended 64 words is at the 12-month 50th-percentile CDI-WG median. The child's DQ would equal 12/17 × 100 or 70.6. Children doing better than expected for their chronologic age would have DQs above 100. Scores below 100 reflect the gap between the child's chronologic age and expected language proficiency, with lower numbers indicating a larger gap. Glennen[22] determined that newly adopted children from Eastern Europe who were home fewer than 4 months averaged English vocabulary comprehension DQ scores of 59. A score of 47 marked the cutoff for the bottom 20th percentile for the peer group. One year later, children whose DQ scores were below 47 were significantly behind their adopted peers when language and speech were assessed. In contrast, those with higher DQ scores were doing well.

In summary, newly adopted children should arrive home with low-average delays in pre-linguistic abilities such as vocalizations, gestures, social interaction, and symbolic play.[3,13] Children with more than mild delays or who are not developing typically should be referred for speech and language intervention. In addition, children aged 12 months and older should quickly learn to comprehend vocabulary in the new language.[3,22] Children who are not rapidly learning to understand new words are at risk and should be referred for EI. In contrast, measures of vocabulary production are not useful for assessing children within the first few months home.[22] When using these pre-linguistic and vocabulary comprehension measures as indicators, Glennen[22] determined that 22% of newly adopted Eastern European children were at risk for language and speech delays and required EI.

Speech-language therapy services can be obtained through private therapists or referrals to area programs for infants and toddlers with disabilities. These programs are federally funded and provide EI services to children younger than 3 years with identified developmental delays.[30,31] Working within federal guidelines, each state sets its own criteria for who qualifies for services.[30] In addition, states can elect to provide services to children who are at risk for developmental delay for biological or environmental reasons.[30] Differences in state criteria mean that children who are internationally adopted easily qualify for infant and toddler services in some states and have difficulty qualifying in others. For example, Hawaii only requires a "team consensus" to qualify for services and works with children who are at risk. In contrast, Arizona requires a 50% or moderate to severe delay in one or more developmental areas to qualify for services and does not serve children who are at risk.[30] Internationally adopted children with mild delays in language or speech would not qualify for infant and toddler services under Arizona guidelines but would qualify in Hawaii.

Children Adopted Before Age 2 Years: The First Year Home

During the first year home, children adopted from abroad as infants and toddlers rapidly make the change from one language to another. Comprehension and articulation of the new language reach age-proficient levels first.[22] One year after adoption, a group of children adopted from Eastern Europe had average English receptive language standard scores of 105 (English normed test average = 100) (Figure 14-1). Only 8% of the children had receptive language standard scores below 80. Similarly, articulation test scores averaged 99 for the same children, with 12% scoring below 80 on standardized articulation measures. After one year home, children adopted before 24 months of age with mild or greater delays in language comprehension or articulation are not progressing typically and should be referred for speech and language intervention.[22]

In the same study of children adopted from Eastern Europe,[22] standard scores from tests of expressive language averaged 94 after one year home, with 15% of the children scoring below 80 (English normed test average = 100) (Figure 14-1). Most professionals recommend using a standard score of 80 as the cutoff criteria for

Figure 14-1.
Language Development in Children Adopted Internationally
Between 12 and 24 Months of Age

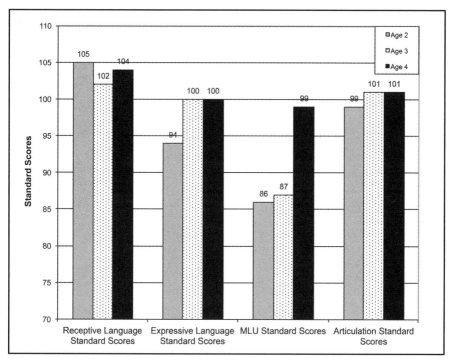

Abbreviation: MLU, mean length of utterance.

speech and language intervention.[32,33] After one year home, children are still in the process of catching up to full expressive language proficiency. However, standardized tests of expressive language can be used to determine which children who were internationally adopted are progressing more slowly. Those who score below 80 are in need of intervention.[22,23]

Two other indicators of expressive language development are vocabulary growth and mean length of utterance (MLU), a measure of sentence length and complexity. Similar to the findings of previous studies,[11,34,35] expressive vocabulary develops rapidly but is not fully emerged to chronologic age expectations after one year home. Communicative Development Inventory: Words and Sentences DQ scores for expressive vocabulary increased from an average of 59 when the children were newly adopted to 81 one year later.[22] As described previously, DQ scores are a measure of the gap between the child's developmental level and chronologic age. A score of 100 indicates that the gap has closed and the child has developmentally "caught up." The fact that scores improved from 59 to 81 indicates that internationally adopted children make rapid strides in vocabulary development during the first year home but not to fully proficient levels. Similarly, MLU was also not fully proficient after one year.[22] Mean length of utterance is a measure of how many words and grammatical endings children use in their sentences. For example, "The doggy's running" would have an MLU of 5 (the + dog + is + run + ing). After one year home, children adopted from Eastern Europe had average MLU standard score equivalents of 84.[22] Like DQ scores, these MLU scores are a measure of the gap between the child's abilities and chronologic age expectations. After one year home, 25 of 27 children (95%) had average MLUs of 2.9 or lower, indicating they were producing English-language utterances that were less complex than expected for their age.[22]

Expressive vocabulary and grammar continue to lag behind 1 year after adoption. Therefore, these 2 components of language cannot be assessed using standard test norms within the first year home.[22,23] However, local norms are available for these 2 measures; they are developed from peer groups of children who were adopted internationally. Using parent survey methods, Glennen and Masters[11] tracked expressive vocabulary development and MLU in children adopted before age 12 months and children adopted between 12 and 24 months of age. Mean length of utterance measures were based on parent reports of the children's 3 longest utterances. These peer norms are listed in tables 14-1 and 14-2. Children who fall below these ranges are progressing more slowly than their internationally adopted peers in expressive language development and should be referred for speech and language services.

In summary, within a year of arrival, children adopted before 24 months of age fully transition between birth and adopted languages in the areas of comprehension and articulation.[22] Any child who has mild or greater delays in these 2 areas

Table 14-1. Expressive Vocabulary Development for Internationally Adopted Children by Age of Adoption

Current Age (Mo)	Adopted 0–12 Mo		Adopted 13–18 Mo		Adopted 19–24 Mo		Adopted 25–30 Mo	
	Average Words	Referral Criteria	Average Words	Referral Criteria	Average Words	Referral Criteria	Average Words	Referral Criteria
15	7	–						
18	34	>2	16	–				
24	116	>40	67	>8	20	–		
30	214	>124	175	>45	132	>51	42	>6
36	272	>221	229	>157	209	>122	181	>111
40			268	>151	251	>184	237	>173

Children who fall below the referral criteria should be referred for speech and language services.

From Glennen S, Masters MG. Typical and atypical language development in infants and toddlers adopted from Eastern Europe. *Am J Speech Lang Pathol.* 2002;11:417–433 should be considered to have a true delay in speech, language, or both and should be referred for speech and language services. One year after adoption, expressive language is not fully proficient; however, children with more than mild delays are not typical and should be referred for speech and language services.[22]

Table 14-2. Expressive Sentence Length (Mean Length of Utterance Average for the 3 Longest Utterances) for Internationally Adopted Children by Age of Adoption

Current Age (Mo)	Adopted 0–12 Mo		Adopted 13–18 Mo		Adopted 19–24 Mo		Adopted 25–30 Mo	
	Average Words	Referral Criteria	Average Words	Referral Criteria	Average Words	Referral Criteria	Average Words	Referral Criteria
18	1.1	–						
24	2.6	>1.0	1.6	>1.0				
30	5.9	>2.4	2.8	>1.0	2.1	>1.0	1.7	>1.0
36	9.5	>6.1	4.8	>3.5	5.5	>5.0	3.8	>1.8
40			9.5	>6.3	5.9	>5.1	5.9	>3.9

Children who fall below the referral criteria should be referred for speech and language services.

From Glennen S, Masters MG. Typical and atypical language development in infants and toddlers adopted from Eastern Europe. *Am J Speech Lang Pathol.* 2002;11:417–433

CASE DISCUSSION: IRINA

The Higgins family adopted Irina from Russia at the age of 18 months. At the orphanage, she was resistant to interacting with her adoptive parents; however, the Higgins observed that she made good eye contact with her caregivers, enjoyed socializing with them, and used gestures such as pointing, showing, and sharing. She also said "no-no" several times while shaking her head. She was below the 10th percentile for weight and height, but other developmental milestones appeared to be normal for her age. During the first few months home she blossomed, gaining weight and becoming increasingly sociable. Within 2 weeks of adoption, she understood a few simple phrases in English. Her comprehension quickly grew by leaps and bounds. However, by her second birthday, she was only speaking 4 words. Her worried parents contacted early intervention to have her speech and language assessed.

The speech-language pathologist visited Irina at home and observed her playing. Irina played appropriately for her developmental level and clearly understood simple commands and words in English. She was content to communicate with gestures and head nods. Irina ate a snack and was observed to have good oral motor abilities. Her parents were asked to complete a vocabulary checklist that confirmed she was only saying 8 to 10 words; however, it also indicated that her play and gestural communication skills were normal. Finally,

CASE DISCUSSION: IRINA, CONTINUED

Irina was given a standardized test to assess receptive and expressive language. She scored a 93 on the receptive language scale, which was remarkable considering that she had only been learning English for 6 months. Expressive language was not as strong, with a standard score of 72.

The speech-language pathologist was familiar with language learning patterns of children who were internationally adopted and explained that during the initial months of language learning, receptive language was the key. The fact that Irina was making rapid progress in language comprehension was a good prognostic sign. If she wasn't talking at all, the speech-language pathologist would be concerned; however, Irina did have a small vocabulary that she used regularly. Although her lack of expressive language was a concern, there were no signs of oral motor weakness, lack of sociability, or other developmental evidence to explain her slow start. It was noted that when her parents played with her, they used long sentences that described past and future events. The speech-language pathologist demonstrated better language modeling techniques and recommended a follow-up visit in 3 months.

Three months later, Irina was communicating regularly in 2-word sentences. When her parents filled out the vocabulary inventory, they indicated she was producing 89 words. The speech-language pathologist told the family that Irina was developing normally for an internationally adopted child and did not recommend further follow-up. By age 3, Irina was fully caught up to English language expectations and continued to do well as she grew through her preschool years.

CASE DISCUSSION: ROBERTO

Roberto was the first child for the Devoe family. He was adopted from Guatemala at the age of 10 months after living in foster care for 4 months. It was unclear where he was living prior to 6 months of age. After bringing him home, the Devoes noticed that he didn't smile or vocalize like other babies and wasn't especially fussy when left alone. By age 14 months, he was walking but didn't speak or understand any English words. His parents simply thought he had an introspective, quiet personality. At a reunion picnic for children adopted from Guatemala, his parents noticed that other adopted toddlers were already understanding and using English words. After conferring with their pediatrician, they set up an appointment with a speech-language pathologist connected with an international adoption team at a nearby children's hospital.

As part of the speech-language pathology assessment, Roberto's parents completed a vocabulary inventory and developmental checklist. These measures confirmed that Roberto understood a few simple commands and words, was not talking, and was delayed in his use of gestures and play abilities. The speech-

CASE DISCUSSION: ROBERTO, CONTINUED

language pathologist then gave a standardized infant-toddler language assessment to directly assess communication abilities. During the test, Roberto made good eye contact with his parents and smiled at them but rarely added gestures or vocalizations to his interactions. He did not understand simple commands, and his symbolic play abilities were delayed. When observed eating and drinking, his oral motor skills appeared normal.

The speech-language pathologist was concerned because Roberto had mild to moderate delays in pre-linguistic communication abilities, which should not be affected by adoption language change. In addition, he was not making rapid progress in learning English. A developmental quotient based on vocabulary comprehension scores indicated that Roberto fell far below age expectations for similarly adopted children. During the assessment, the speech-language pathologist observed that Roberto did not consistently alert or turn toward noises in the environment. The pathologist tested his middle ear status and discovered that both ears were filled with fluid. Roberto's parents stated that he had had multiple colds and ear infections since coming home.

The speech-language pathologist referred Roberto to other team members at the children's hospital to obtain more information about his hearing and developmental abilities. The physical and occupational therapists determined that his gross and fine motor skills were developmentally appropriate. A child psychologist determined that he had low-average to mild delays in most areas and moderate to severe delays in language. Most important, the audiologist determined that Roberto had a moderate sensory neural hearing loss in both ears along with abnormal middle ear pressure. The combination of these 2 sources of hearing loss was a likely factor explaining Roberto's speech and language delays.

During the next month, pressure-equalizing tubes were inserted in both ears to minimize the potential for conductive hearing loss. He was fitted with bilateral hearing aids and referred for early intervention speech and language services from his local infant-toddler program. At age 24 months, Roberto returned to the children's hospital for follow-up visits with the audiologist and speech-language pathologist. His parents reported that he was starting to talk and was more vocal and interactive than before. In addition, he comprehended more than 100 words and many simple commands. His speech and language were still mild to moderately delayed when compared with other internationally adopted children; however, his rate of progress had improved. Although the long-term prognosis was unclear, he was finally headed in the right direction.

Children Adopted Before Age 2 Years: The Preschool Years

Children adopted from abroad at young ages complete the language transition process as preschoolers.[23,24] As discussed in the previous section, language comprehension and articulation catch up after 1 year home. Young children adopted from Eastern Europe had perfectly average receptive language and articulation test scores by age 2, and no further gains were made at ages 3 and 4[23] (Figure 14-1). In contrast, expressive language does not reach full proficiency until age 4.[23] Standard scores on general expressive language tests averaged 94 at age 2, improved to 100 by age 3, and remained at 100 through age 4. However, MLU did not reach age expectations until age 4. Standard score equivalents for MLU averaged 86 at age 2, 87 at age 3, and 99 at age 4. This indicates that the grammatical elements of expressive language take the longest to reach full proficiency. However, a study of the sequence of learning English language morphologic (grammar) elements determined that internationally adopted children learn them in the same sequence as children who learn English from birth.[36] Speech-language pathologists can use this developmental information to track children as they progress through the final stages of reaching full proficiency in the adopted language.

By age 4, children who were internationally adopted before age 2 have abilities that are equal to their non-adopted peers on all tests of language and articulation. This was true for children adopted from China[24] and Eastern Europe.[23,37] Average English-language test scores were well within expected levels by age 4, with several children scoring in the above-average range. Glennen[37] determined that by age 4, 15% of children adopted from Eastern Europe had at least one score on tests of speech and language that qualified for intervention services. These 4-year-olds were not a homogeneous group and had a variety of diagnoses ranging from mild articulation disorders to severe autism spectrum disorder. Using more conservative criteria of 2 or more below-average test scores, Roberts et al[24] determined that 5% of preschool children adopted from China were in need of speech and language services. If the same criteria were used for the Eastern European children studied by Glennen,[37] 4% would qualify for speech and language services. In summary, children adopted before 24 months of age should be fully proficient in their new adopted language by age 4. Any noted delays or differences in speech or language are real, and those children should be referred for services.

Children Adopted Before Age 2 Years: School Age

When children reach school age, they apply their spoken language abilities to the process of reading and writing. Evidence of how well internationally adopted children make this transition is contradictory.[38,39] Some research indicates that internationally adopted children with normal language abilities in the preschool years struggle with the increased literacy demands of language in the upper grades.[40-42] However, evidence from other studies indicates that internationally adopted children with normal language in the preschool years continue to do well when they reach school age.[39] The results of these and other studies are mixed, and there is no clear consensus on the issue at this time.[38]

Initial parent and teacher surveys on language in school-aged children found that internationally adopted children from countries with poor health care systems had worse academic language than non-adopted children.[41] Based on surveys, children adopted from countries such as Romania and Russia were more likely to be diagnosed with speech and language disorders when they reached school age.[40] In contrast, children adopted from countries like South Korea, with good health care and economic resources, had equal, if not better, academic language abilities than non-adopted children.[41] However, more recent information based on direct speech and language assessments has not supported these findings. The majority of children adopted at young ages from China[39] and Romania[43] had average to above-average levels on language and literacy measures when they reached school age. Similarly, Glennen and Bright[44] used the Children's Communication Checklist—2,[45] a standardized parent report measure, to assess speech and language in school-aged children adopted from Eastern Europe. Average scores on all subtests were well within normal limits; however, parents reported that 27% of the same children were receiving speech and language intervention. Indeed, various parent surveys indicate that as many as 47% of internationally adopted children receive speech and language services in school.[40] This discrepancy between reported versus confirmed school-age speech and language issues occurs frequently in the literature, with more children receiving services than actual test scores would predict.[43,44]

It is highly likely that academic difficulties that suddenly emerge when children reach school are not caused by isolated speech or language disorders but are instead the result of other underlying disorders or learning differences. For example, a high percentage of internationally adopted children from Eastern Europe are diagnosed with attention-deficit/hyperactivity disorder (ADHD).[40,44] Glennen and Bright[44] noted that school-aged children adopted from those countries scored lowest on measures of pragmatic, nonverbal, and figurative language. These weaknesses are strikingly characteristic of descriptions of language abilities in children with ADHD.[46] However, although the children scored lowest on these particular test items, they still scored well within the average range. Another factor may be related to the difficulty of testing preschool children. Language abilities that require executive functions such as abstract thinking, sequencing, inferring, comparing, narrating, analyzing, and synthesizing cannot be fully evaluated until school age, when children have the attention span and developmental ability to complete lengthy, complex tasks. Subtle language weaknesses may have been present during the preschool years but did not show up on assessments until the children were older.

In summary, by school age, the evidence is mixed as to the prevalence, type, and cause of speech and language disorders in children adopted at young ages. Speech and language weaknesses during the preschool years often reappear as language literacy weaknesses in school. As previously noted, however, only 5% to 15% of children adopted internationally before 24 months of age had speech or language delays as preschoolers.[23,24] These data do not explain the large numbers of internationally adopted children receiving speech and language services in school. When language literacy weaknesses suddenly emerge in school without a prior history of speech or language delay in preschool, they are likely a symptom of other related causes such as ADHD or executive function disorders. In either case, children experiencing these problems should be referred for a complete neuropsychologic assessment, including an assessment of academic achievement. In addition, they should be seen for a complete speech, language, and hearing evaluation. A complete profile of strengths and weaknesses will aid professionals in developing strategies to help internationally adopted children reach their full language literacy potential.

Children Adopted at Preschool Ages (3 to 5 Years)

Growing up in an orphanage or environmentally deprived setting is a recipe for speech and language delays. Studies and anecdotal reports of preschool children living in orphanages consistently document mild to moderate delays in all aspects of language and speech.[2,4,8,12] Children adopted from abroad at preschool ages will likely have delays in birth language when they first arrive home. These children also have more to learn to rapidly reach proficiency in the new adopted language. Finally, they often begin attending school before the language transition is complete. Unfortunately, language abilities of children adopted from abroad at older ages have not been studied as thoroughly as abilities of children adopted at younger ages. Evidence-based studies tend to group older children with younger children[24,40] or examine academic or cognitive abilities associated with speech and language that are not complete measures of these domains.[5,6,43] Therefore, unlike the preceding section on younger adopted children, this section includes less evidence-based information.

Children Adopted at Preschool Ages: Before Adoption

Parents who are adopting older children from abroad need to collect information about the child's speech and language development from the birth country. Some countries have speech and language professionals who assess and treat children in orphanages.[4,8] Others have doctors, teachers, or others who can provide relevant information. If formal assessment reports are available, parents should request copies of them to bring home. If the child has never been formally assessed, parents should take time to ask caregivers questions about the child's speech and language abilities. Box 14-2 lists questions that can be used to obtain this information. In addition, parents should collect a videotaped language sample of the child conversing with a familiar adult in the birth language. The sample should preferably be

Box 14-2. Language and Speech Development in Children Adopted at Older Ages: Pre-adoption Questions for Orphanage Staff and Caregivers

Expressive Language
- Is the child speaking appropriately for his or her age?
  - — If not, ask for an estimate of the age level of the child's language.
  - — If not, ask what makes the child's speech seem delayed.
- How many words does the child put together in his or her longest sentences?
  - — Ask for translated examples of the child's 5 longest sentences.
- Is the child using grammatical markers such as plurals, verb tenses, or others?
  - — Get a list of the grammatical markers the child is able to use.
- Does the child make grammatical errors in sentences? For example, does the child say the equivalent of "Them is nice"?
  - — If yes, get descriptions of the errors and examples.
- Does the child's vocabulary seem age appropriate?
  - — Ask for examples of advanced words that the child uses.

Receptive Language
- Does the staff know or think the child has a hearing loss?
- Does the child understand language appropriate for his or her age?
  - — If not, ask for an age estimate of the child's comprehension abilities.
- What types of questions or commands does the child understand?
- What types of questions or commands are difficult for the child to understand?
- Does the child need gestures or frequent repetitions of information to understand what to do?

Social Interaction
- Does the child enjoy interacting with familiar adults or children?
- Does the child make eye contact when interacting with others?
- Does the child prefer to play alone or with others?
- When playing with other children, does the child share and play appropriately?
- How friendly or shy is the child?
- Does the child engage in pretend play?
  - — If yes, get examples of the types of pretend play the child enjoys.
- Is the child's pretend play based on everyday life (eg, pretending to cook), community life (eg, pretending to be a firefighter), or fantasy (eg, pretending to be a space alien or princess)?
- Does the child engage in constructive play (eg, building with blocks, coloring, puzzles)?

Articulation Pronunciation
- Does the child pronounce words at an age-appropriate level?
  - — If not, ask for an age estimate of the child's pronunciation level.
- Ask for a list of sounds the child has difficulty pronouncing.
- For each sound that is not pronounced correctly, ask for an example of a word that the child mispronounces. Try to phonetically spell the correct pronunciation and the child's errors.
- Does the child have any difficulty chewing or swallowing food?
  - — If yes, ask for descriptions of the problem.

videotaped when the child is in a comfortable play setting. If possible, tell the adult to refrain from asking the child questions because they lead to short answers. The goal is to videotape examples of the child's best sentences.

Except in conditions of severe deprivation, the majority of children will have mild developmental delays in speech and language in the birth country. Moderate to severe delays are not typical.[25] Any child identified with a moderate to severe delay should be considered at risk and referred for speech and language therapy services soon after arriving home.[25] Documentation of speech and language delays from the birth country is needed to immediately qualify the child for services after arriving home. If needed, the videotaped language sample should be reviewed by a speech-language pathologist or other developmental specialist who speaks the birth language. Assessment of the language sample can provide further evidence of an existing speech or language delay at the time of adoption.

Children Adopted at Preschool Ages: The First Year Home

Most children adopted between 3 and 5 years of age rapidly learn their new adopted language. Within 3 months of arrival, 80% of newly adopted 3- and 4-year-olds were producing more than 100 English-language words, with a few children producing as many as 300 words.[47] Newly adopted preschool children who are not learning new vocabulary at a rapid rate are not typical and should be referred for intervention. Comprehension is another area that develops rapidly. Within 9 months of arriving home, children adopted from Eastern Europe at ages 3 and 4 had average auditory comprehension scores of 91 or higher on English-language standardized tests.[25] Fifty percent of the children scored in the 90 to 110 range, and 90% scored above 80. A score of 80 or lower is the commonly used criterion for diagnosing speech and language disorders.[32] Considering the pre-adoption environment and medical risk factors faced by these children, the fact that comprehension abilities emerge so rapidly is nothing less than incredible. This does not mean that comprehension abilities are fully caught up after such a short time. Evidence suggests that comprehension requires several years to reach full proficiency.[25]

Similar to children adopted at younger ages, expressive language takes longer to reach proficiency in children adopted from abroad as preschoolers. Nine months after arriving home, internationally adopted children scored low on all expressive English-language measures, with standard scores ranging from a low of 50 to a high of 90 and an average of 81.[25] When the same children were tested 6 months later, expressive language test scores improved to an average of 89, with 68% of the children scoring above 80.[25] As seen in younger children, the grammatical elements of expressive language take longer to emerge. After 9 months home, preschool children were producing average sentences of 3.09 units when MLU was used as a measure. Six months later, MLU increased to 4.02. Most sentences consisted of strings of content vocabulary with relatively few grammatical elements such as verb tense or articles.

Children adopted as preschoolers also transition easily into the new speech articulation patterns of their adopted language. After one year home, the average score on standardized articulation tests was 95.[25] Only one preschool child had a standardized score below 80 on this test. Some children adopted at preschool ages can appear to have poor intelligibility; however, the problem is not a speech articulation disorder. Several of the preschool children followed by Glennen[37] used a pattern of producing longer sentences by inserting prosodic or phonologic markers that were not real words. It was as if these 3- and 4-year-olds realized they should be producing longer sentences but didn't have the language ability to do so. Sentences such as "Hmm hmm go hmm a dog" occurred frequently among a small subset of preschool children adopted after age 2. Articulation was always developmentally appropriate for words the children knew well, indicating that the observed unintelligibility was a temporary language-based phenomenon versus a true articulation disorder.

In summary, children adopted at preschool ages make remarkable progress in language development during their first year home.[25,47] Comprehension emerges before production and is a more reliable indicator of who is doing well and who needs EI. After one year home, children who score below 80 on standardized tests of English-language comprehension are not doing as well as their peers and should be referred for speech and language intervention. Articulation should also be developing at age-appropriate levels. Expressive language takes longer to emerge and cannot be validly assessed during the first year home. However, children should be making rapid progress in vocabulary and sentence production. Any child with more than mild expressive delays after one year home is not progressing typically and should be referred for intervention.

CASE DISCUSSION: LISA

The Archer family adopted Li Mei from China in March when she was 3.9 years old. They previously adopted a 14-month-old daughter from China who was now 6. Li Mei was renamed Lisa and quickly adapted to life with her new family. At adoption, she was below the 10th percentile for weight and height but otherwise appeared healthy and developmentally normal. The Archers kept Lisa home through the spring and were amazed at how quickly she began learning the English language. In June, when Lisa turned 4, they signed her up to start preschool the following fall. The Archers' older daughter had attended the same school and they were impressed with its emphasis on early academics and reading. Lisa's sister thrived in the program and was now excelling in the second grade.

Over the summer, Lisa's English-language abilities continued to improve. She communicated in simple sentences and appeared to understand most of what was said to her. By fall, the family had full confidence that she was ready

CASE DISCUSSION: LISA, CONTINUED

for preschool. However, at the first parent-teacher conference, the Archers learned that Lisa was not doing well. When other children listened attentively to stories, Lisa ran around the room. She cried whenever the class worked on alphabet sound/letter activities. When the teacher gave Lisa directions, she nodded her head as if she understood but then would do something else. Lisa also had difficulty socializing with other children during free play, frequently taking their toys or knocking down their activities to get attention. The teacher ended the conference by stating that she was concerned about Lisa's speech and language development and felt that a referral to a speech-language pathologist was warranted.

The Archers contacted the speech-language pathologist at their older daughter's elementary school to find out where to refer Lisa. They were given the referral phone number for the school district's child find identification hotline, which they called. The child find referral specialist stated that Lisa would need to be assessed by professionals who spoke Mandarin and that it would take time to line up the appropriate specialists for the assessment. The Archers explained that Lisa's only language was English but were told that it was school policy to test in the first language. At that point, they consulted an online adoptive parent support group and located a nearby speech-language pathologist who had experience working with children who were adopted internationally.

Lisa's speech and language evaluation took place in November, 8 months after she arrived home. The speech-language pathologist gave several tests of receptive and expressive language, vocabulary, and articulation and collected a sample of Lisa's spontaneous language. In addition, Lisa's hearing was screened and her oral motor abilities were evaluated. Test results confirmed that Lisa had made remarkable progress in learning English but was not fully proficient to a 4-year-old developmental level. Receptive language abilities averaged 94 on standardized testing, but there were subtest areas that were lower. For example, she had difficulty on subtests that involved following complex 2- and 3-part directions and that assessed comprehension of grammatical structures. Expressively, she was communicating in simple 4- to 5-word sentences and could easily use language to discuss people and actions in the "here and now." However, when conversations moved to discussing past and future events, she could not maintain the interaction and appeared confused. Standardized expressive language test scores averaged 84, with wide variability across subtests. Vocabulary was an area of strength, while use of grammatical structures was weak. Lisa's articulation, oral motor abilities, and hearing were all normal for her age.

The speech-language pathologist felt that Lisa was developing typically for a newly arrived child adopted at her age and that many of the behavior issues Lisa was having at school were due to her lack of English-language proficiency.

CASE DISCUSSION: LISA, CONTINUED

The Archers asked the speech-language pathologist to observe Lisa at her preschool and provide consultation to assist the preschool staff. After observing, it was apparent that the level of language expectation in the classroom was at the upper end for normally developing 4-year-olds, much less 4-year-old children who were in the process of learning English. The speech-language pathologist consulted with preschool staff; however, they were not willing to change the curriculum to meet Lisa's needs.

The Archers were counseled to find a new preschool with a play-based experiential curriculum. Such a preschool would allow Lisa to learn to communicate and play with 4-year-old peers without the pressure of an academically focused pre-literacy curriculum. The Archers found a new preschool and transferred Lisa there after the holiday break. When they attended their first parent-teacher conference, they heard glowing remarks about Lisa's ability to function in the classroom. There were times when she had difficulty expressing herself and times when she didn't understand directions, but her teachers were seeing daily improvement and felt that with time, these issues would disappear. By the end of the year, Lisa was doing well. The Archers decided to enroll her in a mixed pre-K program for 4- and 5-year-olds the following year. Lisa easily adapted to the more academic pre-K curriculum and moved into kindergarten the following year. She continued to do well and excelled in school, just like her older sister.

Children Adopted at Preschool Ages: School Age

Children adopted between 3 and 5 years of age typically begin school within 1 or 2 years of arriving home and have to quickly use language for learning. Relatively little is known about outcomes for children adopted as preschoolers when they reach school age. Many studies have found strong correlations between length of institutionalization and eventual language outcomes,[5,21,39,41–43] although other studies have not.[40,48] Although data are clear that adoption before 6 to 8 months of age is preferable, it is not clear whether adoption at older ages causes a steady drop in outcomes with increasing length of exposure to deprived environments or whether there is a steady drop up to a certain point followed by a plateau. That is, we know that children adopted before 6 to 8 months of age have a clear advantage over children adopted at ages 2 or 3, but we cannot state that children adopted at age 2 will have better school-age language outcomes than children adopted at age 3 or that children adopted at age 3 will do better than children adopted at age 4. Unlike their younger counterparts, however, children adopted as preschoolers have to begin using their adopted language in school before they are fully proficient. Without solid language abilities for learning, these children are at risk of falling behind academically.

Data that do exist indicate that the majority of children adopted as preschoolers will have language and speech abilities within the normal range by the time they reach school. In a preliminary report from a longitudinal study, Glennen[25] measured language abilities of 10 children adopted from Eastern Europe between 2 and 5 years of age. Two years after adoption, the children had average receptive language test scores of 100 and expressive language test scores of 101. All of the children had scores above 80 on both measures.[25,47] Croft et al[43] found, however, that by age 6, children adopted from Romania between 24 and 42 months of age did not score as well as children adopted before age 24 months on receptive vocabulary measures and on verbal measures from the McCarthy Scales of Children's Abilities. The differences were slight and the majority of children still scored within the normal range. Finally, children adopted at preschool ages may lag behind classroom peers in school. In teacher surveys of internationally adopted children, Dalen[41] determined that children adopted after age 25 months were not doing as well as classroom peers in comparisons of written language.

By school age, standardized scores on language tests are well within normal limits, although many children continue to make grammatical errors in their conversational speech. Preliminary evidence from conversational samples taken 2 years after adoption indicates that production of the English pronoun system, articles, irregular plurals, and irregular verbs continues to be difficult for children adopted from Russia as preschoolers.[47] Children may differ in the types of grammatical errors produced depending on how closely the birth and adopted language are structured.

In summary, by school age, children adopted as preschoolers tend to perform less well than children adopted at much younger ages on tests of receptive and expressive language. However, data indicate that the majority of children still test in the low-average to average range. Two years after adoption, any child with receptive or expressive language abilities below normal limits should be considered for speech and language intervention services. School systems may attempt to categorize the problem as an English-as-a-second-language (ESL) issue. However, 2 years after adoption, abilities that fall below the normal range for English-speaking children are not typical for internationally adopted children. These children are especially vulnerable to falling further behind as they transition into literacy and require speech and language intervention services that go beyond ESL programs.

Children Adopted at School Ages (5 Years and Older)

Each section of this chapter is shorter than the preceding section because there is less evidence to report. Evidence of language outcomes in children adopted from abroad after age 5 years is scarce. The few studies that include children in this age range tend to group them with children adopted at younger ages, making it difficult to determine differences in outcomes. Because there is little evidence to present, this section will focus on issues related to assessing and making treatment decisions within an ESL framework.

Children Adopted at School Ages: Before Adoption

School-aged children who are adopted from abroad vary widely in their pre-adoption experiences. Some reside in institutions their entire lives, while others reside with families until social conditions lead to placement in an institution. Some children attend school before adoption; others do not. Wide variability in pre-adoption experiences leads to wide variability in language abilities. Parents adopting school-aged children need to collect as much information as possible in the birth country about the child's speech and language. This information can be used to determine if the child has delays or a disorder in the birth language. Similar to the recommendations for younger children, parents should request copies of any formal evaluations and should take time to ask caregivers questions about the child's speech and language abilities. The pre-adoption questions listed for younger children in Box 14-2 are appropriate for older school-aged children. In addition, if the child has attended school, parents should try to collect school records including report cards or teacher reports, copies of written schoolwork, and examples of texts the child can successfully read. Box 14-3 lists additional pre-adoption questions for parents to ask about children who have started school. This information can be used to document the presence or absence of a speech or language disorder and, if necessary, serve as evidence to qualify newly adopted children for speech and language services soon after arrival home.

Children Adopted at School Ages: The First Year Home

Children adopted after age 5 typically enroll in school shortly after arriving home. The school system should immediately identify the child as having Limited English Proficiency (LEP) status and arrange for the child to receive ESL services to facilitate the language-learning process. (Note that some schools use the term English Language Learner [ELL] instead of LEP.) Children with normal cognitive, speech, and language abilities will typically not require any additional services. However, children with previously identified speech, language, or cognitive disorders will require additional services under the Individuals with Disabilities Education Act (IDEA). Most schools will resist this recommendation until the child has been given the chance to benefit from ESL programs.[25] However, if the school waits too long, the birth language will have undergone severe attrition, making it difficult to complete a valid language, speech, or cognitive assessment.[25]

The only way around this dilemma is to have newly adopted children assessed in the birth language within 3 to 4 months of arriving home. These assessments are only recommended for children who were previously identified in the birth country as having speech, language, or cognitive delays[25] or for any child in whom

---

Box 14-3. Language and Speech Development in Children Adopted at 6 Years and Older: Pre-adoption Questions for Orphanage Staff and Teachers

Literacy
- Are the child's reading abilities at, above, or below grade level?
  — If below, how far below? Ask for examples of the types of reading problems that have been observed.
- If possible, videotape the child reading a book out loud. Be sure to zoom in and capture the actual written text on the video.
- Are the child's writing abilities at, above, or below grade level?
  — If below, how far below? Ask for examples of the types of writing problems that have been observed.
- Ask to bring home examples of the child's writing. Be sure dates are noted on each piece.

Academic Abilities
- What subjects are easy for the child to learn? For each easy subject, ask if the child is working at, above, or below grade level.
- What subjects are difficult for the child? For each of these subjects, ask if the child is learning at, above, or below grade level.
- For each area of difficulty, ask why the child has trouble learning the subject.
- How is the child's attention span when compared with classmates?
- Does the child have more or less difficulty sitting still to do work when compared with classmates?
- When compared with classmates, does the child work independently or need frequent assistance or redirection to complete tasks?
- When compared with classmates, does the child keep trying when tasks get difficult? Or does the child easily get frustrated and give up?

---

the degree of delays cannot be determined prior to adoption. Assessments can be completed privately or through the school system under IDEA. As stated previously, the school system will typically resist this request, which is why pre-adoption documents are important. Parents who can produce evidence of a speech, language, or cognitive delay that existed before adoption have solid grounds to request an assessment of those abilities. Parents who cannot produce this evidence will have difficulty proving the need for an assessment under IDEA. In those situations, parents may need to pursue private evaluations.

Individuals with Disabilities Education Act law mandates that children need to be assessed in their primary language.[49] For newly arrived adoptees, that is the birth language. Ideally, professionals who speak the language should conduct the assessment.[50] This allows direct evaluation of the child's ability to understand and communicate. If this is not feasible, an alternative is to conduct the assessment through an interpreter who speaks the language.[50] Professionals conducting the assessment should be skilled in evaluating children with an interpreter. As previously stated, any assessment of the birth language needs to occur within 3 to 4 months of adoption before the language undergoes attrition.[25]

There is little solid evidence about language-learning patterns in children adopted from abroad after age 5. Common sense would indicate that older children should outperform younger adoptees in the pace of language learning during the first year home. However, the effects of long-term institutionalization combined with a wider language gap to bridge means that most children adopted at school age may take longer to fully catch up. Most internationally adopted children are only bilingual for a brief period. However, until more information is available, evidence from second language learning provides the best guide for children adopted at older ages.

Second language learning is divided into 2 major categories: basic interpersonal communication skills (BICS) and cognitive academic language proficiency (CALP).[51] Basic interpersonal communication skills refers to communication in face-to-face social interactions. Anecdotal reports from parents and teachers indicate that most internationally adopted children rapidly acquire proficiency for BICS interactions. Within a year of arriving home, school-aged children should be able to communicate conversationally in sentences, although they may still make errors in pronunciation or grammar. The rapid proficiency in BICS often masks the child's poor grasp of English. Cognitive academic language proficiency refers to language proficiency needed for academic learning. More specifically, it refers to the child's ability to understand and use academic vocabulary, infer meaning from text, and use language in increasingly abstract ways. Language studies of bilingual children indicate that it takes 5 to 9 years for a child to achieve CALP proficiency.[51] What is not clear is whether children adopted from abroad at school age require more or less time to reach this level of proficiency.

The rate of language learning required of newly adopted school-aged children is daunting. Consider Vladimir, a newly adopted 7-year-old from Eastern Europe who starts first grade shortly after arriving home. Vocabulary estimates for typical first-grade children range from 5,000 to 13,000 words.[52] Using the lower estimate of 5,000, Vladimir needs to learn 13 new words per day to fully catch up with his peers within one year of arriving home. However, during first grade, Vladimir's peers are also learning new words at a rate of 3,000 per year or approximately 8 words per day.[53] This means that Vladimir really needs to learn and retain 21 new words per day to catch up to his peers within one year of arriving home.

Most newly adopted school-aged children are placed into ESL programs shortly after arriving home. English-as-a-second-language programs focus on teaching vocabulary linked to the academic lessons children are learning. Studies show that direct vocabulary instruction can teach approximately 400 new words per school year.[54] This means that to catch up, Vladimir needs to learn the remaining 7,600 new vocabulary words on his own. One way that school-aged children learn new vocabulary is through reading.[54] Stories and textbooks are rich in novel words that aren't routinely used in conversational speech. When children encounter new words in a story, they use the context of the surrounding sentences to extrapolate meaning.

This requires an understanding of the grammatical structure of sentences and comprehension of the majority of content words in the text. Children who are in the process of learning English are at a disadvantage in this process because they don't comprehend most of the words they read and get caught in a downward language-learning spiral. They need proficient language abilities to facilitate incidental vocabulary and academic learning from text, yet their inability to do so puts them further behind academically.

These same language-learning factors affect bilingual children who begin learning English when they enter school. However, bilingual children usually retain language proficiency in the first language while in the process of learning English. Concepts and instructions that are not understood in English can be explained using the first language. In contrast, school-aged children who are adopted internationally are not bilingual.[25] After 3 to 4 months at home, they are monolingual in their new adopted language,[27] yet the language is far from proficient. When internationally adopted children need further assistance to understand new concepts, there is no other language to use for instruction. This places them at further academic risk of not catching up to their peers.

Children Adopted at School Ages: Language-Learning Services in Schools

Children adopted at older ages should immediately receive services to assist them in learning English when they start school. As stated in the previous section, schools can offer assistance through ESL programs or under IDEA. The problem is that these 2 programs were designed for specific groups of children, and internationally adopted children don't fit neatly into either category. Most newly adopted children begin receiving services through ESL because they are identified as having LEP. English-as-a-second-language programs are now wrapped into legislation for No Child Left Behind Act of 2001 (NCLB).[55] While the federal government provides funding for ESL programs, it lets each state determine the type and scope of services offered. Because these programs are linked to immigration issues, they are often prime targets for political tinkering. For example, some states, such as Alabama and Vermont, have legislated "English-only" policies and provide all ESL support services in English.[55] Other states allow schools to provide initial ESL services in the first language, then transition the child to English.

The majority of LEP students are enrolled in mainstream classrooms and receive minimal English support services to assist them in learning the regular academic curriculum.[56] This is because more than 60% of students receiving ESL services are in school districts with fewer than 99 LEP students, and half of those districts have fewer than 25 LEP students.[56] Some districts with small LEP populations bus children to a central district school to receive ESL support services. Districts with relatively few LEP students tend to offer less support than those that enroll more. In summary, services for children who are LEP vary widely from state to state and from district to district within states.

■ CASE DISCUSSION: ADINA

Adina was adopted from Ethiopia when she was 8 years old by the Grenn family. The Grenns were told that Adina's parents had died when she was an infant. She was raised by a grandmother who could no longer take care of her. Adina moved into an orphanage when she was 7 years old and was relatively healthy and well-nourished when the Grenns first met her. Records indicated that she spoke a tribal language and did not begin learning Amharic until her arrival at the orphanage one year ago. She attended school at the orphanage 3 days per week, but her teachers indicated that she struggled in school and was not doing as well as other children. When questioned, the teachers said Adina did not pronounce Amharic words clearly, her sentences were short, and she didn't always understand class instructions. The family then went with Adina into the country for one last visit with her grandmother. As part of the visit, they asked questions about Adina's early development. Her grandmother insisted that Adina was a smart child who used many words when she was little.

Adina spent one month adjusting to life at home with the Grenn family before starting school. She rapidly learned new English vocabulary and began communicating in simple 2- to 3-word sentences. However, her word attempts were sometimes hard to understand. In October, the family enrolled Adina in second grade at the neighborhood elementary school, a year below her expected grade level. Adina was 1 of 2 children in the school who were classified with Limited English Proficiency (LEP). The school district assigned an English-as-a-second-language (ESL) specialist to visit the school twice each week for 1-hour pullout lessons. Adina liked going to school, but when her parents observed, it was apparent that she did not understand or participate in most grade-level curricular activities. The ESL specialist told the Grenns about a nearby elementary school with a centralized ESL program where classes were co-taught by teachers and ESL specialists. In January, Adina transferred to a second grade classroom at the new school and began making academic progress. At the end of the school year, the Grenn family met with school staff to discuss plans for next year. They were shocked when the ESL specialist reported that Adina's English-language abilities had improved to the point that she no longer qualified for intensive ESL programming. In addition, she recommended returning Adina to the neighborhood school. When asked to document Adina's progress, the ESL specialist showed them a teacher checklist that was used to determine ESL services.

CASE DISCUSSION: ADINA, CONTINUED

During the summer, the Grenn family hired a tutor to work with Adina on reading and math skills. Her English-language skills continued to improve. She was communicating in 5- to 6-word sentences with good pronunciation on most words. Some words, especially those with 3 or more syllables, were difficult for her. She then entered third grade at her neighborhood school with pullout ESL services twice per week. By October, it was clear that she was struggling. She had difficulty reading aloud and was unable to answer simple comprehension questions. Her writing consisted of a few rote learned sight words surrounded by unintelligible spelling. The Grenns met with Adina's teacher and insisted that more classroom support was needed. They set up a meeting with the principal and Adina's teachers. At the meeting, the ESL specialist stated that Adina's English-language skills qualified her as LEP but were too good to qualify for more intensive ESL support. The Grenns pushed to have Adina referred for more assessment under the Individuals with Disabilities Education Act (IDEA), but the principal stated that she would not qualify for IDEA services as long as she was classified as having LEP. The only option was to refer Adina for assistance from the school reading specialist. The reading specialist began working with Adina in daily 30-minute sessions.

Adina made slow but steady progress through her third grade year; however, by spring she was still academically far behind the other children. In March, the Grenns requested another team meeting to discuss Adina's progress in school. The principal invited the school psychologist and speech-language pathologist to attend. In discussion, it was decided to provide Adina with additional support from the speech-language pathologist through the Response to Intervention (RTI) approach. The speech-language pathologist did not formally assess Adina but began to address weaknesses that were observed watching Adina's classroom reading. She felt that Adina was making good progress learning English but her phonologic awareness abilities were poor. This made it difficult for Adina to sound out and remember new words in reading and affected her spelling and pronunciation of lengthy words. The speech-language pathologist began working on these skills with Adina. However, sessions were frequently cancelled because of school events or field trips. Makeup sessions were only provided for children who had Individualized Education Plans (IEPs), not children under RTI programs. At the end of Adina's third grade year, the Grenns conferred with her teachers. All agreed that she was making good progress but was not ready for fourth grade. It was decided to keep all of the existing supports in place and have Adina repeat third grade with the same teacher. The Grenns once again pushed to have Adina referred for assessment under IDEA and were told to wait until Adina was no longer considered an LEP student.

CASE DISCUSSION: ADINA, CONTINUED

At this point the Grenns were frustrated with the school system's inability to respond to Adina's needs. They were also concerned that Adina would repeat third grade as a 10-year-old. After consulting other adoptive parents, they contacted a nearby hospital that had an interdisciplinary clinic for internationally adopted children. Adina was assessed by the neuropsychologist, speech-language pathologist, and reading specialist. They determined that in addition to having poor phonologic awareness abilities, Adina had difficulty remembering auditory sequences and complex directions. This was true for English-language–based and nonlanguage-based auditory information. She was referred to an audiologist who specialized in auditory processing disorders and had experience with internationally adopted children. Because of Adina's language background, the audiologist worked with the speech-language pathologist to confirm that Adina understood all test instructions and vocabulary before proceeding with each auditory processing task. It was discovered that Adina had an auditory processing disorder and that her abilities were equally poor on nonlanguage-based processing tasks such as remembering high or low musical tones and language-based processing tasks such as discriminating between similar words. Her greatest weakness was listening in noisy environments, such as a classroom.

Armed with this information, the Grenns went back to the school system to request additional support services for Adina. The school finally agreed to develop an IEP that continued ESL services and included additional services from the speech-language pathologist, reading specialist, and special education teacher. In addition, the Grenns purchased an FM listening system for Adina to wear in the classroom. Adina's teacher would speak into a portable microphone and her voice would be conveyed to an earpiece worn by Adina. Adina was initially reluctant to wear the earpiece, but when her mother bought an in-the-ear cell phone and began wearing it around the community, Adina was excited to wear her own "cell phone" at school. The Grenns were hopeful that these additional supports and services would finally get Adina working up to grade level.

In the past, states were able to exclude LEP students from statewide school assessments and only reported test scores based on children who were proficient in English. This changed with the NCLB legislation. Children with LEP must participate in statewide assessments that are used to determine if a school is making adequate yearly progress.[57] In the original legislation, 5% of children with LEP could be excluded from testing each year; all others had to take the statewide tests. The 2007 reenactment of NCLB revised these guidelines slightly; children who have LEP are granted a one-time exclusion from statewide reading and language arts assessments if they have attended school in the United States for fewer than

12 months.[58] However, all LEP students must take the statewide math and science tests, and after 12 months, children who are LEP must take the reading and language arts tests. There are also no standard guidelines on when children no longer qualify as having LEP status.[57] Some states use tests; others use informal processes such as teacher checklists. Under NCLB, children are categorized as "former LEP" for testing purposes for up to 2 years after their LEP status ends.

The purpose of this review of ESL services and assessment policies is to clarify why ESL programs may meet the needs of some newly arrived internationally adopted children and fail to meet the needs of others. Children adopted into school districts and states with large LEP populations will likely benefit from the extensive ESL services offered through the schools. In contrast, children adopted into school districts and states with few LEP children may receive minimal support. In contrast to the wide variability in services available to children who are LEP, special education services mandated under the federal IDEA program are relatively consistent across states and schools. However, obtaining special education services under IDEA for a newly arrived school-aged child is next to impossible unless documents from the birth country indicate a specific qualifying diagnosis, such as hearing impairment, or an assessment within the first few months home indicates the presence of a qualifying diagnosis or a speech, language, or cognitive delay in the birth language. Simply having LEP does not qualify a child for special education services.

School-aged children qualify for services under IDEA, including speech and language therapy, if they have a specific categoric diagnosis.[59] Currently, eligible diagnostic categories are mental retardation, hearing impairment, speech or language impairment, visual impairment, serious emotional disturbance, orthopedic impairment, or specific learning disabilities. In addition, states can choose to qualify children for IDEA if they have a non-categoric developmental delay in one or more areas that meets the state's definition.[59] Each state can determine its own criteria for delay; most states use formulas based on test percentiles or standard deviations. This non-categoric criterion is used for younger children and often has an upper age limit set by the state; all children over the age limit must qualify for services under one of the categoric diagnoses listed previously. Finally, children can only receive services under IDEA when the disability affects academic performance.[59] For example, mild articulation mispronunciations (eg, "wabbit" for "rabbit") often don't qualify for intervention under IDEA rules.

Many children who struggle academically do not meet the strict guidelines of IDEA. In recent reauthorizations of IDEA, the federal government approved using a Response to Intervention (RTI) approach for children who do not meet the strict criteria for categoric diagnoses but still need classroom support services, including speech and language.[60] Response to Intervention allows schools to provide services to children who are struggling academically without formally assessing them to see if they qualify for services under IDEA guidelines. Children who don't improve with RTI are then referred for further evaluation to see if they qualify for services under IDEA. Many school systems are changing their service delivery systems to use RTI as a first strategy before referring children for a full assessment under IDEA. Children who do qualify for special education services under IDEA, including speech and language services, receive an IEP to outline the scope of services or supports that will be put in place and goals for each of the services.[59] Children receiving RTI do not have IEPs. Services and goals in the IEP should focus on facilitating academic performance in the classroom. Once the IEP is approved, school systems are mandated to provide the services indicated in the document.

Some children have known disabilities but fail to qualify for services under IDEA. For example, children with ADHD and normal intelligence often don't qualify for an IEP. However, these children are still covered under Section 504 of the Rehabilitation Act.[61] A 504 plan is a school accommodation plan for a child with a disability. For example, children with ADHD may need to be tested in a quiet room with few distractions. Children with orthopedic impairments may need to dictate answers to test questions rather than write them independently. Unlike an IEP, a 504 plan addresses accommodations that are not necessarily related to academic performance, such as having an escort when changing classrooms or assigning a peer buddy during lunch or recess. However, to qualify for a 504 plan, the child must have a diagnosed disability.

This section of the chapter reviewed information for children adopted from abroad after age 5 years. There are minimal data on typical patterns of language learning in children adopted at these older ages. School-aged children who are adopted with relatively proficient abilities in their first language are not bilingual. However, the initial language-learning process is likely similar to bilingual ELLs. Most schools will provide initial support services through ESL programs. Also reviewed were differences among school support programs offered under ESL, IDEA, RTI, and Section 504. Parents who adopt older children from abroad need to become educated about these programs to advocate for appropriate classroom support services for their children.

Conclusion

Institutional settings are not good places for children to develop language. It is clear that adoption into a nurturing family improves children's language abilities. What is not clear is whether those abilities can return to normal age-appropriate levels. Research evidence indicates that children adopted at young ages respond well to enriched family environments and rapidly learn their new adopted language. Children adopted at older ages need more time to learn a new language to proficient levels, yet most learn to communicate with average proficiency within a few years of arriving home. Parents and professionals who observe the transformation firsthand often marvel at the pace of language learning that takes place, especially in the first year home. Evidence shows that the majority of children who are adopted internationally rapidly transition into using their new language and do well over time; however, some do not. These children need to be identified early and provided with extra speech and language services to boost their language abilities. Professionals need to become familiar with evidence-based information on typical versus atypical patterns of language learning in internationally adopted children and apply that information toward making clinical decisions about internationally adopted children.

References

1. Ames E. *The Development of Romanian Children Adopted into Canada: Final Report.* Burnaby, British Columbia: Simon Fraser University; 1997
2. Dennis W. *Children of the Creche.* New York, NY: Appleton-Century Crofts; 1973
3. Glennen S. New arrivals: speech and language assessment for internationally adopted infants and toddlers within the first months home. *Semin Speech Lang.* 2005;26(1):10–21
4. Johnson DE. Medical and developmental sequelae of early childhood institutionalization in Eastern European adoptees. In: Nelson CA, ed. *The Effects of Early Adversity on Neurobehavioral Development.* Mahwah, NJ: Lawrence Erlbaum Associates; 2000:113–162
5. O'Connor TG, Rutter M, Beckett C, Keaveney L, Kreppner JM. The effects of global severe privation on cognitive competence: extension and longitudinal follow-up. English and Romanian Study Team. *Child Dev.* 2000;71(2):376–390
6. Rutter M. Developmental catch-up, and deficit, following adoption after severe global early privation. English and Romanian Adoptees Study Team. *J Child Psychol Psychiatry.* 1998;39(4):465–476
7. Sigal JJ, Perry JC, Rossignol M, Ouimet MC. Unwanted infants: psychological and physical consequences of inadequate orphanage care years later. *Am J Orthopsychiatry.* 2003;73(1):3–12
8. Muhamedrahimov RJ, Palmov OI, Nikiforova NV, Groark C, McCall R. Institution-based early intervention program. *Infant Ment Health J.* 2004;25:488–501
9. Vorria P, Papaligoura Z, Dunn J, et al. Early experiences and attachment relationships of Greek infants raised in residential group care. *J Child Psychol Psychiatry.* 2003;44(8):1208–1220
10. O'Connor TG, Rutter M. Attachment disorder behavior following early severe deprivation: extension and longitudinal follow-up. English and Romanian Adoptees Study Team. *J Am Acad Child Adolesc Psychiatry.* 2000;39(6):703–712
11. Glennen S, Masters MG. Typical and atypical language development in infants and toddlers adopted from Eastern Europe. *Am J Speech Lang Pathol.* 2002;11:417–433
12. Windsor J, Glaze LE, Koga SF; Bucharest Early Intervention Project Core Group. Language acquisition with limited input: Romanian institution and foster care. *J Speech Lang Hear Res.* 2007;50(5):1365–1381
13. Hwa-Froelich DA. Infants and toddlers adopted abroad: clinical practices. *Perspectives on Communication Disorders in Culturally and Linguistically Diverse Populations.* 2007;14(3):9–12
14. Miller LC, Hendrie NW. Health of children adopted from China. *Pediatrics.* 2000;105(6):e76
15. Miller L, Chan W, Comfort K, Tirella L. Health of children adopted from Guatemala: comparison of orphanage and foster care. *Pediatrics.* 2005;115(6):e710–e717
16. Moorman JR, Hernandez DJ. Married-couple families with step, adopted, and biological children. *Demography.* 1989;26(2):267–277
17. Kreider R. *Adopted Children and Step-children: 2000. Census 2000 Special Reports.* http://www.Census.gov/prod/2003pubs/censr-6.pdf. Accessed February 14, 2014

18. Hoff E. Causes and consequences of SES related differences in parent to child speech. In: Bournstein M, Bradley R, eds. *Socioeconomic Status, Parenting, and Child Development.* Mahwah, NJ: Lawrence Erlbaum Associates; 2003:145–178

19. Horton-Ikard R, Ellis Weismer S. A preliminary examination of vocabulary and word learning in African American toddlers from middle and low socioeconomic status homes. *Am J Speech Lang Pathol.* 2007;16(4):381–392

20. Zeanah CH, Nelson CA, Fox NA, et al. Designing research to study the effects of institutionalization on brain and behavioral development: the Bucharest Early Intervention Project. *Dev Psychopathol.* 2003;15(4):885–907

21. Windsor J. Language skills of Romanian children in orphanage and foster care. Presented at American Speech Language Hearing Association Annual Conference, Boston, MA; 2007

22. Glennen S. Predicting language outcomes for internationally adopted children. *J Speech Lang Hear Res.* 2007;50(2):529–548

23. Glennen S. International adoption speech and language mythbusters. *Perspectives on Communication Disorders and Sciences in Culturally and Linguistically Diverse Populations.* 2007;14(3):3–8

24. Roberts JA, Pollock KE, Krakow R, Price J, Fulmer KC, Wang PP. Language development in preschool-age children adopted from China. *J Speech Lang Hear Res.* 2005;48(1):93–107

25. Glennen S. Speech and language in children adopted internationally at older ages. *Perspectives on Communication Disorders and Sciences in Culturally and Linguistically Diverse Populations.* 2007;14(3):17–20

26. Glennen S. Language development and delay in internationally adopted infants and toddlers: a review. *Am J Speech Lang Pathol.* 2002;11:333–339

27. Gindis B. What should adoptive parents know about their children's language-based school difficulties? Post-Adoption Learning Center. http://www.adoptionarticlesdirectory.com/ArticlesUser/popularArticles_list.php?orderby=aposteddate. Accessed February 14, 2014

28. Wetherby A, Prizant B. *Communication and Symbolic Behavior Scales: Developmental Profile, First Normed Edition.* Baltimore, MD: Brookes; 2002

29. Fenson L, Dale P, Reznick J, Bates E, Thal DJ, Pethick SJ. *MacArthur–Bates Communicative Development Inventories: User's Guide and Technical Manual.* Baltimore, MD: Paul H. Brookes Publishing Co; 2007

30. Shackelford J. State and jurisdictional eligibility definitions for infants and toddlers with disabilities under IDEA. *NECTAC Notes.* 2006;21:1–16

31. Trohanis PL. Progress in providing services to young children with special needs and their families: an overview to and update on the implementation of the Individuals with Disabilities Education Act (IDEA). *J Early Interv.* 2008;30(2):140–151

32. Fey M. *Language Intervention with Young Children.* San Diego, CA: College Hill Press; 1986

33. Olswang LB, Rodriguez B, Timler G. Recommending intervention for toddlers with specific language learning difficulties: we may not have all the answers but we know a lot. *Am J Speech Lang Pathol.* 1988;7:23–32

34. Pollock KE. Early language growth in children adopted from China: preliminary normative data. *Semin Speech Lang.* 2005;26(1):22–32

35. Geren J, Snedeker J, Ax L. Starting over: a preliminary study of early lexical and syntactic development in internationally-adopted preschoolers. *Semin Speech Lang.* 2005;26(1):44–53

36. Glennen S, Rosinsky-Grunhut A, Tracy R. Linguistic interference between L1 and L2 in internationally adopted children. *Semin Speech Lang.* 2005;26(1):64–75

37. Glennen S. A longitudinal study of speech and language outcomes in internationally adopted children: ages 3 and 4. *J Speech Lang Hear Res.* In review

38. Scott K, Roberts J. Language development of internationally adopted children: the school-age years. *Perspectives on Communication Disorders and Sciences in Culturally and Linguistically Diverse Populations.* 2007;14(3):12–17

39. Scott KA, Roberts JA, Krakow R. Oral and written language development of children adopted from China. *Am J Speech Lang Pathol.* 2008;17(2):150–160

40. Beverly BL, McGuinness TM, Blanton DJ. Communication and academic challenges in early adolescence for children adopted from the former Soviet Union. *Lang Speech Hear Serv Sch.* 2008;39(3):303–313

41. Dalen M. School performances among internationally adopted children in Norway. *Adoption Q.* 2001;5:39–58

42. Saetersdal B, Dalen M. Norway: intercountry adoptions in a homogeneous country. In: Alstein H, Simon R, eds. *Intercountry Adoption: A Multinational Perspective.* New York, NY: Praeger; 1991:83–108

43. Croft C, Beckett C, Rutter M, et al. Early adolescent outcomes of institutionally deprived and non-deprived adoptees. II: language as a protective factor and as vulnerable outcomes. *J Child Psychol Psychiatry.* 2007;48(1):31–44

44. Glennen S, Bright BJ. Five years later: language in school-age internationally adopted children. *Semin Speech Lang.* 2005;26(1):86–101

45. Bishop DVM. *The Children's Communication Checklist.* 2nd ed. London, United Kingdom: Psychological Corporation; 2003

46. Humphries T, Koltun H, Malone M, Roberts W. Teacher-identified oral language difficulties among boys with attention problems. *J Dev Behav Pediatr.* 1994;15(2):92–98

47. Glennen S. Language development and disorders in older internationally adopted children. Presented at New Jersey Speech Language Hearing Association Annual Conference; 2007

48. van IJzendoorn MH, Juffer F, Klein-Poelhuis CW. Adoption and cognitive development: a meta-analytic comparison of adopted and nonadopted children's IQ and school performance. *Psychol Bull.* 2005;131(2):301–316

49. Walsh S, Smith B, Taylor R. *IDEA Requirements for Preschoolers with Disabilities: IDEA Early Childhood Policy and Practice Guide.* Reston, VA: Council for Exceptional Children; 2000

50. Goldstein B. *Cultural and Linguistic Diversity Resource Guide for Speech Language Pathology.* San Diego, CA: Singular Publishing Group; 2000

51. Cummins J. *Bilingualism and Special Education: Issues in Assessment and Pedagogy.* San Diego, CA: College Hill Press; 1984

52. Adams MJ. *Beginning to Read: Thinking and Learning about Print.* Cambridge, MA: MIT Press; 1990

53. Nagy WE, Anderson RC, Herman PA. Learning word meanings from context during normal reading. *Am Educational Res J.* 1987;24:237–270

54. Beck IL, McKeown MG. Conditions of vocabulary acquisition. In: Barr R, Kamil M, Mosenthal P, Pearson PD, eds. *Handbook of Reading Research Volume 2.* New York, NY: Longman; 1991:789–814

55. Kindler AL. *Survey of the States' Limited English Proficient Students and Available Educational Programs and Services: 2000–2001 Summary Report.* Washington, DC: National Clearinghouse for English Language Acquisition; 2002. http://www.ncela.gwu.edu/files/rcd/BE021853/Survey_of_the_States.pdf. Accessed February 14, 2014

56. Zehler AM, Fleischman HL, Hopstock PJ, Pendzick ML, Stephenson TG. *Descriptive Study of Services to LEP Students and LEP Students with Disabilities.* Arlington, VA: Development Associates; 2003. http://www.ncela.gwu.edu/files/rcd/BE021199/special_ed4.pdf. Accessed February 14, 2014

57. Wolf MK, Kao JC, Herman J, et al. *Issues in Assessing English Language Learners: English Language Proficiency Measures and Accommodation Uses.* Los Angeles, CA: National Center for Research on Evaluation, Standards, and Student Testing; 2008. http://www.cse.ucla.edu/products/reports/r731. pdf. Accessed February 14, 2014

58. US Department of Education. New No Child Left Behind regulations: flexibility and accountability for limited english proficient students. http://www2.ed.gov/print/admins/lead/account/ lepfactsheet.html. Published September 11, 2006. Accessed February 14, 2014

59. Danaher J. Eligibility policies and practices for young children under Part B of IDEA. *NECTAC Notes.* 2007;24:1–20

60. Griffiths A, Parson L, Burns M, VanDerHeyden A, Tilly WD. *Response to Intervention: Research for Practice.* Alexandria, VA: National Association of State Directors of Special Education; 2007

61. Wrights Law. Section 504, the Americans with Disabilities Act, and education reform. http://www.wrightslaw.com/info/section504.ada.peer.htm. Revised March 2, 2008. Accessed February 14, 2014

CHAPTER 15

Identifying and Accessing Supports: Strategies for Addressing Long-term Issues in Adopted Children

Lisa Nalven, MD, MA, FAAP

Background

This chapter will discuss useful strategies in addressing long-term issues that may be seen in children with a history of adoption. Discussion of "normative" development as well as developmental trajectories seen in children who have had adverse early experiences because of suboptimal care will be detailed. Long-term developmental, behavioral, and emotional concerns need to be viewed within the context of concerns affecting any child, as well as those that are more likely to affect a child who has been subject to early adverse experiences, including negative or absent caregiving or abuse. For any individual child, it is important to consider the child's specific history and current profile in planning for ongoing services and supports. However, summaries of research from cohorts of children with a history of adoption or foster care can serve as a guide and provide insight into the range of issues that need to be considered diagnostically, indications for further evaluation, and development of a plan for intervention. Medical, developmental, and social-emotional perspectives will be discussed to develop a comprehensive approach to providing strategies to support children who are demonstrating chronic difficulties as a result of prior prenatal and postnatal factors discussed in previous chapters of this manual.

Epidemiology

Epidemiologic studies suggest approximately 20% of all children in the United States exhibit some type of developmental or behavioral difficulty, regardless of history of adoption or risk factors. Milder difficulties (eg, weakness in reading, attention, or graphomotor skills) tend to be more common (8%–15%), while more severe disabilities (eg, cognitive-adaptive impairment, 1%–2%; cerebral palsy, <1%) are less common.

Children with a history of developmental risk (eg, family history of a disorder, premature birth, prenatal drug/alcohol exposure, malnutrition, abuse/neglect, institutionalization) are at increased risk of a range of developmental and behavioral challenges that could affect any child (eg, developmental delay, learning disability, attention-deficit/hyperactivity disorder [ADHD]). Literature specifically describing children adopted from orphanages from a variety of countries (eg, Russia, Romania, China) indicate that 50% to 90% demonstrate significant developmental or behavioral issues at initial assessments.[1–5] Similarly, research on children in US foster care demonstrates a similar prevalence (40%–85%) and profile of difficulties.[6,7] In addition to developmental issues that occur in the general pediatric population, children who have had adverse early experiences are at increased risk for other disorders such as toxic stress, reactive attachment disorder (RAD), or post-traumatic stress disorder (PTSD).[8] In many cases, children from these populations have multiple, comorbid developmental and behavioral challenges that will require intervention.

Considerations During Transition to a New Family

When a child transitions to a new family, it is important to comprehensively assess for potential medical, developmental, behavioral, and social-emotional concerns, as well as review current strengths and weaknesses. Medical issues can be acute or chronic and may have resolved or persist by the time a child joins their family. However, research indicates that even treated medical issues can have long-term implications. For example, early protein or calorie malnutrition, iron deficiency, and elevated lead levels can all be treated to achieve a normal range based on laboratory assessments, but the long-term effect of these conditions on neurocognitive function, although at times subtle, is well documented.[9–13] As a result, clinicians must consider the cumulative effects of documented and undocumented influences on development, particularly when a child is demonstrating difficulties. Other chronic medical issues, such as asthma management, chronic ear infections, hearing loss, cleft palate, constipation, spina bifida, and congenital heart disease, all require standard medical interventions. Management of these medical issues, however, calls for consideration of a child's developmental level (vs chronologic age) and emotional status when providing medical care (eg, sedation of a child who has a history of being physically abused for a barium enema). Moreover, simply blaming a child's difficulties on a medical condition without consideration of other factors can result in incomplete intervention (eg, failing to consider the effect of a language-impoverished environment in children with speech delays).

For children leaving foster or institutional care, the transition to family living begins as a significant disruption, hopefully followed by increasing stability. In the case of children who have been previously identified as having medical, developmental, behavioral, or social-emotional issues and are receiving interventions or supportive services, it is important to prepare the child, health care professional(s), and family for the transition and facilitate continuation of indicated services. For those children who are coming from situations without prior interventions (eg, institutions, neglectful home environments), it is important to allow the child and family time to adjust. While doing so, however, everyone involved must remain prepared to make an early assessment and monitor progress to initiate needed interventions in a thoughtful and timely manner.

During the initial transition period to a new family, many adjustments will likely need to occur. The effect of this transition on a child and family and the capacity of adults to understand the underlying cause of a child's behavior are only 2 of the factors that make it difficult to assess a child's developmental level, behavioral issues, and social-emotional function during the transition period. For example, parents adopting internationally typically report rapid developmental gains over the first few weeks by simply providing their child with an opportunity to explore the environment and interact in a positive fashion with others. This does not necessarily mean a child will "catch up" completely, but it does provide some information about a child's potential to learn. Behavioral and social-emotional development may be extremely variable. For example, a child may initially appear calm or withdrawn or be irritable and depressed and act out. These behaviors may gradually evolve into seeking a parent for help and reassurance. Other children make a smooth transition to their new family and after a shorter adjustment period, fall into the flow of family life. Depending on an individual child's prior experiences and individual biology, potential long-term issues may become evident over time, while other issues may resolve.

Developmental Trajectory

When considering impairments with which a child may present, it is important to consider the normal trajectory of development (ie, at what ages do skills/behaviors typically emerge in various domains) and how adverse early experience and toxic stress during sensitive periods of brain development may alter the expected developmental trajectory.[8,14] It is also important to consider what constitutes a normal transition process or acculturation (eg, language delays caused by English as a second language) versus an indication of a possible longer term issue (eg, a 3-year-old who, after he has had time to adapt to the new living situation, does not begin speaking in English or in his native language). In addition, a child's age and previous experiences may lead to very different expectations for the child's transition process to a new family (eg, attachment between an infant vs an older child and a primary caregiver).

The rate of developmental progress in the first few months after joining a new family generally slows down but will typically continue over the next few years. During this time, a pattern emerges as to what a child masters and what continues to pose mild or severe challenges for the child and family. Current evidence suggests that children from foster care and orphanages make rapid gains on joining their families. While many children are resilient and may eventually resolve their pre-existing difficulties, a greater proportion of children than in the typical population will demonstrate mild developmental, behavioral, or emotional difficulties. Finally, a subgroup of children remains who, despite making progress, continues to demonstrate significant difficulties that will require ongoing therapeutic interventions and pose significant challenges for their families.[1,14-26]

Addressing Long-term Challenges

Considerations in Developing a Differential Diagnosis of Developmental and Behavioral Issues

Implementing appropriate interventions to support any child's ongoing development and mental health requires identifying an appropriate diagnosis or diagnoses. However, for many children with backgrounds of abuse or neglect and institutional care, the lack of complete history, dynamic nature of a child's development, suddenness of the transition to a family, and lack of information about a child's likely potential can make the appropriate diagnoses difficult to ascertain. Despite this, using the available information for a specific child in conjunction with an understanding of group data described for children with similar circumstances allows parents and professionals to develop a list of diagnoses that are immediately evident, need to be considered, or may emerge over time. As with the typically developing pediatric patients seen in routine well-child care, the concept of *developmental surveillance and monitoring* remains important in determining if the trajectory of an adopted child's development is reassuring or concerning.[27,28]

Available medical history, physical examination, and routine diagnostic studies (eg, blood work recommended for children adopted internationally or from foster care, routine well-child care) should identify the most immediate and pressing medical issues. If a child is not physically healthy (eg, malnourished, infected with parasites, experiencing chronic ear infections, living with poorly controlled asthma), the child may have limited ability to benefit and respond to a supportive family setting and directed interventions. Physical discomfort can result in irritability and behavioral symptoms that in turn may interfere with family life, attachment, and capacity for learning (eg, gastroesophageal reflux in an infant or dental caries in an older child can be quite disruptive). It is important to treat acute medical concerns and develop a plan for chronic medical issues that will support physical well-being and lay the groundwork for overall optimal development.

When considering developmental, behavioral, and emotional diagnoses, the effect of underlying biology or early experience independently and jointly can be quite significant in producing long-term issues. From a biological perspective, some children are destined to have different developmental trajectories (eg, chromosomal abnormality such as trisomy 21) no matter where they are raised (nurturing home vs institution). However, a child with a known biological predisposition for developmental challenges is more likely to reach her full potential in a nurturing home and may appear more significantly impaired when neglected or in institutional care.[29] Genetic and prenatal and postnatal influences and an individual child's own resilience all contribute to differential outcomes in child development and overall well-being following adverse experiences. The question of nature versus nurture has evolved to an understanding that it is the interface of these influences that account for the differential outcomes seen in individuals subjected to similar life events. For example, a prospective longitudinal study demonstrated that individuals with 1 or 2 copies of the short allele for serotonin transporter (5-HTT) were more likely to develop depressive symptoms in response to life stressors than those who were homozygous for the long allele.[30] Despite the rapid progression of our understanding of the genetic and epigenetic factors that may promote or prevent typical development, far more remains to be learned about potential factors promoting resilience in children or adults with or without a history of adoption.

For many children adopted into families, significant unknowns remain concerning genetic and prenatal factors. However, birth parent and social history (eg, circumstances that led to the child's removal from the birth family; outcomes for other siblings or extended family members) can shed light on possible influences such as parental mental health status and potential for use of drugs or alcohol during or following a child's birth. Anxiety, bipolar disorder, schizophrenia, and learning disabilities have been shown to have genetic contributions. Prenatal exposure to drugs of abuse (eg, cocaine, heroin) or tobacco or nicotine, while possibly not as detrimental as once thought, may result in subtle, long-term differences in self-regulation, attention, learning, and executive function. In addition, some of these outcomes may be more strongly influenced by other associated prenatal exposures and early caregiving environment.[31-36] Extensive literature supports the potential negative effect of prenatal alcohol exposure in terms of primary neurologic deficits and secondary disabilities, which impact all domains of life function.[31,32] Malnutrition and lack of stimulation (eg, learning, social, emotional) during early periods of brain development can have lifelong effects of varying degrees depending on the timing, severity, and duration of the neglect. The impact of abuse, physical and emotional, has long-term ramifications. While some physical injuries may heal, emotional and neurocognitive problems may persist. Abuse and neglect experienced by an immature or developing brain may induce neurophysiologic changes in neurotransmitter levels and structure, which have implications for response to stress, nurturing, and learning.[8,37] For many children, the cumulative effects of genetic, prenatal, and postnatal factors result in significant impairments that require long-term intervention, even though many issues may improve over time.

■ CASE 1: JAYDEN

Jayden is an African American boy who was placed as an infant in foster care with white foster parents and their school-aged birth daughter. He entered foster care reportedly because of voluntary termination of parental rights following the involuntary removal of his older siblings. His birth mother received limited prenatal care, and there was no documentation of prenatal exposures or other perinatal concerns. Jayden remained in the care of this foster family through his toddler years, and they eventually adopted him. He was an active toddler and at 3 years of age, his preschool suggested further evaluation. Preliminary evaluation suggested attention-deficit/hyperactivity disorder (ADHD) symptoms and delays in Jayden's language skills. Referral to his local school district and further testing established his eligibility for a language-based preschool program. Jayden made progress in this program, but his ADHD symptoms persisted at a level that was interfering with his academic and social functioning. Jayden began a trial of stimulant medication and demonstrated gains in his language and pre-academic skills. The following year, Jayden was declassified and transitioned to a mainstream kindergarten setting without any supportive services or classroom modifications.

The following year, Jayden's adoptive mother died of cancer. During the turmoil of that year, Jayden did not continue with developmental follow-up, and his medication was discontinued by the family. A range of behavioral and emotional issues emerged and began to have a negative effect on Jayden's family in conjunction with the impact of the loss of their mother and wife. A case manager became concerned that if immediate support and intervention were not provided, disruption of the adoption could occur. When Jayden returned for follow-up, his father identified the following concerns for Jayden: inattention, hyperactivity, high levels of stress and conflict over repeated bowel accidents, poor school behavior and performance, and absence of supportive services through the school or private counseling. Jayden, who previously presented as a joyful, self-confident child, now appeared depressed and withdrawn.

Given Jayden's prior success with stimulants, medication management was restarted. Based on his prior history of language delay and the high rate of comorbid learning disabilities with ADHD, reevaluation for special education eligibility was requested. Under his state's specific guidelines, the school deferred evaluation but initiated supplemental instructions services and Section 504 accommodations. Simultaneously, a bowel management program, including daily laxatives and a toileting schedule, was used to address his encopresis

CASE 1: JAYDEN, CONTINUED

symptoms. In addition, counseling support for Jayden and his father was provided by a therapist experienced with working with families affected by loss, adoption, ADHD symptoms, and developmental challenges.

Over the course of several months, Jayden's soiling and bowel accidents became infrequent, child care arrangements were stabilized, and the relationship and interactions between Jayden and his father became more positive. School providers had a chance to monitor Jayden's positive response to medication and marginal response to preliminary educational interventions. It was agreed that a full psychoeducational reevaluation was warranted, as identification of significant challenges would allow for implementation of more extensive educational intervention services. With the stress of daily life reduced, effective implementation of supportive services, and the passage of time, the family moved beyond dealing with issues on a crisis basis. Time and emotional energy were spent on developing positive family interactions, settling into a new family rhythm in the absence of Jayden's mother, as well as more common issues that continued to arise with regard to being a single-parent and transracial family expanded by adoption.

Initial Evaluation

Children adopted from foster care or institutional settings or removed from their birth family should be considered at increased risk of developmental and behavioral issues. Pre-placement environment as well as post-placement situation affect the neurobiological and emotional underpinning of a child's development. As a result, it is imperative that children have comprehensive and systematic evaluation of their profile of strengths and weaknesses and review of prior potential influences on their development to arrange for any indicated intervention. If possible, this post-arrival evaluation should be performed by professionals experienced in child development and knowledgeable about the potential effect of pre-adoptive risk factors, including suboptimal care such as abuse and neglect. Often this evaluation takes a multidisciplinary approach, including a pediatrician or pediatric subspecialist (eg, developmental pediatrician, pediatric neurologist) and professionals from other disciplines, including a psychologist or neuropsychologist, an educator, or an occupational, physical, or speech-language therapist. Depending on the age and presentation of any specific child, monitoring or treatment by an age-appropriate school-based or private intervention program may be indicated.

While it is generally recommended that an immediate post-adoption medical evaluation be performed within 3 to 4 weeks of arrival or sooner if a child is acutely ill, a routine developmental evaluation is often best deferred a few weeks. This allows a child time to begin to settle into his new environment and for parents to develop an awareness of whether the child is struggling and what supports the family may need. Initial evaluation should include a review of available history, comprehensive physical examination (if not already performed), and developmental-behavioral assessment. The goal of this evaluation is to establish a child's skill levels in different domains of development (eg, cognitive, fine motor, gross motor, expressive/receptive language, self-help) and identify any behavioral and/or emotional issues that might require intervention. The use of standardized instruments and functional assessment are recommended and can be used during serial evaluations to document rates of progress.

The initial adjustment period for a child entering a new family can be smooth, have episodes of struggle, be a honeymoon period, or be quite overwhelming. Children may need extra time when they enter a family to adapt to their new environment and learn the routine as well as understand any expectations that the family may have for them. For children adopted internationally, hearing a new language, in addition to exposure to new foods, smells, and customs, can be quite overwhelming and adds to the adaptations required of the child. Infants and toddlers may adapt to their new situation more quickly than an older child, who must master home, school, and greater social expectations simultaneously. However, clinical experience indicates that even infants can go through periods of loss and stress associated with the absence of something familiar (ie, be withdrawn, irritable, or have gastrointestinal distress that presents as vomiting or diarrhea). The assistance of qualified professionals can help parents develop strategies to promote bonding, attachment, and skill development during this early period; identify transitional issues; and provide strategies to respond to difficult situations. However, for children who exhibit ongoing difficulties in transitioning to family life or skill development, parents should be encouraged to obtain consultation and support from appropriate professionals.

Initial physical examination should include attention to growth patterns, evidence of prior abuse, dysmorphology, and a detailed neuromotor evaluation. Identifying patterns on examination is essential to directing further evaluation and interventions. Is the child's physical examination consistent with suboptimal caregiving or "organic" factors inherent to the child? Are there physical examination findings suggestive of prenatal alcohol exposure or a chromosomal abnormality as a possible contributor to the child's delays? Children who have been raised in institutions tend to demonstrate low muscle tone caused by poor nutrition and lack of exercise. If the child demonstrates increased muscle tone, microcephaly, macrocephaly, or other focal neurologic findings, additional etiologies for these findings should be explored. This baseline assessment will determine which additional evaluations and interventions are required immediately and which can be deferred. It is also an opportunity to provide guidance to parents to support their child's transition into the family and assist families in prioritizing indicated assessments or services.

Follow-up Evaluation and the Evolution of Interventions

Children who present with developmental delays or behavioral issues at their initial evaluation require continued monitoring to determine if they are making appropriate progress across domains of development. Follow-up visits for these issues (as distinct from those that are medically indicated) should occur within 3 to 4 months, and earlier if concerns arise. For children who exhibit mild delays and where parents are comfortable, it would be appropriate to simply monitor the child without providing specific intervention services. For children with more significant delays, skilled intervention may be deferred for several months while the child is adjusting to family living, as these children still can make progress in skills, self-regulation, and physical health. Additional services may be needed if concerns persist beyond the initial adjustment period. For the child with severe developmental, behavioral, or emotional issues, more immediate intervention with appropriate therapists may be required to support the child and family.

For children who demonstrate developmental catch-up in the early months with their family, it is important to realize that issues may once again emerge when higher order or more complex cognitive skills are required. For example, a child who presents with early language delay and then demonstrates catch-up by kindergarten is still at increased risk for later language-based learning difficulties such as mastering phonemic awareness and decoding skills needed for reading. When problems emerge, even if subtle, it is important to have a low threshold for referring children for further evaluation to identify appropriate interventions (eg, education, therapies, medication, family support).

Accessing Developmental and Behavioral Evaluations and Intervention Services

Services for children with developmental or behavioral issues, aged birth to 21 years, as shown in Box 15-1, can be accessed through public and private educational and health care resources. Privately funded resources include health care facilities such as hospitals, rehabilitation and pediatric therapy centers, and individual practitioners in the community, which may be covered by insurance or require families to self-pay. For example, sometimes an initial consultation or evaluation may be covered by insurance, but interventions or therapies recommended as a result of the evaluation are not. At times, it may be difficult to identify a pediatric practitioner on a family's health care plan, much less one with expertise with a specific age group or particular developmental, behavioral, or mental health profile. To arrange for timely evaluations by appropriate professionals, the cost of the initial evaluation may need to be assumed by the family to confirm and document areas of concern, with the goal of advocating for access to publicly funded resources. The cost of the initial evaluations, although not negligible, is modest compared with the cost of ongoing

---

Box 15-1. Components of Multidisciplinary Evaluations (Private or Public)

- Developmental/cognitive (IQ) testing
- Educational/learning assessment
- Speech-language therapy (eg, communication, feeding)
- Occupational therapy (eg, fine motor, graphomotor, visual motor, visual perceptual, self-help)
- Physical therapy (ie, gross motor)
- Social-emotional
- Medical (May involve pediatrician, family physician, developmental pediatrician, pediatric neurologist, or child psychiatrist.)

---

educational, developmental (speech, occupational, or physical therapy), and mental health (counseling) therapies.

State and federal laws mandate publicly funded resources for children birth to 21 years of age with developmental and behavioral issues under the Education for All Handicapped Act (Public Law [PL] 94-142), the Individual with Disabilities Act (IDEA) (PL 99-457), and their subsequent reauthorizations. These federal laws are administered at the state level; thus, there is significant variability in the guidelines for evaluations, eligibility for services, and services provided. In some cases, the process is handled through government agencies; in others, contracts are held with private providers. Typically, services for children from birth to 3 years of age are provided through an early intervention (EI) program, while children older than 3 years receive developmental and educational supports through their local school systems. Additionally, states vary in their mechanism for providing additional supports for children and adults with severe developmental disabilities (eg, autism spectrum disorder [ASD], intellectual disability) and major mental health concerns. Health care professionals should be familiar with the process and agencies in their local communities.

Early Intervention

Early intervention is a program designed for the identification of children birth to 3 years of age with developmental or behavioral issues. Although evaluations are typically free, the provision of therapeutic services varies by state, ranging from free to requiring only a co-pay, billed on a sliding scale, insurance billed, or no provision of any services. To initiate the evaluation process, a parent or guardian is required to contact the designated agency (typically by phone) and indicate concern about a child's development. The child may be exhibiting delays, be at risk for delays because of medical issues or premature birth, or have a diagnosis associated with delays (eg, trisomy 21). The agency must follow state-specified timelines to complete the intake and evaluation process. A multidisciplinary evaluation of all domains of development is required. Once a child has qualified, an Individual Family Service Plan (IFSP) is written that identifies child-specific goals and objectives and therapies to be provided. This can include therapy by a range of professionals, including an early childhood developmental educator, occupational therapist, physical therapist, speech-language therapist, or social work support. Depending on the state model of intervention, therapies may be provided in the home or child care setting or may be center-based. Periodic reevaluations are usually performed at 3- to 6-month intervals to refine the IFSP and identify needs for further assessment or graduation from a program.

If a child does not qualify for services but is felt to be at risk, some states allow for a child to be enrolled in a tracking program with periodic reassessment of skills. If parents disagree with the results of an evaluation, there is an appeals process. If it is felt that a child will continue to require intervention beyond 3 years of age, a transition plan for working with the child's local school program is initiated. This process is usually initiated at least 90 days prior to a child's third birthday so that that public school system can continue services starting on the child's birthday. Entry into a program after 3 years of age is not based on the start of the academic year but rather should occur immediately after a child's third birthday.

Special Education Services

Beginning at age 3 years and until a child turns 21 years old (22 if the child is already in a program), the public school system becomes responsible for evaluation and provision of services for children with developmental challenges that affect their learning. The process can be initiated by the parent but must be done in writing. If a child is already attending a public school program, the school may notify a parent of concerns and request permission to initiate evaluations. As with EI, there is a state-mandated process and timeline that can be quite lengthy. In some instances, state regulations require that lower level supportive services (eg, basic skills instruction, reading support) be put in place to determine if these are sufficient (known as Response to Intervention) or if formal evaluation for special education services is necessary. For this reason, a parent may choose to pursue private evaluations and present results to the school to expedite the process. A multidisciplinary school-based evaluation usually involves an assessment of a child's cognitive abilities (IQ), educational performance, speech and language abilities, occupational therapy domains, motor skills by a physical therapist, and family and social history and review. Results from standardized testing, in conjunction with a functional assessment, determine if a child is performing at age or grade level and if the differences in performance meet criteria according to state codes to be deemed eligible for special education services. Physician consultation can be included as part of the evaluation process to diagnose medical (eg, diabetes) or emotional (eg, ADHD, depression) issues that negatively affect a child's ability to function at school and therefore qualify for special education services.

Eligibility guidelines for special education services vary from state to state but are based on federal guidelines. These educational categories do not necessarily use the same criteria as medical diagnoses or the *Diagnostic and Statistical Manual of Mental Disorders (DSM)*. Moreover, children with complex histories, including those with a history of adoption or foster care, often do not fit neatly into any diagnostic or educational category, but typically the educational category that best encompasses a child's profile is used. There are 12 basic categories (Box 15-2); however, the specific category does not determine the type of services a child may receive. For example, a child may have severe language delays and milder deficits in attention and fine motor skills. Because the language challenges are the most significant, the child could be classified under "communication impaired" and receive speech-language services and participate in a language-learning–disabled classroom but may also receive occupational therapy services.

If a child is determined to be eligible for services, an Individualized Education Plan (IEP) is created. This document describes the child's profile of strengths and weakness, goals and objectives specific to the child's need with benchmarks for monitoring, and specific interventions or services to be provided. Individualized Education Plans are reviewed and updated on an annual basis, and formal testing or reevaluation is completed every 3 years, or sooner if needed. Federal guidelines mandate that children receive a "free and appropriate education" and that those services should be provided in the "least restrictive environment" that meets the child's needs. The progression of settings begins with modifications within the

---

Box 15-2. Examples of Special Education Categories (Categories of Disability Under the Individuals with Disabilities Education Act)

- Autism
- Developmental disorders/delay
- Emotional disturbance
- Hearing impairment
- Intellectual disability
- Multiple disabilities
- Orthopedic impairment
- Other health impairment (ie, medical issues that interfere with school performance, including attention-deficit/hyperactivity disorder)
- Specific learning disability
- Speech or language/communication impairment
- Traumatic brain injury
- Visual impairment (includes blindness)

classroom setting and can progress to in-class support, pullout instruction for areas of weakness, self-contained classes, and if needed, self-contained schools. Most children do well in a mainstream classroom with appropriate supports within the classroom or specific pullout services for support in discrete areas. However, because of the nature of their learning, physical, or emotional difficulties, some children require placement in a separate school that specializes in providing care for children with complex needs. These programs can be schools run through the public system or private. Of note, some private programs, if approved by the state department of education, can be paid for by the school district when approved by the IEP team and special education director.

If a child is found to have areas of weakness but does not qualify for an IEP under special education guidelines, supportive services may still be provided. Basic skills instruction or supplemental instruction may be provided by the school in subjects such as reading or math without having an IEP. For some children, this is sufficient to allow progress, but it is important to realize that services provided without an IEP may not be at the intensity of or use strategies typical for special education. Because additional state or federal funding is not provided to the school district to provide these resources, there is also no guarantee that these services will continue. If parents disagree with the district's decision to deem the child ineligible for services, they may enter due-process proceedings as outlined in each state's educational code.

For physical and mental disabilities that affect academic function but do not meet criteria for special education, provisions of the Rehabilitation Act of 1973 (PL 93-112) may apply. Section 504 of the Rehabilitation Act represents legislation under the Americans with Disabilities Act, not special education law. The focus of Section 504 is to prevent discrimination by agencies that receive federal funds, against those with disabilities, and requires accommodations so that a disability does not interfere with the ability to perform one's job. Although primarily directed toward physical disabilities (eg, requiring ramps for wheelchair access), Section 504 has been effectively used in school for children with ADHD, a medical condition that can interfere with a child's academic performance. Like an IEP, a Section 504 plan can be written that provides accommodations to support success in the classroom setting (eg, preferential seating, untimed tests). In contrast with special education services, districts do not receive state or federal funding for 504 modifications and different guidelines apply.

In addition to or instead of publicly funded services, parents may choose to provide private academic tutoring or therapies (eg, speech-language, occupation, physical) for their children. These services can be used to augment or reinforce what is being provided in the school. It is critical to realize that private tutoring is not a substitute for support that a child may need during the school day. For example, a weekly session of after-school tutoring or therapy may not address the challenges that a child may face throughout a 6-hour school day. For children with milder or focused areas of impairment, private instruction can be helpful, especially if the tutor and teacher coordinate their approach. With practice and remediation, a child may be able to carry over skills from a private tutor or therapist to the classroom setting. In contrast, children with significant deficits in single or multiple domains of school function require replacement instruction or supportive services in the place where they are required to perform on a daily basis and may require a separate school placement, which can mean significant out-of-pocket costs for parents.

In addition to providing specific educational supports, schools have been mandated by federal laws to address physical issues as well as behavioral and emotional concerns (ie, Education for All Handicapped Act, IDEA, Rehabilitation Act of 1973, and subsequent reauthorizations). Although public schools have developed some resources to address this expanded definition of educational concerns, supports in the domains of learning disabilities, language delays, and slow learning are areas of relative strength within the educational system. Children with milder emotional issues can receive counseling and support within the public school setting, but families often need to provide additional private therapeutic services. Children with more significant issues who require more comprehensive therapeutic support may require an out-of-district placement in a public regional program, private day school, or even residential setting as well as ongoing therapy that may be directed to an individual child and family.

Role of Private Resources

As described previously, public resources exist that can serve as a framework for providing intervention to support a child's overall development and well-being. However, depending on state funding, demographics of the community (ie, urban, suburban, or rural), and a child's specific issues, typically available EI and special education resources may not meet a child's unique needs. In these situations, parents may want to look to private resources in the community to augment and collaborate with pubic resources or possibly provide all interventions. This is often true to obtain evaluations and services in a more timely manner as well as have professionals with specific expertise in working with children with similar histories and complex profiles involved in the diagnostic evaluation and developing a treatment plan. Most school professionals can perform needed evaluations to diagnose a learning disability (eg, dyslexia), graphomotor issues, or attention difficulties. However, many are not versed in the effect of abuse or institutionalization on overall executive function and social-emotional development and may not appreciate how these factors may impact a child's school performance (academic, behavioral, social) and guide specific interventions. Moreover, school systems are not responsible for addressing how these issues may affect home life, family function, and function in the general community.

Across the domains of development, therapists with expertise in different areas can work with children to foster skill development and help them reach their potential. Occupational therapists work on self-care and writing skills, while speech therapists focus on language and communication skills. With younger children, many of these specialists will provide services across domains. For social-emotional and behavioral issues, therapists from distinct but related disciplines can work with a child and family (eg, child psychiatrist, psychologist, social worker). For some children, being in a nurturing family environment is sufficient in supporting them in moving forward. For other children, their genetics, prior experiences, and neurocognitive profiles require directed therapy (or therapies) to allow them to process their prior experiences and begin to move forward. In young children (around 2 to 3 years of age, or when cause-and-effect reasoning is present), therapy may initially take a "play" format; as a child becomes more verbal, "talk" therapy (ie, cognitive, psychodynamic, trauma-focused cognitive-behavioral therapy) may become more appropriate. Therapeutic approaches need to be based on a child's developmental and emotional state (direct discussions or confrontation may be too overwhelming) rather than taking into account only a child's chronologic age and diagnosis. At times, medication may play a role in reducing behavioral and emotional symptoms, making a child more available to participate in and benefit from available therapeutic interventions (eg, pharmacologic management of ADHD, anxiety symptoms).

When identifying potential therapists, it is important to ask about the professional's prior experience with children of similar profiles (eg, age, diagnosis, prior experiences). It is also relevant to ask about therapeutic approach and orientation. For example, is the practitioner using mainstream, evidence-based techniques or trying alternative interventions that are not evidence based?[38] Families also require support and guidance in developing strategies that meet their specific child's profile and needs. Parents often do not come with a skill set that is an ideal match for managing a child's issues, whether they are first-time parents of a typical toddler or experienced parents who have a child with a psychiatric issue. Even parents of children without major delays or behavioral issues can feel overwhelmed by the arrival of a child with whom they have not developed a rhythm for ongoing interactions. Providing a sense of what is normal and directly addressing concerns can provide a stronger foundation for the family to move forward.

Community Resources

Families live in a community and thus should be supported to find ways to participate in and receive appropriate services from their community. This will also prevent families from becoming isolated because of their child's developmental, behavioral, or emotional issues. Family needs can range from acquiring a specific skill set to meet their child's needs to requiring educational, recreational, respite, or developmental disability resources on an ongoing basis. Private organizations such as YMCA programs or religious-affiliated groups may provide recreational activities, while diagnosis-specific resources and support groups as well as state programs (eg, state division of developmental disabilities, adoption subsidy) may provide tangible resources that make day-to-day life easier. There are instances when a child's physical, behavioral, or emotional needs exceed a family's ability to provide the requisite support and care, or a child's behavior may pose a safety threat to themselves or other family members. At these times, a residential placement may be in the best interest of the child and family; it requires collaboration between public and private resources to provide the financial and emotional support for what clearly can be an overwhelming situation.

Psychopharmacology

Who Should Prescribe Medication

For many parents and physicians, the use of medication to help manage a child's behavior, mood, and function poses significant challenges. Parents may be resistant to using medication because of hopes that time and other interventions will be sufficient, misinformation about medication, and concerns about medication safety and side effects. For the general pediatrician, lack of familiarity with the range of medications that may be required as well as the time needed to address complex situations and medication management can be challenging. Subspecialists such as child psychiatrists, pediatric neurologists, and developmental pediatricians are more likely to have expertise in medication management for behavior and mood, as well as prior experience in medicating children with a history of abuse, neglect, or institutionalization. Certainly children can present with a complex profile and may not respond typically to traditional trials of medications. Of note, the number of US Food and Drug Administration–approved medications for the pediatric population for treatment of behavioral and emotional disorders is limited, even in the presence of research literature that supports their use. Thus, off-label use is frequently undertaken to help manage a range of difficulties for this and other pediatric populations. Medical screening is indicated for some medications, particularly in the absence of birth family or prior medical history (eg, baseline electrocardiogram) and some required ongoing medical monitoring (eg, blood pressure, growth, blood work).

When to Consider Medication

In the case of children newly joining their adoptive family, it is usually recommended that the child be allowed time to settle into the family and that some type of behavioral, psychotherapeutic (eg, play therapy, cognitive-behavioral therapy), or educational intervention be initiated prior to considering medication. However, significant difficulties may persist despite a supportive home and school setting and counseling. When professionals and parents working with the child feel that further progress in behavioral, emotional, or academic growth is limited by symptoms that could be responsive to medication, a medication trial may be indicated. In other cases, a child's difficulties may be very severe, or a child may be behaviorally or emotionally unavailable to benefit from educational or other therapeutic interventions (eg, overwhelming anxiety resulting in withdrawal) or a danger to himself or others (eg, irritability, aggression) such that medication is used to enable the child to be available to participate in therapeutic options and family life.

Response to Medication

In some children, there is an immediate and significant response to medication. For example, treatment of ADHD without any other comorbid states (eg, anxiety, developmental delay, learning) can be very rewarding, with up to 80% of children being responsive to one of the stimulant medications. An overflow effect can also be seen; if a child's ADHD symptoms are reduced (eg, more attentive to those around him; less impulsive in responding), the child may have improved peer and family interactions and experience greater success in schoolwork. In some cases, one medication (eg, selective serotonin reuptake inhibitor [SSRI]) can be used to target multiple symptoms (eg, anxiety and depression), although perhaps affecting one symptom more effectively than another. In children with complex profiles and multiple diagnoses, as can be seen in children with adverse life experiences, responses may not be as dramatic, and multiple medications may be required.

When prescribing on- and off-label medications in children (Table 15-1), starting with a low dose and monitoring for side effects and idiosyncratic reactions are crucial. Parents may discontinue a medication trial because of perceived side effects or prior to reaching a therapeutic dose. It is important to have a partnership with parents and children when initiating treatment so that they feel comfortable proceeding with your recommendations, particularly if it takes time for minor side

Table 15-1. Examples of Medication Options Based on Target Behaviors (Including Off-label Uses of Medications)

Target Symptoms	Medication Class and Examples Generic (Brand Name)
ADHD (inattention, impulsivity, hyperactivity)	**Stimulant** • Methylphenidate (Ritalin, Metadate, Methylin, Concerta, Daytrana) • Dexmethylphenidate (Focalin) • Dextroamphetamine (Dexedrine, DextroStat, Vyvanse) • Amphetamine/dextroamphetamine mix (Adderall) **Non-stimulant** • Atomoxetine (Strattera) • Clonidine (Catapres, Kapvay) • Guanfacine (Tenex, Intuniv)

Table 15-1. Examples of Medication Options Based on Target Behaviors (Including Off-label Uses of Medications), continued

Target Symptoms	Medication Class and Examples Generic (Brand Name)
Anxiety	**SSRI** • Fluoxetine (Prozac) • Sertraline (Zoloft) • Escitalopram (Lexapro) • Citalopram (Celexa) • Venlafaxine (Effexor) **Benzodiazepine** • Clonazepam (Klonopin) • Alprazolam (Xanax) • Diazepam (Valium) • Lorazepam (Ativan)
Mood	**SSRI** *Anticonvulsant* • Carbamazepine (Tegretol) • Valproic Acid (Depakene, Depakote) • Lamotrigine (Lamictal) • Gabapentin (Neurontin) • Topiramate (Topamax) • Oxcarbazepine (Trileptal) *Atypical Antipsychotic* • Risperidone (Risperdal) • Aripiprazole (Abilify) • Quetiapine (Seroquel) • Olanzapine (Zyprexa)
Irritability, Aggression, Mood	**Anticonvulsant** • Carbamazepine (Tegretol) • Valproic Acid (Depakene, Depakote) • Lamotrigine (Lamictal) • Gabapentin (Neurontin) • Topiramate (Topamax) • Oxcarbazepine (Trileptal) **Atypical Antipsychotic** • Risperidone (Risperdal) • Aripiprazole (Abilify) • Quetiapine (Seroquel) • Olanzapine (Zyprexa)

Abbreviations: ADHD, attention-deficit/hyperactivity disorder; SSRI, selective serotonin reuptake inhibitor.

effects to resolve (eg, stomach upset) or for a medication to reach a therapeutic level (eg, atomoxetine, SSRIs).

Complex Presentations, Differential Diagnoses, and Intervention

A child's developmental-behavioral profile is the product of multiple influences (Box 15-3). Prioritizing an intervention is not always simple when different causes (eg, prenatal alcohol exposure, anxiety, mild cognitive impairment) may present with a similar behavioral phenotype (eg, inattention).

Children from backgrounds of deprivation, abuse, or neglect may present with a behavioral profile similar to a child with no prior adverse experience or something more familiar to the clinician, such as a history of premature birth. In developing a differential diagnosis, an individual child's prior history as well as knowledge about group data from research reports (eg, effect of institutionalization or prenatal alcohol exposure) may be relevant to a diagnostic formulation. A comprehensive evaluation to identify possible etiologies, comorbidities, and current level of functioning must all be considered in developing a differential diagnosis and an intervention or treatment plan. Pertinent issues and diagnostic considerations can change or become more evident over time, with changing expectations and demands emerging at different ages and with different life situations.

Some children simply do not neatly fit into a diagnostic category. In this case, an accurate description of a child's skills, behaviors, and responses is the first step in identifying targets for therapeutic intervention. For children with complex and confusing profiles, a tiered approach may be used, with the most overwhelming symptom addressed first (eg, anxiety), and the child's ability to perform tasks and behavioral profile reevaluated to tease out contributing or comorbid factors

---

Box 15-3. Observed Behaviors and Possible Diagnoses

Behaviors Exhibited	Diagnoses to be Considered
• Difficulty communicating needs	• Prenatal brain injury
• Poor school performance	• Trauma (physical, emotional)
• Poor eye contact	• Intellectual disability
• Poor or inappropriate social interaction	• Autism spectrum disorder
• Atypical behaviors (eg, self-stimulation)	• Learning disabilities
• Noncompliant/defiant behavior	• Language delay
• Inattention/hyperactivity/impulsivity	• Emotional difficulties (eg, anxiety, attachment
• Aggression	disorder)
• Destruction of property	• Learned behaviors

(eg, learning disability, depression). Once a more complete picture of a child's issues becomes apparent, a more comprehensive and specific intervention plan can be developed. Ongoing follow-up information from parents, teachers, and other intervention providers is critical in refining a child's diagnoses, target behaviors, and intervention. The frequency of follow-up depends on the severity of the issues being addressed, the parents' need for support and feedback, and the time in which one would expect to see a response to the intervention.

Learning Disabilities and Other Cognitive Impairments

A child's early profile of developmental delays may resolve over time but may persist and need to be reformulated as representing a learning disability (ie, difficulty with demonstrating mastery of an academic skill such as reading, despite normal intelligence) or cognitive-adaptive impairment (intellectual disability). A learning disability, intellectual disability (particularly mild), or "slow learner" profile cannot be accurately diagnosed if formal testing is not completed. As noted in the case of Jayden (see page 322), complex histories and changing profiles and circumstances can all affect a child's performance at school.

Interventions for learning issues, whether an isolated issue or more global cognitive deficits, involve initial remediation of skills and ongoing accommodations for continuing areas of difficulty. Research indicates that individuals with dyslexia respond to intensive multimodal intervention (eg, Orton Gillingham) and can become accurate readers. Research also demonstrates that as adults, individuals with dyslexia who have been remediated can become accurate readers; however, they remain slower readers. Therefore, once remediation is completed during early elementary grades, the accommodation of extra time is necessary throughout high school, college, and even work situations.[39] For children with more significant cognitive impairments, appropriate educational supports to maximize academic and life skills are critical to current and future functioning, whether with the family or in a supervised community setting or residential, fully supportive placement.

An important point to remember is that most school environments teach to the mean and by default set a standard that a child should perform equally well at all tasks, independent of interest or ability. For children with milder learning issues or a slower learning profile, school may always be a struggle, but with appropriate supports and expectations, children can still be successful. More importantly, appropriate educational supports will lay the foundation for future opportunities, whether they are educational or vocational experiences that are more tailored to a young adult's specific interests and talents.

Language Delay

Early language delay is one of the more common concerns identified in the toddler or preschool-aged child. When determining etiology, one must consider whether a specific child's language development trajectory is following the trajectory of a late normal bloomer, caused by recent lack of language exposure as seen in orphanage care, due to English being a second language, an early indicator of intellectual disability or ASD, related to selective mutism following trauma, secondary to a hearing impairment, or isolated delays in expressive or receptive language development. A comprehensive history is important but may not be available. Confirming normal hearing is essential for any child with language delays, especially children with relatively unknown family history and past medical history. Establishing baseline language function is essential, as is monitoring early changes in language skills once in a supportive family setting. Young children from neglectful or under-stimulating settings usually increase the frequency and variety of vocalizations when joining a family. Children whose primary language exposure is not English but who have an intact primary language start to pick up English words within a week of arrival and tend to communicate with gestures and nonverbal strategies (see Chapter 14, Speech and Language Outcomes After International Adoption, on page 283 for more information).

The tendency of schools and evaluators to automatically assume that children adopted internationally only require English-as-a-second-language support rather than speech and language remediation is concerning because research has shown that the majority of these children do not have age-appropriate competency in their primary language, and some have no language skills at all.[1-5] Thus, initial evaluations ideally should be done in the child's primary language within several months after arrival, as young children will lose their existing language skills in their primarily language more rapidly than they will acquire English. Some children, depending on age and prior language experience, require 2 to 3 years to master basic conversational language skills, and it may take 4 to 6 more years for a child to achieve cognitive academic language proficiency (ie, language for learning).[40,41] At older ages, language-based issues may emerge and present as a reading difficulty or as difficulties in understanding abstract or complex language.

CASE 2: LILY

Lily was adopted from a Chinese orphanage at 14 months of age. Her history was remarkable for a cleft lip and palate with an initial surgical repair in China and failure to thrive. Due to her overall profile of delay despite significant progress during the first few months with her adoptive family, Lily received early intervention services. Because of more complex speech and language issues, she also received private therapy with a practitioner with experience working with children with cleft lips and palates. By age 3, Lily's global language skills had approached the lower end of age appropriate, but there were continued issues with her willingness to talk and participate in a preschool or child care setting as well as oral-motor and articulation issues related to her cleft repair. Due

CASE 2: LILY, CONTINUED

to her near–age-appropriate language skills, her school district felt that Lily would not qualify for IEP services.

A detailed report from the treating speech-language therapist, including class observation, documented difficulty participating successfully in a mainstream classroom. These findings supported the need for further evaluation, and Lily was later deemed eligible for special education services. Within a few months of participation in a small, self-contained, language-supported classroom, Lily's language, self-confidence, and group participation increased dramatically. The following year she participated in an integrated preschool class with speech and language services and then transitioned to a mainstream kindergarten class with continued speech-language therapy. Because of her early history prior to adoption as well as early language delays and a cleft lip and palate, she will require ongoing monitoring for more subtle difficulties with higher order neurocognitive tasks.

CASE 3: ROBERT

The same family who adopted Lily (see case 2 on page 337) adopted Robert, who also had a cleft lip and palate, from a Chinese orphanage at almost 6 years of age. Robert seemed quite competent with regard to his activities of daily living and demonstrated many age-appropriate play skills. Despite being told he had attended an orphanage school, observation by the parents suggested that Robert did not have any pre-academic or early academic skills. Although he was initially very quiet and watchful, Robert's early transition to his family appeared to be smooth, and he appeared to be acquiring some understanding of English. The school district was contacted to do an evaluation in Mandarin, which was refused with a recommendation to place Robert in a regular preschool (rather than kindergarten) to "see how he did."

Robert was taken for a private developmental pediatric evaluation with a translator present who spoke Mandarin as well as the local dialect that was used in Robert's orphanage. As described by his parents, play skills were fairly well developed. Nonverbal skills, such as puzzles, matching, and fine motor manipulation, were at or close to age appropriate. He learned quickly from demonstration. Graphomotor skills and concepts of quantity were delayed, and he was not familiar with the Chinese symbols for numbers, despite having attended "school" at his orphanage. Most significantly, Robert could not follow a 2-step command, his articulation in his native language was poor, and his language content was immature. This information was taken to the school district, which arranged for a complete evaluation by a bilingual testing service. Robert was enrolled in kindergarten and found eligible for special education services, including small group instruction; speech, language, and occupational therapy;

CASE 3: ROBERT, CONTINUED

and English-as-a-second-language support. A 4-month reevaluation to assess progress was recommended.

Lily and Robert present not only with a history of institutionalization but also cleft lip and palate; both are associated with a range of developmental, learning, and behavioral issues. Although both children present with a resilient profile and many strengths, knowledge of the specific deficits associated with their history (ie, effect of institutionalization and cleft lip and palate on speech and language development) allowed appropriate evaluations and interventions to occur.

Attention-Deficit/Hyperactivity Disorder

Attention-deficit/hyperactivity disorder is reported to affect approximately 5% to 8% of all children.[42,43] Parents may raise concerns during the preschool years about their child's activity and attention level, but often it is not until symptoms interfere with academics, peers, or family interactions that further evaluation or intervention is sought. While ADHD is common in general, symptoms can be manifest in a wide variety of disorders for adopted children. Other diagnoses must also be strongly considered before a child who has experienced adverse early experiences is treated for ADHD (Box 15-4). Pre-adoption history (eg, family, caregiving experiences) can help to delineate possible factors that may mimic ADHD symptoms and determine the most appropriate intervention. Although core symptoms of ADHD—inattention, impulsivity, hyperactivity—can be caused by a primary neurocognitive deficit affecting the prefrontal cortex of the brain, this behavioral presentation can also be a secondary manifestation of or comorbid with other diagnoses. Multidisciplinary evaluations are essential in confirming or ruling out

---

Box 15-4. Differential Diagnosis of Attention-Deficit/Hyperactivity Disorder Symptoms Following Foster Care/Institutionalization

- Age-appropriate behavior in an active child
- Primary attention-deficit/hyperactivity disorder
- Adjustment reaction intellectual disability
- Language delay
- Learning disability
- Anxiety
- Post-traumatic stress disorder
- Depression
- Autism spectrum disorder abnormalities of attachment

other comorbid diagnoses, such as a learning disability, which can affect a significant percentage of children with ADHD.[42,43]

The appropriate use of therapies, including medications, can only be implemented after an accurate diagnosis is made. Typical ADHD medications may be ineffective or may worsen symptoms if the diagnosis is incorrect. Research indicates that appropriate medications can have a significant positive effect independent of other interventions.[44] Stimulant medication also can be effective for children with cognitive impairments. The practitioner and parents, however, need to be realistic about the target symptoms; namely, understanding that underlying cognitive impairments will not change.[45,46] Stimulant medications are the overwhelming preference (vs other drug classes) for treatment of ADHD symptoms because of their high response rate, immediacy of effect, safety profile, and ease of administration, but they should never be considered the sole intervention. In preschool-aged children, behavioral approaches are the recommended first line of intervention, with consideration for the addition of medication when behavioral strategies are not sufficient to manage ADHD symptoms.[43] Multimodal interventions, including providing parent support and behavioral and educational strategies, support better outcomes, especially when there are comorbidities.

CASE 4: TATIANA

Tatiana is a 10-year-old adopted from Russia at 3 years of age. At 6 years of age, Tatiana was evaluated for possible ADHD. At the initial evaluation, physical examination revealed that Tatiana had facial features and growth characteristics consistent with fetal alcohol syndrome (FAS), which had not been previously diagnosed. Tatiana was indiscriminately friendly in social settings, but her parents felt that she was attached to them. Her parents had explicitly taught her to use formal greetings and shake hands, but she needed a reminder not to hug the examiner at the first meeting.

Psychoeducational testing demonstrated Tatiana's intelligence to be in the average range, but she had relative weaknesses with visual spatial and perceptual skills, difficulties with social comprehension, and challenges with aspects of executive function (ie, judgment, organization, inattention, and impulsivity). Based on this assessment, Tatiana was deemed eligible for special education services. Stimulant medication was initiated to address her symptoms of inattention and impulsivity. Behavioral management strategies and information about FAS were discussed with Tatiana's parents.

Because of parental concerns about social skills, safety considerations, and the need for close supervision, Tatiana attended a parochial school through third grade. Although state and federal guidelines require special education services to be provided in this setting, the services were not as extensive as those available in a public school. Because of increasing academic demands, Tatiana could no longer be supported in the parochial school setting, and she transitioned

CASE 4: TATIANA, CONTINUED

to a public school program. Additional academic supports were provided for Tatiana, including resource room supports for some academic subjects, but modifications in her mainstream classroom were not implemented. School staff viewed Tatiana as a child with normal intelligence, ADHD symptoms, and learning weaknesses and did not have an understanding of the larger neurocognitive issues seen in children with FAS. As the year progressed, the need for a classroom aide became evident.

Tatiana remained pleasant and outgoing and made progress in school, but by sixth grade, the effect of her prenatal alcohol exposure on her overall functioning resulted in increasing difficulties. At an age when children are expected to begin to exhibit more independence and require less adult supervision, Tatiana increasingly demonstrated poor judgment and did not learn from her prior experiences. In middle school, it was necessary for her teacher to supervise her packing her backpack at the end of the school day; Tatiana would put work back in her locker if she did not like the assignment or thought that it was already completed. Her teachers thought that because Tatiana was in middle school, she should be more "responsible" and not need additional support or supervision from parents or teachers. They did not understand that having 6 different teachers and needing to organize her locker and school supplies was an overwhelming task for her. Tatiana's parents and private professionals continued to advocate for ongoing academic and behavioral support at school, including appropriate modification of her work assignments, support for organizational skills, and increased supervision.

Although growing, Tatiana remained smaller than her peers, was excluded by the other girls, and frequently got into trouble by doing something that other students told her to do. To reduce the chances of Tatiana causing more trouble, her parents limited her social activities to those at their church with adult supervision. Tatiana's parents were provided with information and resources to help mitigate the secondary morbidities (eg, school failure, trouble with the law, substance abuse) seen in individuals with FAS.[32] Despite normal intelligence, Tatiana will require lifelong support. Comprehensive evaluation revealed that Tatiana's inattentive and impulsive behaviors, which were thought to represent only ADHD symptoms, had much broader implications for diagnosis and intervention plans.

Attachment Disorders

The diagnosis of reactive attachment disorder (RAD) is one of the most confusing and misrepresented diagnoses by parents and many practitioners. Many children adopted internationally from orphanages and domestically from foster care settings may experience attachment difficulties. The lack of a consistent caregiver in a child's early life can make it difficult for that child to feel attached or bonded to caregivers. When a child is adopted, she may experience behaviors that present obstacles for the new family to develop closeness with the child. While these behaviors are very common when a child arrives, severe reactive attachment issues are, fortunately, rare.

As per the *DSM, 5th Edition (DSM-5)*, the diagnosis of RAD is a "trauma and stressor-related disorder." Reactive attachment disorder should be considered in children who present with "a consistent pattern of inhibited, emotionally withdrawn behavior towards adult caregivers"; "persistent social and emotional disturbance" (eg, minimal social responsiveness, lack of positive affect, unprovoked irritability or sadness during interactions with caregiver); prior experience of "extremes of insufficient care"; a developmental age of at least 9 months; and onset at younger than 5 years.[42]

The *DSM-5* also distinguishes between children who meet criteria for RAD and are unable to form selective attachments with their caregivers and those who have disinhibited social engagement disorder and are attached to their caregivers. Children with disinhibited social engagement disorder exhibit the following profile: indiscriminately approach and interact with adults; have experienced "extremes of insufficient care"; and socially disinhibited behavior not due to ADHD or impulsivity.[42]

Insufficient care can include abuse, neglect, or lack of a stable primary caregiver. This type of history is nearly universal in children adopted from an orphanage and can also be a significant factor for children adopted from foster care. Although challenges to bonding and attachment are expected as a child becomes part of a family, a small number of children who experience pathologic care develop RAD symptoms. However, children who have been maltreated or exposed to violence frequently exhibit aggressive, oppositional behaviors or other challenging behaviors. Although a child's outward behaviors may suggest the possible diagnosis of RAD, the underlying issue may not be the child's inability to form selective attachments but another developmental or behavioral disorder such as ASD or PTSD. Thus, consideration of the diagnosis of an attachment disorder requires careful evaluation of a child's pre- and post-adoptive history, current levels of function across domains, past and current behaviors, and review of medical issues (Box 15-5).

Box 15-5. Differential Diagnosis of Reactive Attachment Disorder

Adjustment reaction	Learning disability
Parent-child relational problem	Cognitive impairment/intellectual disability
Depression	Autism spectrum disorder
Anxiety	Attention-deficit/hyperactivity disorder
Post-traumatic stress disorder	Oppositional defiant disorder

Considerable controversy exists concerning not only assessment but also treatment of children with attachment disorders. There are a variety of therapeutic models available for approaching attachment problems as well as RAD. Key components include a stable caregiving environment with an appropriate attachment figure, creating positive interaction opportunities between child and caregiver, and treatment of comorbid disorders. Concerns have been expressed about more controversial therapies that involve "holding" and coercive strategies.[42,47]

CASE 5: SASHA

Sasha is a 7-year-old adopted from a Russian orphanage at approximately 3 years of age. At his initial evaluation, shortly after joining his adoptive family, he presented with mild delays in his nonverbal skills and more significant delays in his primary language (Russian) skills. Sasha participated in a special education preschool program for 2 years; because of gains in his overall skills, he was no longer deemed eligible for special education services. Sasha was then enrolled in a private kindergarten program.

Sasha returned for evaluation during first grade at 6 years of age. Sasha lived in a family with 2 working parents, an 11-year-old birth daughter of the parents, and a nanny who had been with the family for 10 years. Concerns were expressed about Sasha's inattentive, impulsive, and explosive behaviors at home and at school and his learning being at a "standstill." There was significant sibling rivalry, and Sasha "always appeared to be angry." At the evaluation, Sasha appeared sullen, anxious, and uncooperative. A recommendation was made for comprehensive psychoeducational testing and counseling. Private testing and emotional evaluation were completed and demonstrated average IQ but persistence of a language-based learning disability, in addition to emotional dysregulation, anxiety, and concerns about attachment. It was not felt that the private school he was attending had the resources to continue to meet Sasha's needs, and it was recommended that Sasha return to the public school and be reassessed for special education services. Given Sasha's emotional profile, it was felt that it would be best to finish the last few months of the year at his current school and focus on family-based interventions.

The family began weekly counseling with an experienced psychologist. Initially, the therapist met with the parents and provided them with strategies to promote more positive interactions and feedback, as well as a behavior plan for managing unacceptable behaviors. The child care provider was also able to use these strategies. This helped to improve Sasha's self-esteem and reduce conflict in the home. Sasha attended a specialized camp program in the summer, which assisted in building Sasha's self-confidence through appropriately structured and supervised activities. In the fall, Sasha entered the second grade in public school with an IEP to support his learning weaknesses and behavioral profile. During the course of these interventions, Sasha was also started on

CASE 5: SASHA, CONTINUED

medication to address his mood, anxiety, and impulsivity (risperidone and ato-moxetine) with a significant positive response.

As Sasha began experiencing increasing success during his interactions at home and school, he became more available to participate in therapy individu-ally and with other family members. Despite his significant gains in learning, mood, and behavior, attachment issues were still felt to be significant. Sasha was able to articulate that his anger toward his sister was caused by the fact that she was the birth child of their mother and, therefore, there was no way his mother could love him the same way. The family continues to use an inter-disciplinary team to address Sasha's complicated profile. Through successive evaluations and monitoring of response to multimodal intervention, diagnostic considerations and treatment plans will continue to be refined. Learning and attachment issues are unlikely to resolve entirely; however, Sasha and his fam-ily have supports in place and are learning strategies to better negotiate the demands of family and community life.

Post-traumatic Stress Disorder

In the category of trauma and stressor-related disorders in *DSM-5*, PTSD is the result of overwhelming anxiety that is precipitated by a traumatic event or series of events that result in a real or perceived threat to an individual's or another's safety. This event can be directly experienced or witnessed. Individuals with PTSD experience symptoms of intrusion (eg, distressing memories or dreams, flashbacks, physiological reactions to cues). There is also a "persistent avoidance of stimuli associated with the traumatic event" (ie, certain places, people, or activities that are reminders and result in feelings of distress). There are "negative alterations in cognition and mood" and "alterations in arousal" (eg, hypervigilance, sleep distur-bance, poor concentration).[42]

In preschool-aged children, alternate criteria for PTSD, which adjusts manifesta-tions for children's developmental level, have been reviewed (eg, regression in previ-ously attained skills such as toileting or language, changes in play behaviors, extreme temper tantrums). Studies using these criteria for PTSD suggest that this disorder is more prevalent in the high-risk pediatric population than previously reported.[48,49] The *DSM-5* has included modified criteria for the diagnosis of PTSD in children younger than 6 years to reflect these developmental differences in expression of emotional distress. The *DSM-5* also describes a range of trauma- and stress-related disorders that affect behavior but do not meet criteria for PTSD.

Foster and adoptive parents may not be aware of prior trauma in their child's history and the risk of PTSD. As a result, they may misinterpret a child's behavior as being willfully oppositional for not complying with a request when, in fact, the child may be paralyzed by overwhelming anxiety. A young child may have previously seemed "fine," but as the child reprocesses experiences at different developmental ages and the demands of functioning in a family and community become more complex, symptoms may become more apparent. For example, although a child is being successfully toilet trained at home and in public places, he refuses to use the white-tiled, institutional-appearing bathroom at school and has extreme tantrums to avoid entering the bathroom. Similarly, symptoms of PTSD may not be evident until a child experiences an event that triggers a memory or is able to act on or verbalize past experiences and emotions. For children who come from backgrounds of risk (eg, institutionalization, subject or witness to abuse, violence, catastrophic events) or with an unknown history, PTSD and the continuum of behaviors seen as a result of toxic stress should be included in the differential diagnosis when being evaluated for ADHD, RAD, or other difficulties such as anxiety, developmental regression, or oppositional behaviors.

It is important to remember that often a child's history is incomplete and may not mention any traumatizing events. More importantly, it is the child's perception of events (as a threat to himself or others) that influences development of these symptoms. Interventions should be evidence based and directed at helping a child feel safe and process his past experiences. In some cases, medication management may be necessary.

■ **CASE 6: SYLVIA**
Sylvia is an 8-year-old girl adopted from foster care. She was orphaned at 4 years of age after she witnessed her mother being murdered by a boyfriend. Limited information was available about Sylvia's history and profile prior to coming to the attention of child protective services. Sylvia was placed in the custody of an elderly aunt, who cared for her for 1 year, but due to a combination of factors, she was unable to continue in this placement. Sylvia was adopted by a single, professional woman and enrolled in kindergarten and seemed to be able to do grade-appropriate work. Because of the circumstances of Sylvia's life, her mother initiated a relationship with a therapist experienced in working with families affected by adoption. Despite individual and family counseling over several years, slow progress was observed, and Sylvia began demonstrating increasing behavioral and emotional difficulties in home and at school.

In third grade, because of continued behavioral issues at home and in school, Sylvia and her mother came for psychiatric evaluation. School providers indicated that Sylvia's academic performance was not significantly below grade level and that any academic and social difficulties she exhibited were caused by ADHD and oppositional defiant disorder (ODD) and, therefore, no intervention was required by the school. Review of behavioral rating scales completed by her teacher indicated that Sylvia was disruptive in class and verbally aggressive toward peers, had not developed good peer relationships, and was

■ **CASE 6: SYLVIA, CONTINUED**

noncompliant with teacher's instructions. In the home setting, Sylvia displayed a range of behavioral extremes—calm and wanting to be held, humorous and playful, unable to fall asleep, oppositional behaviors, and screaming fits.

A coordinated team of professionals evaluated Sylvia over 3 separate sessions. Psychoeducational testing revealed above-average verbal and nonverbal cognitive abilities, with academic performance in the low-average range. Sylvia was somewhat coy and resistant but responded to the structure of the testing format and complied with the examiner's requests. At the second evaluation, Sylvia arrived in a fancy holiday dress and party shoes; her mother indicated that she was not willing to fight with her daughter over clothing. Sylvia's demeanor alternated between very engaging and animated and being withdrawn. For the final visit, Sylvia arrived in a black pant shirt that had leopard-spotted trim and a headband with ears. She appeared disorganized and fearful. She crawled around the waiting area, climbed on furniture, acted like a cat, and refused to comply with any requests.

Sylvia's history, current behavior, and cognitive profile were felt to be most consistent with PTSD with dissociative features. The ADHD and ODD symptoms reported by her school providers overshadowed the underlying cause of her behaviors and the need for intensive therapeutic intervention, rather than a simple behavioral plan or stimulant medication. Sylvia's mother engaged an advocate and pursued due process to have her daughter enrolled in an approved private therapeutic school, at the district's expense. This school had the resources to meet her daughter's academic and emotional needs. A trial of medication, which included an SSRI and mood stabilizer, was also initiated.

In Sylvia's case, initial behavioral presentation, without consideration for the child's entire history, initially lead to the wrong diagnosis and resulted in ineffective intervention. Sylvia's adoptive parent's knowledge of her daughter's prior experiences and their implications enabled her to effectively advocate for more appropriate evaluations and services.

Autism Spectrum Disorder

Autism spectrum disorder, as defined in *DSM-5*, includes the range of pervasive developmental disorders (ie, autism; pervasive developmental disorder, not otherwise specified; and Asperger syndrome) described in the previous version of *DSM*. The diagnosis of ASD is made based on the presence of a pattern of behaviors that present as persistent deficits (including qualitative differences) in the domains of communication and social interaction and restricted and repetitive behaviors, interests, or activities (including play).[42] In the past, most children identified with autism demonstrated significant delays consistent with mental retardation. More recently, the prevalence of ASDs has increased significantly (from 1 in 10,000 in the 1980s to 1 in 55 in the most recent National Survey of Children's Health parent questionnaire) in part because of changing criteria and identification of milder cases in which significant delays may not be present.[50] Autism spectrum disorder is the result of difference in brain development and function, and there is a body of literature that supports a significant genetic component (as in fragile X, 15q duplication, higher reoccurrence rates in biological siblings). Although the cause of ASD remains unclear, there may be a role for other triggers, including environmental causes, in those who may have a genetic risk.

Literature describes children who present with an ASD behavioral profile as a result of neglect associated with institutionalization or poor caregiving situations. Children in these settings do not learn to interact with others (eg, avert eye gaze, do not initiate or respond to interactions) and may entertain or soothe themselves with self-stimulatory behaviors (eg, rocking, staring at their fingers). For many children, these atypical patterns fade quickly when placed in a nurturing environment but may reappear during times of stress. There are other children in whom the autistic profile persists, despite gains in skills, which raises the question as to whether environmental factors alone caused autistic behaviors or if the child would have been autistic no matter where he had been raised. The work of Michael Rutter on children adopted from Romanian orphanages found that children with prolonged symptoms of ASD were more likely to have been in the orphanage longer and had a greater degree of cognitive impairment.[17]

Independent of the etiology of ASD, which remains largely unknown, intensive behavioral intervention is effective in helping affected individuals develop new skills and reduce atypical patterns. Depending on a child's age and the organization of local resources, these services are typically provided by EI for children younger than 3 years and by public schools and public mental health programs for older children. Depending on a child's individual profile, other therapeutic formats can also be implemented, such as occupational therapy, speech therapy, and social skills training. Depending on the reason for a child's ASD profile as well as the child's inherent potential, children can make significant gains in their functioning.[51,52]

CASE 7: SUSAN AND KAREN

Susan and her twin sister Karen were adopted from a Chinese orphanage at 2 years of age. Six months after arrival, they presented for evaluation because of continued delays in their development. However, while Karen was making significant strides in her development and was making a smooth transition to family living, Susan was experiencing significant difficulties—she was not acquiring language and would only vocalize open vowel sounds; she would bang her head, pull hair (hers or her mother's) for attention; and she did not engage in eye contact, explore toys' functionally, or join her sister in play. She would flex her right index finger and stare at it when she became overwhelmed or did not want to do something. Susan was slightly smaller than her twin; her head

CASE 7: SUSAN AND KAREN, CONTINUED

circumference was at the second percentile. Hearing and vision evaluations were recommended. Susan was found to have significant visual acuity deficit, but glasses did not improve her eye contact or overall profile. The family was hopeful that Susan only needed more time to catch up and deferred additional diagnostic testing, including genetic studies (eg, karyotype, fragile X, microarray) and magnetic resonance imaging of the brain.

Early intervention services were initiated, including applied behavior analysis for 20 hours per week. Susan continued to make slow progress and at 3 years of age transitioned to a specialized preschool program. Her sister entered a different classroom to address what was determined to be a mild residual language delay.

By kindergarten, Susan had learned to use limited sign language to make requests. She was able to follow home routines and seemed more aware of family members but still did not interact reciprocally. When she became upset, she would revert to gazing at her finger or pull at someone's hair to gain attention. She continued in a self-contained classroom with a one-to-one aide. By this time, Karen had entered a mainstream kindergarten and appeared to be following a trajectory of normal development but remained at risk for later learning disabilities.

This case of twin children raised in the same orphanage setting highlights the need to evaluate children with reference to normal developmental trajectories and the emerging research data on children raised under adverse circumstances. Simply blaming a child's profile on prior caregiving environment without considering patterns that point to underlying genetic or biological mechanisms compromises the ability to determine an accurate diagnosis, perform appropriate medical evaluations, and advocate for appropriate intervention services to maximize a child's long-term outcome.

Summary

Children who join their families from foster care, international orphanages, or other adverse early life environments can present with a complex history and clinical profile. Children who have experienced early abuse, neglect, or other adverse situations are at increased risk of a range of developmental, behavioral, and emotional issues that also can affect the general pediatric population. Developing a complete history (as much as possible) and using available individual and relevant information from research about this population is the first step in determining which factors may be contributing to a child's difficulties. Multidisciplinary evaluations by professionals with expertise working with this pediatric subpopulation can determine a child's profile of strengths and weakness and incorporate available history to develop a comprehensive differential diagnosis and treatment plan.

Most children do well despite their high-risk background and the fact that their history prior to and following the process of adoption will always be part of their lives. There are children who require no or only short-term interventions, those who may require ongoing low-level services for ongoing areas of weakness that are manageable within the context of family and public or private resources, and a subset of children with complex profiles who have significant ongoing issues that require substantial and specialized support. Accurate and comprehensive diagnosis of medical, developmental, and behavioral issues is critical in developing the most appropriate intervention plan that supports the child and family. Periodic reevaluation should review a child's progress, the possibility of alternative or additional diagnoses, the need for further diagnostic testing, and the appropriateness of existing intervention services. Pediatric health care professionals are uniquely positioned to assist children and families in obtaining an appropriate diagnosis and treatment such that children can achieve their full potential while promoting the most functional outcome possible for everyone involved.

Educational, Special Needs, and Mental Health Resources

Special Needs/Educational Resources

National Dissemination Center for Children with Disabilities
www.nichcy.org

Council for Exceptional Children
888/232-7733
www.cec.sped.org

Learning Disabilities Association of America
412/341-1515
www.ldaamerica.org

National Center for Learning Disabilities
888/575-7373
www.ncld.org

Children and Adults with Attention-Deficit/Hyperactivity Disorder
800/233-4050
www.chadd.org

Fetal alcohol spectrum disorders (FASDs)
www.cdc.gov/ncbddd/fasd

Autism spectrum disorders (ASDs)
www.cdc.gov/ncbddd/autism

Mental Health

Substance Abuse and Mental Health Services Administration
www.samhsa.gov

American Academy of Pediatrics Mental Health Initiatives, Key Resources
www.aap.org/en-us/advocacy-and-policy/aap-health-initiatives/Mental-Health/
Pages/Key-Resources.aspx

Pediatrics: "Appendix S7: References for Evidence-Based Programs for
Young Children"
http://pediatrics.aappublications.org/content/125/Supplement_3/S155.full.pdf

Evidence-Based Child and Adolescent Psychosocial Interventions
www.aap.org/en-us/advocacy-and-policy/aap-health-initiatives/Mental-Health/
Documents/CRPsychosocialInterventions.pdf

Toxic Stress/Trauma and Trauma-Informed Care

National Child Traumatic Stress Network
www.nctsnet.org

National Center for Trauma-Informed Care
www.samhsa.gov/nctic

Healthy Foster Care America: Trauma Guide
www.aap.org/traumaguide

References

1. Ames EW, Chishom K, Fisher L, et al. *The Development of Romanian Children Adopted to Canada: Final Report.* Burnaby, British Columbia: National Welfare Grants Program, Human Resources Development Canada; 1997
2. Miller LC, Kiernan MT, Mathers MI, Klein-Gitelman M. Developmental and nutritional status of internationally adopted children. *Arch Pediatr Adolesc Med.* 1995;149(1):40–44
3. Miller LC, Hendrie NW. Health of children adopted from China. *Pediatrics.* 2000;105(6):E76
4. Benoit TC, Jocelyn LJ, Moddermann DM, Embree JE. Romanian adoption: the Manitoba experience. *Arch Pediatr Adolesc Med.* 1996;150(12):1278–282
5. Johnson DE, Miller LC, Iverson S, et al. The health of children adopted from Romania. *JAMA.* 1992;268(24):3446–3451
6. Szilagy M. The pediatrician and the child in foster care. *Pediatr Rev.* 1998;19(2):39–50
7. Leslie LK, Gordon JN, Meneken L, et al. The physical, developmental, and mental health needs of young children in child welfare by initial placement type. *J Dev Behav Pediatr.* 2005;26(3):177–185
8. Shonkoff JP, Garner AS; American Academy of Pediatrics Committee on Psychosocial Aspects of Child and Family Health; Committee on Early Childhood, Adoption, and Dependent Care; Section on Developmental and Behavioral Pediatrics. The lifelong effects of early childhood adversity and toxic stress. *Pediatrics.* 2012;129(1):e232–e246
9. Lozoff B, Jimenez E, Smith JB. Double burden of iron deficiency in infancy and low socio-economic status. *Arch Pediatr Adolesc Med.* 2006;160(11):1108–1113

10. Algarin C, Nelson CA, Peirano P, Westerlund A, Reyes S, Lozoff B. Iron-deficiency anemia in infancy and poorer cognitive inhibitory control at age 10 years. *Dev Med Child Neurol.* 2013;55(5):453–458

11. Galler JR, Barrett LR. Children and famine: long-term impact on development. *Ambulatory Child Health.* 2001;7(2):85–95

12. Liu J, Raine A, Venables PH, et al. Malnutrition at age 3 years and lower cognitive ability at age 11 years: independence from psychosocial adversity. *Arch Pediatr Adolesc Med.* 2003;157(6):593–600

13. Yan W, Holland SK, Cecil KM, et al. Impact of early childhood lead exposure on brain organization: a functional magnetic resonance imaging study of language function. *Pediatrics.* 2006;118(3):971–977

14. Weder N, Kaufman J. Critical periods revisited: implication for intervention with traumatized children. *J Am Acad Child Adolesc Psychiatry.* 2011;50(11):1087–1089

15. Loman MM, Wiik KL, Frenn KA, Pollak SD, Gunnar MR. Postinstitutionalized children's development: growth, cognitive, and language outcomes. *J Dev Behav Pediatr.* 2009;30(5):426–434

16. Rutter M. Developmental catch-up, and deficit, following adoption after severe global early privation. English and Romanian Adoptees Study Team. *J Child Psychol Psychiatry.* 1998;39(4):465–476

17. Rutter M, Andersen-Wood L, Beckett C, et al. Quasi-autistic patterns following severe early global privation. English and Romanian Adoptees Study Team. *J Child Psychol Psychiatry.* 1999;40(4):537–549

18. O'Connor TG, Rutter M, Beckett C, Keaveney L, Kreppner JM. The effects of global severe privation on cognitive competence: extension and longitudinal follow-up. English and Romanian Study Team. *Child Dev.* 2000;71(2):376–390

19. Verhulst FC, Althaus M, Versluis-den Bieman HJ. Problem behavior in international adoptees: II. Age at placement. *J Am Acad Child Adolesc Psychiatry.* 1990;29(1):104–111

20. Verhulst FC, Althaus M, Versluis-den Bieman HJ. Problem behavior in international adoptees: III. Diagnosis of child psychiatric disorders. *J Am Acad Child Adolesc Psychiatry.* 1990;29(3):420–428

21. Verhulst FC, Althaus M, Versluis-den Bieman HJ. Damaging backgrounds: later adjustment of international adoptees. *J Am Acad Child Adolesc Psychiatry.* 1992;3(3):518–524

22. Nickman SL, Rosenfeld AA, Fine P, et al. Children in adoptive families: overview and update. *J Am Acad Child Adolesc Psychiatry.* 2005;44(10):987–995

23. Howe D. Parent-reported problems in 211 adopted children: some risk and protective factors. *J Child Psychol Psychiat.* 1997;38(4):401–411

24. Rushton A, Dance C. The adoption of children from public care: a prospective study of outcome in adolescence. *J Am Acad Child Adolesc Psychiatry.* 2006;45(7):877–893

25. Brand AR, Brinch PM. Behavior problems and mental health contact in adopted foster and non-adopted children. *J Child Psychol Psychiat.* 1999;40(8):1221–1229

26. Fergusson DM, Lynskey LM, Horwood LJ. The adolescent outcomes of adoption: a 16 year longitudinal study. *J Child Psychol Psychiat.* 1995;36(4):597–615

27. American Academy of Pediatrics Council on Children With Disabilities, Section on Developmental and Behavioral Pediatrics, Bright Futures Steering Committee, Medical Home Initiatives for Children With Special Needs Project Advisory Committee. Identifying infants and young children with developmental disorders in the medical home: an algorithm for developmental surveillance and screening. *Pediatrics.* 2006;118(1):405–420

28. King TM, Glascoe FP. Developmental surveillance of infants and young children in pediatric primary care. *Curr Opin Pediatr.* 2003;15(6):624–629

29. Rosenberg DR, Pajer K, Rancurello M. Neuropsychiatric assessment of orphans in one Romanian orphanage for unsalvageables. *JAMA.* 1992;268(24):3489–3490

30. Caspi A, Sugden K, Moffitt TE, et al. Influence of life stress on depression: moderation by a polymorphism in the 5-HTT gene. *Science*. 2003;301(5631):386–389

31. Barth RP, Freundlich M, Brodzinsky D, eds. *Adoption and Prenatal Alcohol and Drug Exposure*. Washington, DC: Child Welfare League of America; 2000

32. Streissguth A. *Fetal Alcohol Syndrome: A Guide for Families and Communities*. Baltimore, MD: Paul H. Brookes Publishing Co; 1998:95–119

33. Warner TD, Behnke M, Eyler FD, et al. Diffusion tensor imaging of frontal white matter and executive functioning in cocaine-exposed children. *Pediatrics*. 2006;118(5):2014–2024

34. Frank DA, Augustyn M, Knight WG, et al. Cognitive outcomes of preschool children with prenatal cocaine exposure. *JAMA*. 2001;285(12):1613–1625

35. Ornoy A, Segal J, Bar-Hamburger R, Greenbaum C. Developmental outcome of school-age children born to mothers with heroin dependency: importance of environmental factors. *Dev Med Child Neurol*. 2001;43(10):668–675

36. Ackerman JP, Riggins T, Black MM. A review of the effects of prenatal cocaine exposure among school-aged children. *Pediatrics*. 2010;125(3):554–565

37. Stirling J, Amaya-Jackson L. Understanding the behavioral and emotional consequences of child abuse. *Pediatrics*. 2008;122(3):667–673

38. American Academy of Pediatrics. Evidence-based child and adolescent psychosocial interventions. In: American Academy of Pediatrics. *Addressing Mental Health Concerns in Primary Care: A Clinician's Toolkit*. Elk Grove Village, IL: American Academy of Pediatrics; 2010. http://www.aap.org/en-us/advocacy-and-policy/aap-health-initiatives/Mental-Health/Documents/CRPsychosocialInterventions.pdf. Accessed February 14, 2014

39. Shaywitz SE, Shaywitz BA. Dyslexia (specific reading disability). *Pediatr Rev*. 2003;24(5):147–152

40. Cummins J. *Bilingualism and Special Education: Issues in Assessment and Pedagogy*. San Diego, CA: College Hill; 1984

41. Ochoa SH, Rhodes RL. Assisting parents of bilingual student to achieve equity in public schools. *J Educational and Psychological Consultation*. 2005;16:75–94

42. American Psychiatric Association. *Diagnostic and Statistical Manual of Mental Disorders, Fifth Edition*. Washington, DC: American Psychiatric Publishing; 2013

43. American Academy of Pediatrics Subcommittee on Attention-Deficit/Hyperactivity Disorder, Steering Committee on Quality Improvement and Management. ADHD: clinical practice guideline for the diagnosis, evaluation, and treatment of attention-deficit/hyperactivity disorder in children and adolescents. *Pediatrics*. 2011;128(5):1007–1022

44. Jensen PS, Arnold LE, Swanson JM, et al. 3 year follow-up of the NIMH MTA study. *J Am Acad Child Adolesc Psychiatry*. 2007;46(8):989–1002

45. Peason DA, Santo CW, Roache JD, et al. Treatment effects of methylphenidate on behavioral adjustment in children with mental retardation and ADHD. *J Am Acad Child Adolesc Psychiatry*. 2003;42(2):209–216

46. Handen BL, Breaus AM, Janosky J, et al. Effects and noneffects of methylphenidate in children with mental retardation and ADHD. *J Am Acad Child Adolesc Psychiatry*. 1992;31(3):455–461

47. American Academy of Child and Adolescent Psychiatry. Practice parameters for the assessment and treatment of children and adolescents with reactive attachment disorder of infancy and early childhood. *J Am Acad Child Adolesc Psychiatry*. 2005;44(11):1206–1219

48. Newman L, Mares S. Recent advances in the theories of and interventions with attachment disorders. *Curr Opin Psychiatry*. 2007;20(4):343–348

49. Sheering MS, Zeanah CH, Myers L, Putnam P. New findings on alternative criteria for PTSD in preschool children. *J Am Acad Child Adolesc Psychiatry*. 2003;42(5):561–570

50. Blumberg ST, Bramlett, Kogan MD, et al. *Changes in the Prevalence of Parent–Reported Autism Spectrum Disorder in School-Aged U.S. Children: 2007 to 2011-12. National Health Statistics Reports; No. 65.* Hyattsville, MD: National Center for Health Statistics; 2013

51. Myers SM, Plauché Johnson C; American Academy of Pediatrics Council on Children with Disabilities. Management of children with autistic spectrum disorders. *Pediatrics.* 2007;120(5):1162–1182

52. Plauché Johnson C, Myers SM; American Academy of Pediatrics Council on Children with Disabilities. Identification and evaluation of children with autistic spectrum disorders. *Pediatrics.* 2007;120(5):1183–1215

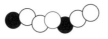

CHAPTER 16

Working With Schools: Considerations for Adopted Children and Their Families

Lisa Albers Prock, MD, MPH, FAAP

Children with a history of adoption or foster care are at increased risk of developmental, behavioral, or emotional concerns related to their pre-adoptive experiences that may affect their functioning in any school setting. While the exact percentage of children with a history of adoption or foster care receiving school-based services is unknown, it has been estimated to be at least twice that of the general population (See Chapter 11, Long-term Developmental and Behavioral Issues Following Adoption, on page 217). As children join their pre-adoptive or adoptive families, the need for support within an educational environment may range from minimal to extensive. In addition, the needs of children evolve as they settle into family and school settings. As a result, parents and professionals including pediatricians, psychologists, speech-language pathologists, and occupational and physical therapists may be interacting with school providers to address a range of treatment needs over time for children with a history of adoption.

This chapter will provide an overview of public school–based services, including the legal background for these services and process that families and children follow to request services. The process of assessment for and creation of an Individualized Education Plan (IEP) for children who qualify for special education supports will be outlined. Additional supports that may be available for children through their school systems (including a Section 504 plan) will also be discussed. Case-based discussions will highlight the role of school systems and ancillary services that may be helpful for children and their families in maximizing children's long-term success.

Legal Background for the Role of School Systems

Federal and state laws mandate publicly funded resources provided through school systems for children from birth to 21 years of age with developmental or behavioral issues affecting their learning based on federal regulations included in the Education for All Handicapped Act (PL 94-142) and the Individuals with Disabilities Education Act (IDEA) (PL 99-457) and subsequent revisions of these acts.[1] As these federal laws are administered at the state level, some variability exists in the guidelines for each state in providing for evaluations and services.[2]

Prior to age 3 years, children typically receive support for developmental challenges through their local early intervention (EI) program, which may provide a range of services in home- or center-based settings and often in collaboration with parents. When children turn 3 years of age and until they graduate from high school or are 21 years of age, they transition to their local public school system to receive services for developmental or emotional challenges that may affect their learning. Although states must meet minimum federal criteria with respect to education of all children, state statutes vary greatly from one to the next.[3]

For children receiving EI support prior to turning 3 years of age, transition to the public school system is typically facilitated by the EI team working with a child and family. However, if children have not previously received developmental services, parents or guardians need to initiate the process of receiving services through the school system. Parents may initiate the evaluation process on their own, or school providers may suggest an evaluation, but parents typically must sign a request for evaluation.[4] United States federal law outlines explicit expectations of school systems with respect to providing an adequate education for all children.[4] *Italicized items* in the following paragraphs discussing the process are the exact words used in federal mandates for childhood education; however, these laws are interpreted by each state and implemented differently in each school district.[2]

School systems are legally mandated to provide children identified with disabilities *free and appropriate public education*. In other words, no child can be refused access to education regardless of physical or emotional disability. Each child identified as having a disability (broadly defined federally; states may include additional disability classifications) is required to be provided with *special education and related services*. Schools are expected to provide children with access to a *general education curriculum*. If requested, school systems are expected to assess children for possible disorders that may be *impacting a child's ability to make educational progress*.

In compliance with federal requirements, each state has its own mandated process and timeline for applying for evaluation of a child for services through the public school system (ie, IEP).[3] It is noteworthy that there may be significant variability among the processes and services provided from state to state. As a result, health care professionals and others working with families to access services through their local school system on behalf of their child should be familiar with the exact process, requirements, and agencies in their local communities.[3]

Many children who struggle academically do not meet the strict guidelines to qualify for an IEP. In recent reauthorizations to IDEA, the federal government approved using a Response to Intervention (RTI) approach for children who do not meet strict criteria for categoric diagnoses but still need classroom support services, including educational or speech and language services.[5] Response to Intervention allows schools to provide services to children who are struggling academically without formally assessing them to see if they qualify for services under IDEA guidelines. Children who don't improve with RTI are then referred for further evaluation to see if they qualify for services under IDEA. Many school systems are changing their service delivery systems to use RTI as a first strategy before referring children for a full assessment under IDEA.

Children who do qualify for special education services under IDEA, including speech and language services, receive an IEP to outline the scope of services or supports that will be put in place and goals for each of the services.[6] Children receiving RTI do not have IEPs, and children with IEPs are not eligible to receive RTI. Services and goals in the IEP should focus on facilitating academic performance in the classroom. Once the IEP is approved, school systems are mandated to provide the services indicated in the document. In addition to the option of pursing school-based evaluations, parents may choose to pursue private evaluations instead of, commensurate with, or following the school-based assessment process (often at their own expense) and present the results to the school to expedite the process.

The Individualized Education Plan Process

After parental/guardian consent is obtained, school systems are responsible for ensuring each child receives a multidisciplinary and nondiscriminatory IEP eligibility assessment for potential disability affecting a child's learning and access to a general education curriculum. A multidisciplinary assessment including parent consultation is completed within the time frame specified by specific state guidelines. Mechanisms for ensuring due process throughout the evaluation and service provision process allow for parents/guardians to pursue further opinions or judgments about their child's needs and provided services via independent evaluations, mediation, or even litigation to ensure a child receives appropriate services in the *least restrictive environment.* The definition of an educational disability does vary greatly from state to state.

Although components of the multidisciplinary assessment are not mandated, evaluation of a child in *all areas of suspected disability* is required. For example, if concerns are raised about a child's math abilities, an assessment is not complete if there is no assessment of math abilities, even if all other measures of ability and function suggest no concerns. Typical components of an IEP evaluation may vary from one school system to another, but in brief, cognitive abilities, educational achievement, speech and language abilities, fine motor skills, gross motor skills, and current psychosocial setting and stressors are reviewed (Table 16-1.)

Assessment is *not to be biased by culture, language, or disability*. Clearly, this requirement is important for many children, including those with physical challenges or hearing or vision impairments, and ensures comprehensive and appropriate assessment. Interestingly, for many children with a history of adoption into families in which they need to learn a new primary language, this can be a challenging requirement, as many school systems consider children with such a history to be bilingual when in fact they are transitioning from one primary language to another. In addition, the timeline of losing one's first language if not continually exposed can be quite rapid (eg, within several months), and often, school systems do not have access to competent evaluators in a child's native language with accessibility in a timely fashion.

After members of the IEP assessment team complete their evaluations, a meeting is held to review the results of the assessments and determine whether a student meets eligibility for a disability category. Each state has a required time frame (typically 30 to 45 days) from the point a parent requests an IEP evaluation to completion of the team meeting discussing the outcome and any IEP recommendations. If a child is found to be *making effective educational progress*, typically an IEP is not provided.

Table 16-1. Examples of Typical Individualized Education Plan Assessment Components

Evaluation Domain	Examples of Tools Used
Psychologic assessment	Cognitive scales (WPPSI, WISC, DAS)
	Parent and teacher reports of behavior, emotions (BASC, CBCL)
Educational assessment	Academic assessment (WIAT; Woodcock Johnson; GORT; CTOPP)
Developmental history	Interview by psychologist, social worker, school nurse
Psychosocial history	Interview by psychologist, social worker, school nurse, other
Medical data	Hearing assessment
	Vision assessment
	Neurologic assessment

Abbreviations: BASC, Behavior Assessment System for Children; CBCL, Child Behavior Checklist; CTOPP, Comprehensive Test of Phonological Processing; DAS, Differential Ability Scales; GORT, Gray Oral Reading Test; WIAT, Wechsler Individual Achievement Test; WISC, Wechsler Intelligence Scale for Children; WPPSI, Wechsler Preschool and Primary Scale of Intelligence.

As the result of an IEP assessment, children who are found to *not be making effective educational progress* may qualify for services through an IEP if they have specific categoric diagnoses affecting their educational performance. Based on federal standards stated in IDEA, current eligible diagnostic categories used in all states include autism spectrum disorder (ASD), sensory impairments (hearing, vision), mental retardation (now intellectual disability), speech or language impairment, serious emotional disturbance, orthopedic impairment, other health impairment, traumatic brain injury, or specific learning disabilities. In addition, states can choose to qualify children for an IEP if they have a non-categoric developmental delay in one or more areas that meets the state's definition.[6] Each state can determine its own criteria for delay; most states use formulas based on test percentiles or standard deviations. This non-categoric criterion (called developmental delay in many states) is typically used for younger children and often has an upper age limit set by the state, generally 8 to 10 years of age. All children older than the state's specific age limit must qualify for services under one of the categoric diagnoses listed previously. Importantly, although children may have a categoric diagnosis, they can only receive services under IDEA when their disability affects academic performance.[6] For example, children with attention-deficit/hyperactivity disorder (ADHD) symptoms or relatively mild speech and language concerns often don't qualify for intervention under IDEA rules.

If the decision of the team is to create an IEP, specific goals with benchmarks to assess the child's progress and a service grid outlining necessary services will be created. As part of the IEP process, transportation needs (to and from school; other services) and length of the school year (eg, full-year services to prevent regression of skills) are also considered. A routine schedule is established for communicating about a child's progress with parents. The IEP is formally reviewed annually, but parents or school providers may request an interim meeting to review additional results or discuss concerns or needs for a change in services. Routinely, children are reassessed every 3 years, but this may be done more frequently, if needed. Children may receive services via an IEP whether or not they attend their local public school system, but typically services are provided at the local school system.

Some children with known disabilities do not qualify for an IEP under IDEA because their challenges do not affect their educational progress significantly. For example, a child with ADHD, relatively manageable behavioral challenges, typical intelligence, and average academic skills may not qualify for an IEP. However, services may be covered under Section 504 of the Rehabilitation Act.[5] A Section 504 plan is a school-based accommodation for a child with a disability that typically provides for behavioral and procedural accommodations in a classroom. Unlike an IEP, a Section 504 plan provides accommodations that are not necessarily related to academic performance, but a diagnosed disability is still required. For example, preferential seating in class or for testing or an escort when changing classrooms for a child with ADHD, accommodations for an FM system for a child with hearing loss, and the capacity to dictate answers to questions for children with orthopedic impairments may all be provided via a 504 plan if a child does not have an IEP. Children have an IEP or a 504 plan, although some children may not initially qualify for an IEP but receive a 504 plan and later qualify for an IEP as academic demands increase. In contrast with special education services, school districts do not receive state or federal funding for 504 plan modifications.

Certainly, options exist for providing educational and associated services beyond those offered in public school settings; however, options may be limited based on geography or financial considerations. In addition to or instead of publicly funded services, parents may choose to provide private academic tutoring or therapies (ie, speech-language, occupational, physical) for their children, or even seek private placement at their own cost. Even for families with substantial resources, it is critical to consider that intensive tutoring is not a substitute for the support a child may require to learn in his or her classroom. For example, even several sessions per week of excellent tutoring do not remediate the challenges a child may face during each school day. However, for children with more mild or focused areas of impairment, private instruction may be quite helpful, especially if the tutor and teacher coordinate their approach. With practice and remediation, children with relatively discrete or mild challenges can learn to carry over skills learned in tutoring sessions to the classroom. In contrast, children with significant challenges in single or multiple domains of school functioning require replacement services or instruction wherever they are doing the bulk of their learning and may require a separate school placement, which can be extremely expensive to self-pay.

In addition to mandates to address educational supports and physical disabilities, federal laws also address behavioral and emotional concerns for children. Children with milder emotional challenges can receive counseling and support within public school settings, but this is not the appropriate single venue for children with major mental health diagnoses. Children with more significant mental health issues affecting their functioning in school and other settings may require a specialized or even an out-of-district or regional placement.

Role of Families in Working With Schools

As advocates for their child's well-being in educational settings, parents are often in a challenging and potentially adversarial position when working with school systems to provide educational services for their child. While parents are focused on obtaining optimal services to promote a child's long-term educational success and well-being, school systems are required to provide services necessary for adequate educational progress. For many children affected by adversity prior to joining the family, including exposure to neglect, trauma, abuse, institutional care, or poor nutrition and health care, diagnostic categories and treatments available through school providers may not adequately capture or address their complex educational, emotional, or behavioral needs. For example, a child transitioning to a new family at school age may be in need of educational remediation because of lack of educational exposure or learning disabilities, specific developmental therapies such as speech-language or occupational therapy, behavioral support and strategies at home and school given behavioral challenges, and some degree of individual or family therapy related to previous trauma, attachment vulnerabilities, or symptoms of anxiety or depression.

School services are legally required and should be expected to address educational, emotional, and behavioral needs in the school setting, but additional community-based or private services are routinely required to support children and their families, especially related to evolving emotional and behavioral needs. Ideally, services between school and community providers are well coordinated and complementary; practically, parents are essentially case managers who often drive the diagnostic process and identify treatment providers in the community while needing to learn about the idiosyncrasies and complexities of educational, mental health, and health delivery systems.

Practical Considerations for Families

While local school systems and services available in communities are extremely variable, the following considerations are suggested for families:

- When beginning collaboration with a school system, parents with concerns about their child's educational, emotional, or behavioral performance at school will do well to start by *understanding the IEP process*.[1-4]
- Although further support (eg, educational advocate, lawyer) may eventually be necessary, parents should consider *bringing family and friends only to initial meetings* with school providers to discuss possible need for services.
- If parents are unsatisfied with services offered for their child, it may be helpful to engage an *educational advocate* who ideally has had some training about and experience with the IEP process with children with similar issues.
- Appreciate the *scope of services reasonable for a school to provide* (eg, academic support, in-class behavioral plan, coordinated school and home-based supports for children with ASDs) as opposed to those services best provided in a community-based or private setting (eg, treatment of anxiety symptoms, parental guidance on behavioral concerns, family therapy to address attachment vulnerabilities or parent-child interaction difficulties).
- Know your *health insurance coverage options* with respect to potential coverage for mental health, speech-language, occupational, and physical therapy services. Up-to-date coverage policies, including additional fees for out-of-network providers, are typically available by calling customer service centers (insurance cards usually list phone numbers).

- *Document all communication* to and from school providers about an IEP process and child-specific information. Especially for children who have recently joined families, frequent reassessments of children's needs should be expected and planned for as part of the IEP process.
- *Appreciate that a child's needs may be dynamic,* especially around the time of transitioning to a new family and school system, and therefore will require frequent adjustment of services.
- *Realize that limited capacity and expertise for service providers may exist* in a child's school system. If a child's progress appears modest, consider supplementing with select private services (eg, speech-language supports) if feasible and available.
- Even with excellent school-based or private assessments, well-crafted IEP goals, benchmarks, and a service grid, the *quality of services* provided ultimately depends a great deal on the *actual service providers* rather than the IEP itself. If children are not making progress, *in-class observation* may be helpful.
- *Creativity with respect to service provision* should never be underestimated. For example, a shorter day may not be proposed by an IEP team but may be well received by the team if a child is having significant regulatory or anxiety concerns that can be moderated by a shorter period of school attendance.
- *Appreciate the limits of professionals with whom you are working.* For example, most teachers and other service providers may not have intimate knowledge of the long-term effect of early malnutrition, trauma, or institutionalization; in fact, they may not even appreciate the importance of using appropriate terms when discussing a child's history of adoption (eg, birth or adoptive parents rather than "real" or "natural" parents.)
- *Don't hesitate to identify professionals to assist you with the process* (potentially, educational advocates, lawyers, developmental-behavioral pediatricians, neuropsychologists, or psychiatrists).
- *Private schools or homeschooling are options* but can be challenging for children with complex issues and parents or teachers with limited experience or knowledge.

Special Considerations for Internationally Adopted Children Joining Families at an Older Age and Learning a Second Language

Children who are internationally adopted after age 5 years may enroll in their local public school system shortly after joining their adoptive family and well before developing fluent English-language skills. In this situation, school providers should immediately identify the child as having *Limited English Proficiency (LEP) status* and arrange for English-as-a-second-language (ESL) services (also known as English Language Learner services in some states) to facilitate the language-learning process. For children with typical cognitive, speech, and language abilities, additional services may not be required. In contrast, children with previously identified speech, language, or cognitive disorders typically require additional services based on IDEA. Many schools will resist this recommendation until a child has been given the chance to benefit from ESL programs.[7,8] However, if the school waits too long, a child's first primary language will have undergone severe attrition, making it difficult to complete a valid language, speech, or cognitive assessment.[7,8]

As described by Glennen, the only way around this dilemma is to have newly adopted children assessed in the birth language within 3 to 4 months of arriving home.[7] Such an assessment is only recommended for a child who has been previously identified in his or her birth country as having speech, language, or cognitive delays or for any child in whom the degree of delays cannot be determined prior to adoption.[7] Assessments can be completed privately or through the school system under IDEA. Given logistic and financial constraints, local school systems often resist this request, which is why pre-adoption documentation of developmental challenges is important. Parents who can produce evidence of a speech, language, or cognitive delay that existed before the child's adoption have solid ground to request an assessment of those abilities per routine IEP processes. Parents who cannot produce this evidence may have difficulty proving the need for an assessment under IDEA, and as a result, parents may need to pursue private evaluations.

Regardless of known disabilities, IDEA law mandates that children need to be assessed in their primary language.[9] For newly arrived international adoptees, that is their primarily birth language. Ideally, professionals who speak the language should conduct the assessment.[10] This allows them to directly evaluate the child's ability to understand and communicate. If this is not feasible, an alternative is to conduct the assessment through an interpreter who speaks the language. Professionals conducting the assessment should be skilled in evaluating children with an interpreter. As previously stated, any assessment of the birth language needs to occur within 3 to 4 months of adoption before the language undergoes attrition.

Clearly, children adopted at older ages should immediately receive services to assist them in learning English when they start school. As described previously, schools can offer assistance through ESL programs by providing an IEP or through a Section 504 plan. Interestingly, there are no standard guidelines for when children no longer qualify as having LEP status. Some states use tests; others use informal processes such as teacher checklists. In addition, based on the number of children receiving ESL services in a district, there is wide variability in services available to children who are LEP. In contrast, special education services mandated under the federal IDEA program are somewhat more consistent across states and schools. However, obtaining special education services under IDEA for a newly arrived school-aged child is next to impossible unless documents from the birth country indicate a specific qualifying diagnosis, such as hearing impairment, or an assessment within the first few months home indicates the presence of a qualifying diagnosis or a speech, language, or cognitive delay in the birth language. Simply having LEP does not qualify a child for special education services, nor should it.

Conclusion

Working with school systems to support the needs of children with a history of adoption or foster care requires parents to have an understanding of the legal framework for and practical aspects of their local educational system as well as other community resources. Although all children with a history of adoption may not need to access school-based supports, many appropriate services may be accessed through the educational system to support children in achieving their full potential. On the other hand, parents will benefit from appreciating the role of additional private and community-based services when needed.

Parent Resources

Center for Parent Information and Resources
www.parentcenterhub.org
Central resource of information and products to Parent Training Information Centers and the Community Parent Resource Centers, so that they can focus their efforts on serving families of children with disabilities

Wrightslaw
www.wrightslaw.com
Up-to-date and reliable information about special education law and advocacy for children with disabilities

Individuals with Disabilities Education Act (Public Law 94-142)
www.scn.org/~bk269/94-142.html

References

1. Public Law 94-142 – Education of All Handicapped Children Act, now called Individuals with Disabilities Education Act. http://www.scn.org/~bk269/94-142.html. Accessed February 14, 2014
2. Center for Parent Information and Resources. Find your parent center. http://www.parentcenterhub.org/find-your-center. Accessed February 14, 2014
3. FindLaw. State education law. http://statelaws.findlaw.com/education-laws. Accessed February 14, 2014
4. Wrightslaw. Section 504, the Americans with Disabilities Act, and education reform. http://www.wrightslaw.com/info/section504.ada.peer.htm. Accessed February 14, 2014
5. Cummins J. *Bilingualism and Special Education: Issues in Assessment and Pedagogy.* San Diego, CA: College Hill Press; 1984
6. Danaher J. Eligibility policies and practices for young children under Part B of IDEA. *NECTAC Notes.* 2007;24:1–20
7. Glennen S. Speech and language in children adopted internationally at older ages. *Perspectives on Communication Disorders and Sciences in Culturally and Linguistically Diverse Populations.* 2007;14(3):17–20

8. Gindis B. Children left behind: international adoptees in our schools. http://www.bgcenter.com/BGPublications/ChildrenLeftBehind.htm. Accessed February 14, 2014
9. Walsh S, Smith B, Taylor R. *IDEA Requirements for Preschoolers with Disabilities: IDEA Early Childhood Policy and Practice Guide*. Reston, VA: Council for Exceptional Children; 2000
10. Goldstein B. *Cultural and Linguistic Diversity Resource Guide for Speech Language Pathology*. San Diego, CA: Singular Publishing Group; 2000

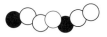

CHAPTER 17

Adoptive Identity and Children's Understanding of Adoption: Implications for Pediatric Practice*

David M. Brodzinsky, PhD

Introduction

Adoption offers the opportunity of stability, loving care, security, and lifetime family connections for boys and girls whose birth family cannot or choose not to raise them for a variety of reasons. In fact, research strongly supports the belief that adoption protects children, especially when one considers the alternatives for many of these youngsters—namely, remaining in neglectful and abusive homes, in long-term foster care or orphanages, or with parents who are unprepared to care for them.[1-5]

At the same time, research and clinical experience also suggest that being adopted is a risk factor associated with many challenges and complications in the lives of children, as well as in the lives of those who parent them. Adopted children are significantly overrepresented in outpatient and inpatient mental health facilities[6-9] and are more likely than their non-adopted peers to be diagnosed with a range of externalizing and internalizing psychological symptoms,[10] substance abuse,[11] and learning difficulties.[12] Adjustment differences between these groups, when significant, are generally small to moderate in effect size, with the exception of mental health utilization rates, for which the effect size is relatively large. Yet many of the difficulties affecting adoptees and their families have less to do with adoption per se than with various life complications that predate children's placements, such as the legacy of genetically based problems, adverse prenatal experiences (eg, exposure to drugs and alcohol), and adverse pre-placement experiences (eg, malnutrition, neglect, abuse, exposure to parental psychopathology and domestic violence, institutional rearing).[10,13–16] In many cases, experiences of deprivation and early life trauma undermine children's physical and emotional well-being through their negative effect on brain development and functioning.[17]

Nevertheless, having a history of adoption can color children's self-esteem and identity[18,19] as well as parent-child relationships, potentially leading to adjustment difficulties. Beginning with the work of Kirk,[20] adoption professionals have identified a number of challenges associated with adoptive family life that affect children and parents at each stage of the family life cycle.[21–23] Of the many challenges noted, one of the most important is sharing of adoption information with children and the way children and young adults come to understand the meaning and implications of being adopted. In this chapter, developmental changes in children's understanding of adoption will be examined, along with the implications of these changes for children's identity and psychologic adjustment. Particular focus will be placed on children's experience of adoption-related loss. Finally, given that adopted children are at increased risk of psychologic problems and parents frequently consult their pediatrician for advice on managing adoption-related concerns, guidelines will be offered for helping parents discuss adoption issues with their children. Throughout the chapter, case vignettes, as well as the voices of adoptees and their parents, are used to highlight the issues being discussed. All identifying information, including quotes, have been altered to protect the confidentiality of these individuals.

Developmental Changes in Children's Understanding of Adoption

Parents usually begin talking about adoption with their children prior to or during the preschool years.[22,24] Typically, they begin with very basic background information and gradually build on their child's adoption story as children get older. Often, children's books are used as way of introducing or expanding the basic adoption story. Of critical importance, however, is the way children interpret the information provided, the manner in which their understanding of adoption changes with age, and how this understanding affects their adjustment, self-esteem, identity, and family relationships.

Infant and Toddler Years

Although children may have a limited understanding of conversations during infancy and childhood, parents can begin the discussion of adoption with their child as soon as they begin changing their diapers. *Adoption* is a concept far in the future in terms of a child's full understanding, but even toddlers may perceive differences between themselves and others around them. For example, many children with a history of interracial adoption or with same-sex parents may ask questions about perceived differences between themselves and peers or parents. During these years, parents can practice discussions with their children affected by adoption and respond to questions with a limited amount of factual information.

Preschool Years

As parents begin to share adoption information, their 3- to 5-year-olds gradually learn parts of their adoption stories. They often are able to label themselves as being adopted as well as talk about having a birth mother and/or birth father. Sometimes they can identify another place as the origin of their birth and may learn a fragmentary story about how they came to their new family. Yet the capacity of preschool-aged children to understand all of the larger implications of being adopted is limited by their developmental understanding of the world at large.[25] Similar to many situations, each child's capacity to understand his or her complete story varies greatly. For the most part, children initially learn the language of adoption; in other words, they learn to talk about being adopted, without fully understanding what this aspect of their life implies. In some cases, children confuse being adopted with being born or believe that all children are adopted; in other cases, their wish to be born to their parents leads them to misconstrue how they came into their family. Consider Ellie, a 4-year-old girl placed for adoption soon after birth.

"Mommy told me that when I was in her tummy she wanted me...so she told the doctor to make me adopted...so then I was adopted.... (What do you mean you were adopted?) Well, mommy told the doctor to take me out of her tummy and to make me adopted. (How did the doctor make you adopted?) I don't know."

Although limited in their understanding of adoption, the vast majority of boys and girls adopted in infancy will have quite positive views of their family status as preschoolers. Their feelings are based on the fact that during this period, most parent-child conversations focus on the positive aspects of being adopted—namely, being loved and having caring parents and a "forever family"—rather than the more difficult aspects of their experience, including the circumstances surrounding separation from their birth family. Preschool-aged children's positive views about adoption are reflected in research findings showing little or no differences in psychologic adjustment of these children compared with their non-adopted peers—at least for those placed as infants.[26] Only as children enter the school-age years does research suggest an increased risk among adopted individuals of psychologic, behavioral, and academic difficulties.

Interestingly, parents of preschool-aged children who were adopted in infancy often overestimate the extent to which their children comprehend the meaning and implications of being adopted.[27] Listening to their children talk about being adopted or about their birth mother often leads parents to assume that their boys and girls have a reasonably clear understanding of their family status. Parents of children adopted during toddler or preschool years may find that past experiences may be recalled by children and may come up at various times during discussions with their child. This misunderstanding can result in parents curtailing discussions about adoption prematurely, especially for those individuals who were initially quite anxious about sharing adoption information. Pediatricians and other professionals working with families need to caution parents about assuming too much understanding about adoption on the part of their preschool children and to encourage them to remain attuned to their children's need for additional information about their history of adoption. They also need to support parents in creating a family atmosphere that makes it easier for children to ask relevant questions about their background and current family status.

Middle Childhood

Children between 6 and 12 years of age undergo many changes in cognitive and socio-emotional development that have significant implications for their understanding of and adjustment to adoption.[18,22,25,28] For one thing, their capacity for problem solving becomes more sophisticated, leading them to realize that birth parents may have had options other than adoption to choose from. For example, a 9-year-old who previously was told that her birth mother was too poor to raise a child and had no one to help her now can recognize the possibility of the birth mother getting a job or perhaps asking someone in her family for help. Although still somewhat limited in their reasoning and certainly without any realistic understanding of the difficult circumstances facing most birth parents, school-aged children's ability to conceptualize multiple solutions for a given problem may lead them to reject, or at least challenge, the previous explanations offered by adoptive parents about the circumstances of their placements. As a result, in attempting to understand the birth parent's decision for adoption, some children now begin to question whether they were ever wanted by the birth parents in the first place, which can undermine their view of themselves and their origins.

"Maybe the real reason I was given up was that she just didn't want me…maybe she just didn't care."
~ Eight-year-old boy adopted domestically at birth

"I can't really understand how she could give up her own baby…even if she was poor.…I don't think most poor people do that…it makes me mad to think that she just wouldn't keep me." ~ Nine-year-old girl adopted from Guatemala at 8 months of age

Another cognitive change affecting adoption awareness and adjustment is the way children understand the nature of family. Children adopted during infancy gradually develop an awareness of the meaning of adoption throughout childhood and adolescence. For children adopted beyond infancy, memories of their past positive or negative circumstances, caregivers, and family may be relevant to their current understanding of their adoptive family constellation, but for children with limited pre-adoptive memories, their understanding of the world gradually evolves over time. During the preschool years, most children define *family* in terms of geographic and emotional criteria. In short, for young children, the people who live with them and love them (and who are loved in return) are considered family. Biological relatedness plays a limited role in the young child's conception of family. By 6 to 8 years of age, however, children are beginning to understand the importance of biological connections among family members.[29] For many children, this new knowledge raises questions as to the nature of their family membership. As one 7-year-old boy, adopted as an infant, said,

"Do I have one family or two? My mom and dad didn't make me…I was born to another lady somewhere…so is she my mother too? …[I]t gets kind of confusing sometimes."

The struggle to understand and accept one's connection to 2 families, one of which may be unknown, fully emerges when children can conceptualize the nature of family in a more sophisticated way than when they were younger.

Middle childhood also is a time when logical thought emerges. This new capacity affects adoption awareness and adjustment in profound ways. As children develop the ability for logical reasoning, they automatically recognize that gaining a new family through adoption also means having been separated from a previous family. This insight sensitizes them—perhaps for the first time—to the reality of adoption-related loss, which is viewed by most adoption professionals as a core issue in the emotional adjustment of adopted individuals[22,28,30-33]—one that helps explain the emergence of increased adjustment difficulties among adoptees during this developmental period.[26]

The capacity for understanding another's perspective, as well as feeling empathy for another's plight, also undergoes significant advancement during middle childhood. These achievements help adopted children conceptualize the problems faced by birth parents and the possible implications of adoption for these individuals. Often, school-aged children begin to wonder whether they are the object of their birth parents' thoughts and, if so, whether they are unhappy about, or even regret, the decision they made. This insight into the inner world of their birth parents may give rise to confusion, anxiety, and sadness in the child.

> *"Last night, when I put my daughter to bed, she asked me whether her birth mother ever thinks about her….She asked if her birth mother might be sad about not being with her….She started crying and said that she worried that her birth mother misses her and doesn't know where she is. I didn't know what to say. We both cried, and finally I told her that I was sure her birth mother did think about her sometimes, just as she thinks about her too….I tried to help her understand that a person can make a decision that she knows is right and still be sad about it. I don't know if she really understood what I meant….She [daughter] really seems to be struggling with this idea of her birth mother being unhappy about the adoption."* ~ Mother of a 9-year-old girl adopted domestically soon after birth

As children develop a more comprehensive understanding of adoption, they naturally begin to examine what being adopted means to them, as well as its meaning for others. Exploring thoughts and feelings about their birth family and circumstances of their own adoption is a normal and inevitable developmental process for adopted children. However, in the absence of specific information about their birth family or contact with them, it is common for children of this age to develop fantasies about them that can be quite distorted, positively or negatively. For example, Mrs R, the mother of an 11-year-old boy placed from Mexico at 2½ years of age, reported that her son, beginning around 5 years of age, became "fixated" on the idea that his birth father was a famous soccer player. She noted that they had no information that supported this belief. Nevertheless, her son identified with the fantasized birth father and began playing organized soccer when he was 7 years old. Four years later, he had become an excellent soccer player, one of the stars on his team. She noted,

> "Although there's no reason to believe that his birth father played professional soccer or was famous, [he] has turned the fantasy into something positive for himself. It's given him the determination to be like his birth father…he's identified with him…which has turned into something good for him…something he's proud of…something we're all proud of."

In contrast, Lila's beliefs about her history have been more disturbing, with recurring fantasies that she was stolen from her birth family.

> *"Beginning around 6 or 7 years, she began to have nightmares that someone stole her from her birth mother…it's been a preoccupation over the years…sometimes she's blamed us or the adoption agency for being part of it…it's been difficult for her to accept that she was removed from her birth mother because of drugs and other problems…she thinks that being separated from her child destroyed her mother's life."* ~ Mother of a 13-year-old girl placed for adoption at 2 years of age

Pediatricians need to emphasize the normality of children's curiosity about their origins as well as help adoptive parents validate and support their children's efforts to understand their pasts and find healthy connections to them. They also need to help parents find ways of discussing birth family issues with their children in a positive light. This is especially true when the information about birth parents involves sensitive and emotionally charged matters (eg, neglect, abuse, parental psychopathology) or when there is a limited amount of information about them, as is the case in many international placements.

> "Some parents I know worry about how to talk with their children about their family history because the birth mother used drugs or the birth father was in jail....I understand that this might be difficult for them...what they sometimes don't understand is that it's just as difficult, and maybe more difficult, for us because we have virtually no information about our daughter's birth family or what really happened to her...all we know is that she was abandoned soon after birth and lived in an orphanage for over a year...we know nothing about what her birth parents were like...what they looked like or why they didn't keep her....[She] keeps asking us what we think her birth mother might be like...where she lives...whether she has any brothers or sisters...all sorts of questions which we simply can't answer....I don't know what's worse, knowing things about your family that are difficult to accept, or simply not knowing anything at all...all I know is that we often feel helpless in the face of our daughter's questions." ~ Mother of a 10-year-old girl adopted from China at 14 months of age

Adolescence

With the emergence of adolescence and the development of abstract thinking, the capacity for understanding the meaning and implications of adoption deepens. For one thing, teenagers begin to understand the legal permanence associated with adoption. This awareness can reduce anxiety found in some younger boys and girls who occasionally worry about having to return to, or be reclaimed by, their birth family. For example, I worked with a 14-year-old girl who reported that when she was younger, perhaps 7 or 8, she often would get anxious when someone showed up at the house unexpectedly. She expressed worry that it was her birth mother coming back to get her. Although curious about her birth mother and definitely wanting more information about her, the child was clear that she did not want to leave her family. Now that she was older, she reported realizing that her birth mother did not have the right to "take her back," which gave her a sense of security that previously was missing.

Yet even adolescents sometimes fail to understand that adoption involves a legally binding relationship between parents and child. For example, I was asked to consult on a case involving a 17-year-old African American boy who lived with his single adoptive mother. Placed from foster care at 4 years of age, James had an excellent relationship with his adoptive mother, as well as a history of academic success and few adjustment problems. However, beginning in his senior year of high school, his grades began to slip and he was reported to be staying out late on school nights and the weekend as well as hanging out with what his mother called the "wrong crowd." When interviewed, James acknowledged that he was less focused on schoolwork and admitted that he had developed new friendships. He reported that he was very anxious about turning 18 and having to "fend for himself." When asked what he meant by this comment, he indicated that when he turned 18, he would no longer be a minor and, therefore, would not be adopted anymore. He recognized that he needed to develop more "street smarts" to survive on his own and, consequently, had found new friends who could help him learn these skills. It was obvious that James, despite his above-average intellect, somehow had misunderstood the implications of being adopted. When it was explained that being adopted meant that he was legally a part of his family forever, and when his mother reaffirmed her lifelong commitment to him, James was visibly relieved. Over the next few months, he was able to refocus on schoolwork, improve his grades, and give up inappropriate friends in favor of the previous ones who had served him well. This case is a reminder that even bright teenagers, on the verge of adulthood, can sometimes misunderstand aspects of their adoption.

The capacity for understanding other people's thoughts and feelings also matures during the adolescent period. This achievement allows the teenager to have a more realistic and empathic view of the birth parents' states of mind and life situations. They are also better able to conceptualize adoption from a societal perspective, which has positive and negative implications. On the positive side, teenagers begin to recognize the role of adoption as a social service system geared toward bettering the lives of needy children. And yet they also become increasingly aware that, for most people, adoption is still viewed as a "second-best" route to parenthood. In other words, although viewed as an admirable way of forming a family, teenagers are now becoming aware that most people prefer to have children through procreation rather than adoption, which sometimes leads them to question how they are viewed by others.

"My friends say it's cool that I'm adopted…you know, having 2 sets of parents…2 moms and 2 dads…but I also know that they're glad that they're not adopted and that makes me feel a little uncomfortable…it feels like they're saying one thing, that adoption is cool, but really thinking that it's not…that they're glad it didn't happen to them…that makes me think that they feel sorry for me….I hate that." ~ 16-year-old boy adopted from Colombia at 18 months of age

Like all adolescents, adoptees are in the process of trying to define themselves and find their place in the world. This process is more complicated for adopted individuals, however, because of their connection to 2 families, one that gave birth to them and one that is raising them.[19,22,34] In their search for self, adoptees must find a way of integrating aspects of both families into their emerging identity. In discussing these issues with adoptive parents, pediatricians should emphasize the following points:

- Interest in adoption and efforts to integrate this aspect of one's life into an emerging sense of self is a normal and healthy process.
- Adolescents are highly variable in the extent to which they are interested in their adoption. Some are intensely interested in their birth origins and are helped by contact with birth family members; others show little interest in adoption and their birth heritage.
- The role of adoption in a person's identity is influenced by many different factors, including those within the individual (eg, temperament, self-esteem), those within the family (eg, parents' attitudes and child-rearing style, quality of parent-child attachment), and those outside of the family (eg, experiences with birth family, peers, schoolmates, and the broader community).
- Parents who are more open, supportive, and empathic in their communication about adoption are more likely to have children who are able to integrate this aspect of their lives into a positive sense of self.
- Access to information about one's birth family and the circumstances surrounding the adoption, as well as contact with birth family, generally facilitate positive adoptive identity development.
- Adoption across racial lines adds another layer of complication for adoptive identity development; however, with support and access to appropriate role models, most transracially placed youngsters, including those placed from abroad, are able to negotiate this developmental task successfully.
- Adolescents going through the process of adoption, although relatively uncommon, need to address a range of adoptive identity issues while attaching to an adoptive family and simultaneously developing independence.

Although the process of searching for one's origins usually begins in middle childhood in the form of children's curiosity and questions about their birth family, it is closer to adolescence that this process intensifies as a result of the many physical, sexual, cognitive, social, and emotional changes that are occurring.[18,19]

"I don't know who I look like….I don't know where my traits come from…it's different for my brother because he was born to my parents…but for me, it's harder…there are lots of questions that I would like answered…but the people who can answer them aren't around…if I could find them, I could get answers." ~ Eric, a 16-year-old Hispanic teenager placed from El Salvador at 22 months of age

With the advent of the Internet, children may be searching for family members well before adolescence; social networking sites such as Facebook can make communication between extended birth family members and those with a history of adoption far less predictable. Historically, it was during adolescence that we first began to see adopted individuals thinking about and even planning a search for birth family, although for most, putting these plans into effect usually does not occur until the adult years. Although certainly not the intention of all adopted individuals, research suggests that the number of people searching for more information about their origins, as well as for birth family members, is increasing.[35] Yet this process can be quite stressful for the adopted person and adoptive parents. In discussing this possibility with adoptive family members, pediatricians should emphasize that a child or adolescent's need for information about his or her heritage is common and normal; it is not a reflection of emotional disturbance or dissatisfaction with the adoptive family, nor does it reflect disloyalty to the adoptive parents. Pediatricians also should note that, whenever possible and appropriate, the adolescent's desire to search should be supported by parents. However, professional preparation of children or adolescents and their families often is advisable before undertaking a search to ensure that realistic expectations are maintained and appropriate safety measures are considered.

Role of Loss in Adoption Adjustment

Of the many psychologic issues associated with adoption, none has received as much attention by the professional community as loss.[28,31–33] The experience of loss is universal among adopted individuals, although certainly the way it is experienced varies significantly from one person to another.[36,37] At one extreme are individuals who experience infrequent and rather mild feelings of confusion, sadness, or other grief-related emotions associated with separation from birth family; at the other extreme, however, are individuals for whom grief-related reactions are nearly constant and deeply, sometimes traumatically, felt. Most adoptees, however, fall in the middle of this continuum, periodically thinking about their adoption and reacting with varied emotions that are usually coped with quite well.

"I usually think about my birth family on my birthday or on Mother's Day or Father's Day....I wonder where they are and what they are doing....I wonder what they are like...sometimes it makes me a little sad to think about them, but not too much...when I was younger, I sometimes cried when I thought about them...not now, though." ~ 11-year-old boy adopted domestically soon after birth

"I miss my younger brother the most...we lived together when we were with Mrs _____...but he was adopted by another family that lives pretty far away...not sure why they didn't adopt me too....I was really angry at first when he left...got into a lot of trouble with my foster mom then....I've seen him a few times since I was adopted by my parents...usually in the summer when he comes here or I go

there to visit....I really like seeing him...but when the visit is over it's really sad for me...he's the only one of my real family that I know...can't remember my real parents....I really hate it that we couldn't grow up with them." ~ 12-year-old African American boy placed in foster care at 3 years of age and adopted at 7 years

"[He] came to us when he was 6 years old...he had been removed from his birth family, along with his 2 older sisters, when he was 2 because of neglect and maybe abuse...he was separated from his sisters and went through 3 foster homes before coming to us...he's never known any stability in his life...he trusts no one and when you think about it, why should he...up to now, everyone has let him down...he's difficult to manage at this point...angry and oppositional...but underneath there's a very deep sadness." ~ Adoptive mother of an 8-year-old Hispanic boy

Nature of Adoption-Related Loss

Although most people, professionals and laypersons alike, recognize that adoption inherently is connected to loss, few realize the full extent of loss experienced by those who are adopted. Some of these losses are experienced in middle childhood; others don't appear until adolescence. Moreover, the variability in the ways in which adopted individuals experience loss is associated with a range of intrapersonal, interpersonal, experiential, and contextual factors, including age, cognitive level, temperament, pre-placement history, attachment patterns, current family relationships, and current support systems.[26] Among the various losses associated with adoption are

Loss of Birth Parents

The first and most obvious loss experienced by adopted children is the one associated with separation from birth parents. For those youngsters placed as babies, this sense of loss emerges slowly as they begin to understand the meaning and implications of being adopted—usually at around 6 to 7 years. It is seldom the case, however, that early placed children experience birth parent loss as traumatic, primarily because they have never formed attachments to them. However, for those placed beyond infancy, the loss of birth parents is likely to be experienced more immediately and acutely because of its association with the severing of attachment relationships.[38] For these youngsters, birth parent loss can be quite traumatic, at least in the early stages following placement into substitute care.

"She cries almost every night...thrashes around...not sleeping well...isn't eating...she started soiling herself too....She just doesn't understand what happened and why she's no longer with her mother." ~ Foster mother of a 4-year-old girl removed from her birth family 3 months earlier

Loss of Siblings and Half Siblings

Although current best practices in child welfare make placing siblings together a priority, it is quite common for adopted children to experience the loss of full or half sibling relationships.[30,39] Too often when children enter foster care, they are separated, sometimes permanently, from their brothers and sisters, which can be quite traumatic. Moreover, it is common for birth parents who have placed an infant for adoption to give birth to other children. As adopted children mature, they become increasingly aware of these possibilities and often wonder about their brothers and sisters. When they believe that their birth parents possibly kept other siblings but placed them for adoption, it can create great confusion and anger and possibly undermine self-esteem.

> *"It makes me wonder if she thought there was something wrong with me...because she didn't keep me but kept my brother and sister."* ~ Eric, a 10-year-old boy placed for adoption at 5 days of age. His birth mother subsequently gave birth to and raised 2 other children.

Loss of Extended Birth Family

As children get older, they come to recognize that that they not only have been separated from their immediate birth family but also the entire extended birth family—grandparents, uncles and aunts, cousins. Although this may not have as much meaning for younger children, when adoptees reach adolescence they are much better able to understand their place within a family system and across generational lines. Consequently, the sense of loss, at least for some, deepens. Furthermore, for those individuals placed at older ages, the loss of extended family can be quite devastating because it often involves the severing of strong and secure attachments to grandparents, uncles and aunts, and cousins.

Loss of Previous Nonbiological Caregivers and Supports

Children who enter foster care, as well as those who reside for periods in orphanages, often form very meaningful and supportive relationships with individuals who are not part of their biological family, eg, foster parents, foster siblings, orphanage staff, friends, teachers, coaches, therapists. Removing children from these temporary residences and supports and placing them in adoptive homes may provide boys and girls with increased residential permanency, but it often does so at the expense of terminating important relationships for children. Too little attention is often given to finding ways of maintaining children's relationships with these nonbiological caregivers and supports. Yet these individuals often are sources of emotional security for children, perhaps the first ever experienced by them. In making and supporting adoption plans, professionals need to consider children's relationship histories and seek to preserve those relationships that have served them well.

Loss of a Meaning Maker

Parents and other early caregivers are *meaning makers* for children. They are the repository of childhood memories and the gatekeepers to artifacts that represent children's early lives. As children develop, these memories and early childhood representations (eg, pictures) are shared by parents, creating moments of emotional family connection and supporting identity development. In adoptive families, parents may not have shared the early years with their children and do not have much high-quality information about their history. In addition, limited information about potentially challenging topics in a child's history may need to be shared with children by adoptive parents with limited access to answer questions children may ask. In such cases, they are at a disadvantage in helping children understand who they are, where they came from, and what happened to them prior to adoption— in short, to give meaning to children's early years.

> *"With our older child, who was adopted at 2 weeks, I've able to talk with him about what he was like as a baby….I have lots of pictures of him with us from when he was just 2 weeks old…he loves to hear stories about when he was just a baby….With our second child, however, it's been different and more difficult….He came to us from Russia when he was almost 3 years old, and we weren't given much information about him….I can't answer his questions about when he was very little…which upsets both of us."* ~ Mother of 7- and 5-year-old adopted boys

Loss of Status

Although most people view adoption positively, there is still at times an undercurrent of opinion suggesting that adoption is a "second-best" route to becoming a family. As children mature cognitively and socially, they become increasingly aware that their peers do not envy them for being adopted. This recognition can undermine self-esteem and identity.

> *"Sometimes the kids at school tease me because I'm adopted…when we fight they sometimes say, 'You don't even know who your mother is!'"* ~ Becky, an 8-year-old adopted girl

Loss of Stability in the Adoptive Family

Before adolescence, few children truly recognize the legal basis for adoption. As a result, they sometimes worry that their birth parents can return to reclaim them or that their adoptive parents can send them back to their birth family. For these children, the sense of stability in their adoptive family can be fragile, at least until they better understand the nature of adoptive family life. Moreover, for children who have experienced multiple foster placements, anxiety about residential stability and parental commitment is even greater.

> *"He's lived in so many homes and had so many people reject him that I can only imagine that he must be waiting anxiously for the time when we will reject him too....I imagine this must be something he thinks about whenever my wife or I get upset with him or punish him for some inappropriate behavior."*
> ~ Adoptive father of an 8-year-old boy placed from foster care at 7 years of age

Loss of Fit in the Family

As they are growing up, most children probably take for granted their degree of fit in their family, that is, whether or not they are similar to their parents and siblings in relation to various personal traits. Only when there are distinct differences among family members in physical, psychologic, or behavioral characteristics is it likely that children will begin to question the extent to which they "fit in." This experience, however, is much more common for adopted individuals. Because of the lack of a genetic link to their parents, it is a common experience for adopted children to recognize that they do not look like others in the family or that their interests, personality traits, temperament, talents, skills, and behaviors may not be similar to their parents and siblings. This recognition, however, is experienced in quite varied ways by adopted children and adolescents. For some youngsters, it's just a matter of being different, with no inherent value attached to that fact. For others, however, the observed differences are unsettling. This is often true for those placed across racial lines.

> *"Looking so different from my parents and brothers is something that's bothered me a lot for a long time....I don't want to be white like them...but I wish I just didn't stand out so much...it makes me feel different, like I don't really belong here."* ~ Thomas, a 14-year-old African American teenager living with his white parents

The lack of a genetic link between parents and children in adoptive families and the resulting differences that are experienced among family members often affect parental expectations. One of the most frequent areas in which this occurs is related to children's academic performance. When adoptive parents are well educated, they often place a high value on academic success in raising their children. Yet adopted children are at increased risk for learning problems.[12] Faced with a child with learning disabilities, adoptive parents may have difficulty altering their expectations related to school performance, which can create significant tensions in the parent-child relationship and undermine children's sense of being accepted or "fitting into the family."

> "I have dyslexia...it's a problem with reading...have always had a problem reading...and my dad just doesn't seem to understand...it's not my fault that I don't read very well...but he believes I just don't try very hard....I don't think I'll ever be able to satisfy him...not like my sister who always gets As or Bs." ~ William, a 15-year-old boy adopted from Korea

Loss of Genealogic Continuity

Because teenagers are better able to conceptualize their place in a family line than younger children, it usually isn't until adolescence that adoptees become especially sensitized to the fact that they have been "cut off" from a biological family line—their intergenerational heritage—leading to what Sants[40] referred to as "genealogical bewilderment." Awareness of this type of loss often leads adopted individuals to begin questioning their parents about the source of certain personal traits or characteristics and sometimes leads them to consider the possibility of searching for birth family members.

> "I'm curious to know who I look like...do I get my features more from my birth mom or my dad... where do my musical interests and abilities come from...certainly not from my [adoptive] parents, who can't play any musical instruments....I don't know too much about them [birth parents], but I'm really interested to find out what I can." ~ 18-year-old adopted girl placed in infancy from Colombia

Loss of Racial, Ethnic, and Cultural Heritage

In domestic and international adoption, children are often placed across racial and ethnic lines. When this happens, children sometimes are cut off from others or experiences that represent their racial, ethnic, or cultural heritage. Although children as young as 3 years display awareness of racial differences between themselves and their parents, it isn't until later in childhood or adolescence that most individuals typically begin to experience heightened interest in, and sometimes a sense of confusion about, their racial, ethnic, and cultural origins.[18,19,41] This interest and confusion is tied to normal questions about identity development.

Research and clinical experience suggest that when children are exposed to appropriate racial and ethnic role models and when adoptive parents provide positive messages about their children's birth heritage, transracially placed adoptees generally are quite successful in integrating this aspect of the self into a healthy and secure identity. In the absence of these experiences, however, there may be ongoing confusion, bewilderment, and a sense of loss about their racial and ethnic heritage. Daniel, a 17-year-old African American boy transracially placed in infancy, reported,

> "I look black, but I can't even dance….I'm not interested in rap music….I don't like to hang out….I'm an Oreo…black on the outside, white on the inside."

Referring to his 16-year-old sister who also was adopted in infancy by his parents, Daniel further stated

> "It's easy for Samantha to fit in, but not for me…she has plenty of [black] people to hang out with, but not me…she feels black; I don't."

Thomas, a 28-year-old African American man placed with his white parents when he was 1 year old, echoes some of the same difficulties as Daniel because of inadequate racial role models during his childhood years.

> "I grew up in a community where there were very few blacks like me…most of my knowledge of what it meant to be black was gained through television and other forms of media…at least until I went to college…then it hit me…I really didn't know anything about a very important part of who I was…it took quite a while for me to really understand and feel comfortable about being a black man."

Yet not all transracially placed adopted individuals feel cut off from their racial or ethnic origins. Consider Sean, a 17-year-old African American boy placed transracially at the age of 2 years.

> "I grew up in a very integrated community and went to very integrated schools….I've always had both African American and white friends…and some Asian friends too…being black has never been an issue for me….I'm very comfortable with who I am…my parents are very open and supportive….I feel good about being adopted by them…the fact that they aren't African American hasn't prevented me from feeling proud that I'm black…they've helped me with that."

Loss of Privacy

Unless they choose to share their adoptive family status with others, most in-racially placed adoptees can keep their adoption a private matter; not so for those placed across racial lines. In transracial placements, the ability to keep the adoption a secret is lost. Racial differences between parents and children are not only obvious to all but often a matter of speculation and questioning by others, which can be disconcerting and even embarrassing for parents and children. This is especially true during adolescence, when feelings of self-consciousness and the need for privacy often are intense.

> *"When I'm out with my parents…walking down the street, in a restaurant, at school, or whatever, I sometimes feel that people are looking at us…and then they know I'm adopted…it's not that I'm ashamed to be adopted…what bothers me is that I can't control who knows or not…if I was [white] like my parents, or I lived with a Chinese family, then people wouldn't automatically know that I was adopted."* ~ 14-year-old girl adopted from China at 20 months of age

Loss of Identity

Adolescence is the time when most adopted individuals begin the process of integrating adoption into their developing sense of self. This process is an extension of the more universal task of identity development.[19] Exploring connections to birth family and origins and understanding the meaning of adoption, from personal, familial, and societal contexts, are all part of this process. Adoptive identity development may also include plans for searching for more information about one's origins or making contact with birth family members.

In the course of normal adolescent identity development, many adopted individuals come to feel that part of themselves is missing. This is typically connected to a lack of relevant information about their birth family and origins. They often use spatial metaphors to express their sense of loss.

"The most difficult thing about being adopted is that there's no real information....I have scraps here and there but nothing that seems real to me....I often feel empty inside." ~ 17-year-old girl adopted as an infant

"It's as if something is absent...there is a hole in me." ~ 18-year-old girl adopted as an infant

"I feel like I've been cut off from something that is truly a part of me....I think of it as if I've experienced an amputation...just like an amputee experiences the pain from a phantom limb, I experience emotional pain because of what I've lost." ~ 21-year-old man adopted as an infant

Uniqueness of Adoption-Related Loss

Grieving is a normal and universal response to loss, one that involves a complex array of emotions and behavior.[42] Adopted children are like all other children who experience loss; as they grieve, they can be expected to manifest an array of emotions and behaviors, including confusion, anxiety, sadness, crying, anger, and acting-out behavior. There is no correct way to grieve, and there is no specific timetable that defines appropriate grieving. Some types of loss, however, are more complicated than others, making them more difficult to resolve.[43] Adoption may fit this pattern for a variety of reasons.[28,30]

First, relatively few children are adopted. In fact, only about 2% of children in the United States are non-related adoptees, that is, children who have been adopted by individuals with whom they have no biological connection. As a result, adopted children and teenagers who are struggling with adoption-related loss are at risk of feeling different, ie, feeling that there is no one else around who really understands what they are going through. In turn, this feeling of difference can undermine self-esteem and identity and complicate the resolution of loss.

Adoption-related loss also is unusual in that it is not necessarily permanent, unlike death, creating a sense of ambiguity surrounding the loss.[43] As children mature, they recognize that birth parents, birth siblings, and other birth family members may be alive. Moreover, it is extremely common for adoptees to fantasize about meeting these individuals—and in fact, they often do. The potential for searching for birth family and the possibility of reunion with these individuals makes it more difficult, at least for some adopted people, to find a comfortable resolution for their grief and feelings of loss. Moreover, open adoptions, which are becoming increasingly routine in the United States,[44] do not eliminate, although they may reduce, the sense of confusion, dismay, and loss experienced by adopted individuals.

Circumstances surrounding separation from birth parents and the nature of their relationship with these individuals also complicate the resolution of grief for some adoptees. Children who were placed as newborns or infants have never had relationships with their birth parents, but this reality does not preclude them from experiencing loss. As they mature cognitively and emotionally, children begin to fantasize about their birth parents, wondering who they are, what they are like, and what they may be doing with their lives, as well as about the circumstances surrounding the adoption placement. Children who believe their birth parents made a voluntary choice not to raise them sometimes interpret this decision in terms of negative self-characteristics. Consider Annie, an 8-year-old Chinese girl, placed for adoption at 14 months of age.

> "Maybe she didn't want a girl…maybe she didn't like something else about me…it makes me upset to think that maybe she wanted a baby, just not me."

For those children who were removed from their birth families by child protective services, the implications associated with their placements in care can negatively affect their view of their birth parents as well as their self-image.

> "They use to hit me and my brother…a lot.…I remember when the police finally came…they arrested my parents and put us in foster care.…I was glad to leave them.…I hate them for what they did to us.…I hate everything about them…but sometimes I think that maybe I deserved it…maybe I was partly to blame." ~ 12-year-old Hispanic boy placed for adoption with his brother when he was 9 years old

Finally, unlike death and many other forms of loss, adoption-related loss too often goes unrecognized by society. Emphasis is placed on what is gained by children through adoption—eg, legal permanence; a caring, capable, and "forever" family—but not on what is lost. However, from the child's perspective, adoption also involves substantial loss, some parts of which are obvious and readily observable and other parts more subtle and slower to emerge over time. Appreciation of adoption-related loss, like understanding of many concepts, is developmentally determined and may evolve over time. When loss is unrecognized by others, there is the risk that the individual will feel ignored, misunderstood, and unsupported, leading to what Doka[45] referred to as "disenfranchised grief." This type of grief is much more difficult to resolve than grief that is more openly acknowledged and socially supported through recognized rituals and public mourning. In the latter situation, the bereaved person is able to share grief-related thoughts and feelings openly, have those thoughts and feelings understood and validated, and in so doing, find comfortable ways of integrating the loss into a healthy sense of self. But when these conditions of grieving are not present, especially when the bereaved person believes that significant others do not understand or accept what he or she is thinking and feeling, grieving can be blocked or distorted, increasing the risk of adjustment difficulties such as depression. Such is the experience with some adopted individuals.

"It seems to me that few understand what I have gone through....I haven't found others, except for one or two people, who can listen to me, understand my pain, and not just try to cheer me up or tell me that I'm being silly or overly dramatic...that I should be grateful for being adopted and not dwell on the sad parts...it was so different when my [adoptive] mother died...then everyone seemed to understand what I was going through....I felt their support...but it's been so different regarding my adoption...few people really get it." ~ Sharon, a 38-year-old adoptee placed as a newborn

Guidelines for Discussing Adoption With Children

As noted previously, some of the more important responsibilities for parents involve sharing adoption information with their children, helping children to understand the meaning and implications of being adopted, and supporting them in their efforts to cope with feelings related to their family status, including those connected to loss. In concluding this chapter, I would like to offer some guidelines that pediatricians can share with adoptive parents in helping them with this process.

- *Discussing adoption with children is a process, not an event.* Because of anxiety related to talking with their children about adoption, often linked to a history of infertility or previous child loss,[46] some adoptive parents approach this task as if it were a one-time event, flooding their youngsters with too much information and attempting to avoid further discussions unless pressed by their children. Parents need to recognize that providing information should be an ongoing process that unfolds over time, often beginning in infancy, and one that is geared toward their children's readiness, cognitively and emotionally, to assimilate what they are learning and make appropriate use of it.

- *Adoption revelation is a dialogue, not a process of talking to children.* Although the initial information about adoption is provided by parents, adoption revelation should be an active give-and-take process between parents and children. By asking children questions and normalizing their curiosity, parents can ensure that their understanding of the information presented is reasonably accurate; if it is not, they can then take steps to correct any misperception or misunderstanding. Developing a parent-child dialogue also ensures that parents are kept reasonably apprised of how the child is coping emotionally with the information provided and whether there is a need for additional support, including professional help, for their son or daughter during this process.

- *Early telling has advantages over late telling.* Although there is no right or wrong time to begin sharing adoption information, most professionals believe that beginning the process relatively early in life has distinct advantages. In fact, most parents begin sharing details of adoption information between 2 and 4 years of age[18] or earlier. Although early telling may not accomplish the goal of fostering a realistic understanding of adoption in children, it normalizes the word for them, provides them with positive messages about their family status, and helps parents become desensitized to this sometimes anxiety-arousing process, prior to the time when most boys and girls begin to ask more direct and difficult questions about their origins and the reasons for their adoption.

- *Be emotionally available for the child and listen.* It's not enough for parents to be physically present while discussing their child's history of adoption; they must be emotionally present as well. Parents are notoriously good advice givers but not always the best listeners. This is especially true when their children are facing a challenge, manifesting distress, or having some type of difficulty coping. Parents need to remember that when they share information about adoption, it may result in unanticipated thoughts and feelings in their children, some of which can be unsettling. To help their children cope in healthy and normative ways with their adoptions, parents need to be attuned to what children are thinking and feeling. Engaging in active listening is essential to achieving this goal.

- *Begin the adoption story with birth and family diversity, not adoption.* One of the most frequent questions asked by adoptive parents is what information should be presented first and how the information should be shared. Although there are no right and wrong answers to these questions, it is generally helpful to begin this process by emphasizing that children, regardless of what kind of family they live in, are created through a biological process. Once the "simple" facts of reproduction and birth are explained, parents can then go on to talk about how families are formed. For example, parents may begin by explaining that all babies start out the same way and that a man and a woman make a baby and it grows in a special place in the woman's body called a uterus. To further reinforce the idea that adopted children are similar to many, if not most, of their peers, parents should then begin to talk about the different types of families that exist in ways that make clear that they are all equal (even if different). For example, parents can explain that sometimes the man and woman are not able to take care of a baby, so they look for other adults to be the baby's parents. In short, before even identifying adoption as the means by which the child entered the family, adoptive parents should normalize, and even celebrate, family diversity, with adoption being just one of many different types of families that exist. Normalizing diversity reduces the risk that children will feel that only their family is different.

- *Keep in mind the child's developmental level and readiness to process specific information.* Children vary in their intellectual capacity and emotional maturity, even at young ages. Parents need to consider what their children are likely to understand and be able to cope with emotionally as they allow the adoption story to unfold. Pediatricians should emphasize the use of age-appropriate language in discussing adoption issues. In addition, they should encourage the use of one or more of the many children's books on adoption that are readily available as a means of facilitating children's interest in the adoption story, as well as supporting their understanding and coping in relation to the information being presented. It is especially helpful if such books are integrated into other reading material rather than saved for "special discussions," which can further normalize the adoption process.

- *Validate and normalize children's curiosity, questions, and feelings about their adoption, birth parents, and heritage.* As children begin to be exposed to their adoption stories, they often show significant curiosity about their birth parents and the circumstances surrounding their placements, as well as about adoption itself. Although questions about these issues are common, they sometimes create anxiety for adoptive parents. This is especially true when children appear to be preoccupied with adoption-related issues, show ambivalence about being adopted, or begin to deal more openly with adoption-related loss. Children very often become aware of their parents' anxiety, and when they do, they sometimes wonder whether their parents disapprove of their questions and interest in their backgrounds. This can leave children feeling caught in the middle between the family they love and the family they want to know more about. Adoptive parents can be especially helpful to their children by validating and normalizing their youngsters' curiosity and questions about their origins, specifically by encouraging adoption-related questions, finding ways of bringing up the topic themselves, and talking about their children's birth heritage in a positive and respectful manner.[47]

- *Be aware of your own feelings and values related to birth parents and the child's history.* Before embarking on the specifics of a child's adoption history, parents need to consider their own feelings related to their connections to the birth family as well as the specific information known about the birth parents and their child's history with them. Too often, information associated with a child's history can challenge the values and beliefs of adoptive parents—eg, mental illness or criminality in the birth family, incest or rape as the means of a child's conception, or neglect and abuse during the child's earlier years. Working through conflicted feelings associated with these issues will help adoptive parents become better prepared emotionally to discuss their child's origins in a truly supportive way.

- *Avoid judgmental comments about birth parents or the child's heritage.* To feel worthy as a human being, children need to believe they come from worthwhile beginnings. This principle suggests that when their children are young and the adoption story is just beginning to be told, parents should avoid negative descriptions or derogatory comments about birth families; otherwise, there is a risk of undermining children's self-esteem and identity. Such comments can also undermine any contact the adoptive family may have with birth relatives, which in turn could further compromise children's psychologic adjustment. In short, adoptive parents must find ways of discussing their child's history so as to be supportive of connections with their origins.

- *Discuss "difficult" background information.* Adoptive parents often feel confused and stymied about how to discuss certain information related to their child's history that could be interpreted in a negative way, eg, inappropriate parenting, substance abuse, parental psychopathology.[24] Pediatricians can be helpful to parents by providing the following guidelines for managing difficult information:
  — First, do not lie! It is better to acknowledge that one has background information, some of which will be shared at the present time and some when the child is older, than to avoid discussing certain topics because the information is emotionally charged. Secrets are difficult to keep and can undermine family relationships. For example, parents too often deny knowing specific information about the birth parents or their child's history, only to reveal it later. When this happens, it undermines a child's ability to trust parents.
  — Adoptive parents also should be encouraged to differentiate between a birth parent's intent and desire and actions. It is probably safe to assume that virtually all birth parents wanted the best for their children and, if they could have, to have been good parents to them. Nevertheless, intent and desire are not always translated into loving and competent behavior. When developmentally appropriate, adoptive parents should help their children recognize that despite the birth parents' desire to be nurturing and effective caregivers, they could not do so. In explaining the reasons, adoptive parents may need help in translating their knowledge of the birth parents' circumstances into more neutral, less value-laden terms. One example is the use of an illness model. Birth parents who cannot meet their children's basic needs because they abuse alcohol or drugs or because of some form of psychopathology can be described as suffering from an illness that could not be overcome quickly or easily. Similarly, neglectful or abusive behavior can be reframed in terms of judgment problems, impulsive control problems, or other difficulties that are related to personality problems that are very difficult to correct. When parents suffer from these types of life problems, their children suffer too, even if that is not the adults' intent. Consequently, a difficult but necessary decision must be made in the best interests of the children—namely, removing them from the care of the birth parents and placing them in a more stable, nurturing, and capable family. Empathy, affection, calmness, self-confidence, and openness to children's needs and views are the key traits needed by adoptive parents during these discussions.

- *Be prepared to help the child cope with adoption-related loss and grief.* In counseling adoptive parents, pediatricians need to educate them about adoption-related loss and normalize children's reactions to it. Too often, when parents see the confusion, sadness, anxiety, and anger that sometimes are manifested by their children, they panic and interpret those reactions in a pathologic way. This reaction probably accounts, at least in part, for the fact that adoptive parents are quicker to use mental health services for their children compared with non-adoptive parents, especially when symptoms are still relatively mild.[48] Adoptive parents can be helped when pediatricians reinterpret children's reactions, when appropriate, in terms of a grief model. By doing so, children's responses to adoption-related loss are normalized and put into a more familiar context. Moreover, this type of reframing also helps parents feel more empowered to manage their children's distress.

- *Foster open, honest, and respectful parent-child communication about adoption.* The ability to grieve adoption-related loss is tied to a family environment character-ized by openness, honesty, and respect.[47] In counseling adoptive parents, pedia-tricians need to emphasize the importance of working toward these goals. When children feel understood and accepted, even in the midst of their confusion, sadness, and anger related to adoption, they will eventually find ways of integrat-ing this aspect of their life into a healthy and secure sense of self. The type of family emotional and communicative environment created by parents is a key for achieving this goal.

Conclusion

Adoption offers children the promise of nurturance, emotional stability, and lifetime family commitment. As children learn their adoption story from their parents, including their connections to their birth origins, their lives take on new meaning as well as new challenges and complications. Finding ways of understanding and inte-grating this new information into a healthy sense of self is an important develop-mental task for adopted children, and supporting this process is a vital responsibility for adoptive parents. Pediatricians are often the first professionals outside of the adoption agency who parents turn to in seeking answers about childhood stress and parenting challenges. Being aware of normative developmental changes in children's understanding of adoption, as well as common reactions to adoption-related loss, will allow pediatricians to offer timely and useful guidance and support for parents as they seek to meet the challenges of raising their adopted children.

References

1. Hoksbergen RAC. The importance of adoption for nurturing and enhancing the emotional and intellectual potential of children. *Adoption Q.* 1999;3:29–42

2. Selwyn J, Quinton D. Stability, permanence, outcomes, and support: foster care and adoption compared. *Adopt Foster.* 2004;28(4):6–15

3. Triseliotis J. Long-term foster care or adoption? The evidence examined. *Child and Family Social Work.* 2002;7:23–33

4. van IJzendoorn MH, Juffer F. Adoption is a successful natural intervention enhancing adopted children's IQ and school performance. *Curr Dir Psychol Sci.* 2005;14(6):326–330

5. van IJzendoorn MH, Juffer F. The Emanuel Miller Memorial Lecture 2006: adoption as intervention. Meta-analytic evidence for massive catch-up and plasticity in physical, socio-emotional, and cognitive development. *J Child Psychol Psychiatry.* 2006;47(12):1228–1245

6. Elmund A, Lindblad F, Vinnerljung B, Hjern A. Intercountry adoptees in out-of-home care: a national cohort study. *Acta Paediatr.* 2007;96(3):437–442

7. Howard JA, Smith SL, Ryan SD. A comparative study of child welfare adoptions with other types of adopted children and birth children. *Adoption Q.* 2004;7:1–30

8. Keyes MA, Sharma A, Elkins IJ, Iacono WG, McGue W. The mental health of US adolescents adopted in infancy. *Arch Pediatr Adolesc Med.* 2008;162(5):419–425

9. McRoy RG, Grotevant H, Zurcher S. *Emotional Disturbance in Adopted Adolescents.* New York, NY: Praeger; 1988

10. Juffer F, van IJzendoorn MH. Behavior problems and mental health referrals of international adoptees: a meta-analysis. *JAMA.* 2005;293(20):2501–2515

11. Marshall MJ, Marshall S, Heer MJ. Characteristics of abstinent substance abusers who first sought treatment in adolescence. *J Drug Educ.* 1994;24(2):151–162

12. Brodzinsky DM, Steiger C. Prevalence of adoptees in special education populations. *J Learn Disabil.* 1991;24(8):484–489

13. Cadoret RJ, Yates WR, Troughton E, Woodworth G, Stewart MA. Adoption study demonstrating two genetic pathways to drug abuse. *Arch Gen Psychiatry.* 1995;52(1):42–52

14. Crea TM, Barth RP, Guo S, Brooks D. Behavioral outcomes for substance-exposed adopted children: fourteen years post-adoption. *Am J Orthopsychiatry.* 2008;78(1):11–19

15. Gunnar MR, van Dulmen MH; International Adoption Project Team. Behavior problems in post-institutionalized internationally adopted children. *Dev Psychopathol.* 2007;19(1):129–148

16. Rutter M, Beckett C, Castle J, et al. Effects of profound early institutional deprivation. An overview of findings from a UK longitudinal study of Romanian adoptees. In: Wrobel GM, Neil E, eds. *International Advances in Adoption Research for Practice.* New York, NY: Wiley; 2009:147–167

17. Lanius RA, Vermetten E, Pain C. *The Impact of Early Life Trauma on Health and Disease: The Hidden Epidemic.* Cambridge, England: Cambridge University Press; 2010

18. Brodzinsky DM, Schechter MD, Henig RM. *Being Adopted: The Lifelong Search for Self.* New York, NY: Doubleday; 1992

19. Grotevant HD. Coming to terms with adoption: the construction of identity from adolescence into adulthood. *Adoption Q.* 1997;1:3–27

20. Kirk HD. *Shared Fate: A Theory and Method of Adoptive Relationships.* New York, NY: Free Press; 1964

21. Brodzinsky DM. Adjustment to adoption: a psychosocial perspective. *Clin Psychol Rev.* 1987;7(1):25–47

22. Brodzinsky DM, Pinderhughes EE. Parenting and child development in adoptive families. In: Bornstein M, ed. *Handbook of Parenting: Children and Parenting (Vol 1).* Mahwah, NJ: Lawrence Erlbaum Associates; 2002:279–311

23. Rosenberg EB. *The Adoption Life Cycle: The Children and Their Families Through the Years.* New York, NY: Free Press; 1992

24. Melina LR. *Raising Adopted Children: Practical, Reassuring Advice for Every Adoptive Parent.* Rev ed. New York, NY: Harper Perennial; 1998

25. Brodzinsky DM, Singer LM, Braff AM. Children's understanding of adoption. *Child Dev.* 1984;55(3):869–878

26. Brodzinsky DM, Smith DW, Brodzinsky AB. *Children's Adjustment to Adoption: Developmental and Clinical Issues.* Thousand Oaks, CA: Sage Publications; 1998

27. Brodzinsky DM. *Adjustment Factors in Adoption.* Rep No. MN34549. Washington, DC: National Institute of Mental Health; 1983

28. Brodzinsky DM. A stress and coping model of adoption adjustment. In: Brodzinsky DM, Schechter MD, eds. *The Psychology of Adoption.* New York, NY: Oxford University Press; 1990:3–24

29. Newman JL, Roberts LR, Syre CR. Concepts of family among children and adolescents: effect of cognitive level, gender, and family structure. *Dev Psychol.* 1993;29(3):951–962

30. Brodzinsky DM. The experience of sibling loss in the adjustment of foster and adopted children. In: Silverstein DN, Smith SL, eds. *Siblings in Adoption and Foster Care.* Westport, CT: Praeger; 2009:43–56

31. Leon IG. Adoption losses: naturally occurring or socially constructed? *Child Dev.* 2002; 73(2):652–663

32. Nickman SL. Losses in adoption: the need for dialogue. *Psychoanal Study Child.* 1985;40:365–398

33. Silverstein DM, Kaplan Roszia S. Lifelong issues in adoption. In: Coleman L, Tilbor K, Hornby H, Baggis C, eds. *Working with Older Adoptees.* Portland, ME: University of Southern Maine; 1988:45–53

34. Grotevant HD, Dunbar N, Kohler JK, Esau AML. Adoptive identity: how contexts within and beyond the family shape developmental pathways. In: Javier RA, Baden AL, Biafora FA, Camacho-Gingerich A, eds. *Handbook of Adoption: Implications for Researchers, Practitioners, and Families.* Thousand Oaks, CA: Sage Publications; 2007:77–89

35. Müller U, Perry B. Adopted persons' search for and contact with their birth parents I: who searches and why? *Adoption Q.* 2001;4:5–37

36. Smith DW, Brodzinsky DM. Stress and coping in adopted children. *J Clin Child Psychol.* 1994;23(1):91–99

37. Smith DW, Brodzinsky DM. Coping with birthparent loss in adopted children. *J Child Psychol Psychiatry.* 2002;43(2):213–223

38. Bowlby J. *Attachment and Loss: Vol 2. Separation.* New York, NY: Basic Books; 1973

39. Silverstein DN, Smith SL, eds. *Siblings in Adoption and Foster Care.* Westport, CT: Praeger; 2009

40. Sants HJ. Genealogical bewilderment in children with substitute care. *Br J Med Psychol.* 1964;37:133–141

41. Baden AL, Steward RJ. The cultural-racial identity model. In: Javier RA, Baden AL, Biafora FA, Camacho-Gingerich A, eds. *Handbook of Adoption: Implications for Researchers, Practitioners, and Families.* Thousand Oaks, CA: Sage Publications, 2007:90–112

42. Bowlby J. *Attachment and Loss: Vol 3. Loss, Sadness and Depression.* New York, NY: Basic Books; 1980

43. Boss P. *Ambiguous Loss: Learning to Live with Unresolved Grief.* Cambridge, MA: Harvard University Press; 1999

44. Grotevant HD, Perry YV, McRoy RG. Openness in adoption: outcomes for adolescents within their adoptive kinship networks. In: Brodzinsky DM, Palacios J, eds. *Psychological Issues in Adoption: Research and Practice.* Westport, CT: Praeger; 2005:167–186

45. Doka KJ. Disenfranchised grief. In: Doka KJ, ed. *Disenfranchised Grief: Recognizing Hidden Sorrow.* Lexington, MA: Lexington Books; 1989:3–23

46. Brodzinsky DM. Infertility and adoption: considerations and clinical issues. In: Lieblum S, ed. *Infertility: Psychological Issues and Counseling Strategies*. New York, NY: Wiley; 1997:246–262

47. Brodzinsky DM. Reconceptualizing openness in adoption: implications for theory, research, and practice. In: Brodzinsky DM, Palacios J, eds. *Psychological Issues in Adoption: Research and Practice*. Westport, CT: Praeger; 2005:145–166

48. Warren SB. Lower threshold for referral for psychiatric treatment for adopted adolescents. *J Am Acad Child Adolesc Psychiatry*. 1992;31(3):512–527

CHAPTER 18

Working With Adoptive Families: What Every Professional Should Know

Joyce Maguire Pavao, EdD, MEd, LCSW, LMFT

Editors' note: This chapter is in essay format.

It is estimated that adoption affects the lives of 40 million Americans. This is startling, considering that there are approximately 5 million adopted people living in the United States. Importantly, for each adopted person, there are also birth parents, adoptive parents, birth and adopted siblings, grandparents, and a whole array of extended family members who are affected by adoption as well. Given these numbers, it is important for professionals to be skilled in working with the unique issues that face adoptive family systems. Adoption has the potential of being a very positive way to create a family. One must remember, however, that there are feelings about having surrendered a child to adoption, about having adopted a child—especially when one cannot bear children—and about being adopted that pose special concerns for those involved throughout their lives.

Until recently, much discussion in the literature addressing families of adoption has been based on the perspective that most issues of the adoption triad (birth parents, adoptive parents, and adopted persons) are pathologic rather than normative. For example, the depression, anger, and shame of the birth parent have often been seen as an unhealthy response to be conquered. The pain of infertility that adoptive parents often face is too frequently transformed into the sense that there is a "problem" with them, especially in the realm of parenting. The adopted person is overrepresented in treatment facilities and often seen as having learning disabilities and emotional difficulties at best and even more pathologies and diagnoses at worst. In other words, these 3 groups are often perceived as having problems that are not "normal" and raising questions such as

- Is it normal not to be able to have a child?
- Is it normal not to keep a child?
- Is it normal not to be kept?

Several important concepts are critical to consider when working with adoptive families.

- Entering a new family system causes disequilibrium.
- Losing a family member causes pain and loss, which is hard to resolve—if ever.
- Birth parents never fully resolve the loss of their children to adoption, and infertile couples or individuals never resolve the loss of the children they might have had by birth.
- Adoption does not "fix" these problems, and the adopted person develops with these losses as the very foundation of his or her life.

All parties to adoption try to make their present family work in ways that remind them of the ghosts of histories past, with expectations of self and others in mythic proportions. Anniversaries and other rites of passage of developmental stages specifically bring crises to a head. Some of these families (in whole or part) may present as angry, blaming, depressed, paralyzed, confused, or rejecting of a family member, and most often it is the adopted person—a child or an adolescent—who is the focus. Some of these families may seek nontherapeutic and preventive consultation so that they can work hard to avoid the pain.

Society has promulgated the interpretation that these adoption issues are pathologic and has made the very real problems of untimely pregnancy and surrender, of infertility and adoption, more of a stigma and wound than they already are in and of themselves. There are ethical and philosophic issues relevant to untimely pregnancy, infertility issues, and adoption that are critical to consider when working with families affected by adoption.

Throughout this chapter, I will highlight my research completed at Harvard University, *The Normative Crisis in the Development of the Adoptive Family,* and describe a model for treatment and training I developed, which explores the special issues and concerns that birth parents, adoptive parents, and adopted people face. The model presumes that there are "normal" developmental crises that occur in adoptive systems. Although all families and individuals go through developmental stages, the special circumstances that adoption creates add issues and complexity to the process of identity development. These issues are normal and healthy under the circumstances that surrender and adoption create. This normative model proposes that a systemic approach is needed to work with adoptive family systems. There is no "identified patient" in this model; the whole system (from the wider context of adoption practices to the intricate relationships in the adoptive and birth families) is regarded as the client. Crises can be normal and can even lead to transformation. To truly understand and work with this complex system, the pediatrician must be familiar with, and empathetic toward, each member of the adoption circle, including the birth family, whether it is known or not.

This chapter will simply reflect on the complex concerns for individuals and families that arise after adoption is the path chosen or otherwise decided by birth and adoptive parents. It will address the ways that open adoption (which can happen at the time of adoption or at any time in the life span when there is a search and then a reunion) can dispel some of the myths and missing links in adoption.

Birth Parents

Choice of words is important. Birth parents feel discounted when referred to as "biological parents" because they are far more than just "baby-making machines." Adoptive parents feel discounted when birth parents are referred to as "real" or "natural." Some birth parents like to be called "first parents," and no birth parent is a birth parent until the adoption has been finalized—they are the parents to that child during the 9 months of pregnancy and during the interim while the adoption is being finalized.

When working with women and their partners who are dealing with an untimely pregnancy and are trying to make a decision about whether or not to surrender a child for adoption, it is essential that all involved in the decision be educated about the posttraumatic effects that will be permanent, especially for the birth mother. In most cases, surrender is a no-win situation. The pain of loss is likely to be great, but the issues that make the question of adoption a serious one indicate that being a parent might also be a very difficult choice for this person or these 2 people at this time. Pediatric health care professionals may be involved with an adolescent or young adult who is about to be a birth parent.

Beyond the decision to place a child for adoption, birth parents need to be prepared for additional implications for their family over time. For example, issues are common for families having "next children" born to them, especially those referred to as the "second first child," ie, the child born first after the surrendered child. For older birth parents who surrendered a child many years ago, there are several stages of treatment that may be helpful, including psycho-education, confronting the shame, allowing the anger, acknowledging and grieving the loss, and finally the empowering and accepting stages, which are crucial to the mastery and emotional development that is often arrested at the time of surrender. In addition, there are post-search issues created by initiating a search or being searched for by the adopted person.

For those who are able to work with couples prior to surrender of an infant or child, it is useful to educate and expose prospective birth parents to the experiences of those who have made this decision in the past and to birth parents who have more recently surrendered. Please see Resources on page 410.

It is important to acknowledge that there are also many birth parents who have had their children removed because of abuse or neglect. Perhaps domestic violence, drug abuse, mental illness, or other circumstances contributed to the need for an authority to make a decision to remove a child or children from parental care, and after working toward reunification with the birth family, another permanent decision such as kinship placement, guardianship, or adoption was necessary. In these cases, older children who have suffered abuse and neglect are often placed in a family that may or may not be fully prepared to deal with their posttraumatic issues and concerns. Ongoing relationships between birth parents and children who are connected to them but are no longer in their care require special consideration and family support.

Pre-adoptive Couples

The majority of pre-adoptive couples have been struggling for years with issues of infertility. (This is not to exclude single adopters, but infertility is presently the most common cause for beginning the road to adoption.) The pain and loss that result from constantly hoping for a birth child coupled with the invasive experiences of medical, pharmacologic, and surgical procedures, as well as the strain on a couple's relationship that these procedures may produce, can make the process of adoption seem like more hoops to jump through to attain the goal to be parents. For parents experiencing infertility who have previously been pregnant and chosen to terminate a pregnancy or those who are no longer involved in a previous birth child's life, the decision to adopt may be especially poignant. Just like birth parents, adoptive parents may feel like victims of the situation. Birth parents are victims of untimely pregnancy and lack of support from a partner, family, and society, leading to a life-long experience of pain, shame, guilt, and loss. Most pre-adoptive parents are victims of the situation of infertility, lack of understanding by some family and friends, and society, often also resulting in a lifelong experience of pain, guilt, shame, and loss, a portion of which may be seemingly "fixed" by adoption. Of course, adoption does not "fix" the challenges of infertility. It does, however, make available the experience of parenting.

Pre-adoptive couples and individuals are subject to a variety of stresses that non-adoptive parents do not experience in parenting a child. For example, prospective adoptive parents need to be involved in agency assessments and home studies, process the variety of types of adoption includes varying degrees of openness, and make choices that will affect the rest of their lives—often while lacking support and information from people who understand the process or specific concerns for specific children. Groups like Resolve can provide support and education about these issues (see Resources on page 410.)

Because they are making a lifelong decision, couples and singles considering adoption of a child need education about the varying degrees of openness in adoption and the various types of adoption. Prospective adoptive parents are often quite surprised to hear that, just as in a marriage in which the in-laws and families are present (like a Greek chorus) whether they live next door or 3,000 miles away, so too in adoption are the birth parents and birth families present in the lives of the adopted ones, whether the adoption is closed or open. Education of the pre-adoptive couple or individual about the issues of adoption and how they affect the whole family (extended birth and adoptive families), the kind of adoption that is best for them, and the empowerment that is so important for them to be strong and caring parents are components of this very specialized clinical work.

It is important to keep exploring, not ignoring, the effect of infertility on the whole family and the individuals involved. Infertility affects the whole family system. Infertility is a life crisis. Infertility is a lifelong issue.

In my experience, we hear from many adoptive parents, but we most often hear about their parenting challenges and their children—not about themselves. We rarely hear about how the ongoing issues of infertility affect their parenting and identity. If we could have a more intimate voice about this in the world of adoption, it would help older children and adolescents in adoption to have better insight into the challenges of their birth family and adoptive family. As a result, children would understand that their lives are founded in love and loss. Strength and healing is important, and it requires acknowledgment and openness. Professionals working with children and their families who are tuned into these issues can help adults to deal with their own losses and not assume that all of the issues of attachment and loss belong only to the child.

Adoptive Families

Adoption can be a very positive way to create or expand a family. However, linked with the process of adoption are ongoing issues related to adoption for the whole family to address, including how to tell the child, what to tell the child, when to tell the child about his or her adoptive history, how to deal with extended family members and neighbors, and how to work with schools and professionals who have little or no experience with learning disabilities, attention-deficit/hyperactivity disorder, and emotional difficulties within the context of an adopted child's history. Things that root families take for granted, such as knowing their medical history, may pose serious dilemmas for adoptive families. Some physicians describe dealing with an adopted person like dealing with a coma victim, in the sense that critical and current family history information is often missing and impossible to get.

In adolescence, a variety of issues emerge for the adopted person and adoptive family (see Chapter 17, Adoptive Identity and Children's Understanding of Adoption: Implications for Pediatric Practice, on page 367). Adopted children, like all adolescents, begin to look at themselves more carefully. For the adopted person, looking in the mirror may lead to the realization that he does not know another human being in the world who is related to or looks like him. The fact of adoption complicates issues of identity, sexuality, trust, self-esteem, and individuation, just to name a few.

As adolescence brings on a search for identity, adoptive parents are often faced with the confusing task of helping their child integrate a complete sense of self when pieces of the child's heritage may be problematic or even missing entirely. Simultaneous with the adolescent doing her search, adoptive parents are often subconsciously or consciously dealing again with their own issues of loss. They may be wondering what their birth child might have been like and about the preparation for their adopted child's move toward adulthood and intense feelings about the loss of this child, who will soon be an adult.

There are also effects on the adopted person and family if a search for birth parents is undertaken. The search brings up issues of conflicting loyalties for the adopted person between adoptive parents and birth parents. It also brings up fear and fantasies for everyone that are often difficult to manage. It is at this time that issues of loss arise again for all members of the adoption circle. For the adopted person, there is fear of loss and rejection by the adoptive family and possible rejection by birth parents. Adoptive parents must confront the fear of losing their adoptive child to the birth family, and birth parents have the pain and loss associated with surrender of a child for adoption brought back into their lives. It is important to note that although search brings up difficult and painful issues, it is an integral part of the healing process of identity development and capacity for intimacy that is essential to making whole all of these broken connections.

Search (for birth family members) is different than reunion with them. It is possible to search without having a reunion. Every human being has a need to search and learn more about himself, often through his ancestors, and adopted people are no different. If parents have not pursued a semi-open adoption in the child's youth, adolescence is the parents' last chance to be fully involved in the search process; once a child is an adult, she may or may not include the adoptive parents in her search or in the reunion with birth family members. In my experience, I feel that it is in the better interest of the child or adolescent to have adoptive parents on the voyage into the past with him or her, to fully integrate all that is learned into the child's future.

Health care practitioners and other professionals working with children and their families must understand the importance and intricacies of adoption and the search for birth family. They must recognize that it is a healing journey, no matter what is found. Adoption is an ongoing issue throughout the life cycle and beyond, affecting not only generations past but the ones to come as well. There are complexities for an adopted person as parent, for birth parents' past or future children who are parented by them, and with open adoption evolution.

Families affected by adoption may have intermittent needs for working with professionals in a therapeutic way. To address the experiences of adoptive systems throughout the life span, I have developed a therapeutic approach in the Pavao model called *brief long-term therapy*. In this model, a family and various constellations (family as a whole and different subsystems) are seen during a crisis, and the work is in transforming the crisis into an empowering experience. Coming back for further counseling at another point in the development of the family is not seen as failure but rather as a success in working through yet another stage of development. There is a completion of each stage of therapy but no termination. The word *termination* is too loaded for those who have suffered losses associated with adoption. An approach that incorporates *normative crisis* allows professionals to see the difficult times in a way that is not based in pathology. This creates opportunities for clinicians to act in ways that lead to the empowerment of individuals and families affected by the issues of adoption.

Professionals involved with children affected by adoption and their families can normalize and demystify the process of adoption so that the family involved can be treated honorably and be prepared to handle the complex issues that should be considered normal under the circumstances of adoption. As would be expected, adoption issues can be magnified by factors contributing to adoptions of older children or transracial or international adoptions.

Most adoptive parents become adoption educators and learn that they have to stop and educate all of their extended family and community to understand what it is they are doing and why. They work to help people in schools and churches understand some of the very common and expected problems that a child (especially an older placement child) encounters because of early trauma and many moves. The belief that in days of old, the panacea for infertility was adoption is one that people may still think about. But we are now aware that the pain and loss of infertility is ongoing, and although a family and a wonderful life can be crafted by adoption, the loss of the child one would have had is continually mourned. We know now that adoption does not "fix" infertility. It fixes the loss of parenting, and adoption is a wonderful way to become a parent. However, the issues of never seeing a child of "one's own" continue to exist. These issues exist for extended family members as well, grandparents in particular.

Adoption Sensitivity and the Role of Psycho-education

Psycho-education, even many years after the legal act of adoption, can help an entire family. Psycho-education and counseling prior to adoption for the parents of the couple or individual adopting (ie, the grandparents) and the extended family or community will lead to more support for the adoptive family, along with greater understanding of the participants' own feelings.

A knowledgeable pediatric health care professional can help families discuss and make sense of these issues in the pre-adoptive process. Single parents and gay and lesbian parents who adopt will also benefit from adoptive psycho-education about the added complexities that their families will face.

If professionals who are working with birth and adoptive families are not fully trained to understand all aspects of adoption—intergenerational, systemic, and developmental—and if they are not trained to understand that adoption is more than one thing, they are not providing what the family truly needs.

Adoption is so many things. It is public and private; domestic and international; open, semi-open, and closed; in-racial and transracial; infant and older child; and foster, kinship, and guardianship.

Adoption Is Forever—and So Is One's Past: Differentiating the Role of *Secrecy* From *Privacy*

We want adoption to be forever. We want permanent plans for all of the children who are in the situation of needing parents other than those who gave them birth. Along with that, we want children to feel connected and whole as well as protected and loved. It is possible that a person who cannot parent can still love and be of importance to a child. We have a responsibility to keep children whole and to work hard to cut them off only from danger and harm, not from the truth. However, even well-intended families who support their children in all ways possible may find themselves wondering how to support their children (or extended family members) as they seek to integrate the history of adoption into their own identity.

The following 2 de-identified clinical vignettes illustrate key issues for all affected by adoption, specifically the issues of secrecy versus privacy, and identify incorporating past and present lives.

Seth's Story: Secrecy Versus Privacy

Several years ago, I received a phone call from a woman named Linda. She was concerned about her father, who she said was not sleeping or eating. She felt that he needed to see someone for therapy. She mentioned that she thought this was a unique issue and that I might be able to help. I asked what had happened.

Three days before, the telephone at her home rang. She picked up one extension, and her 85-year-old father, Seth, who lived in an in-law apartment in the house, picked up another. At the other end of the line was a young woman who wanted to speak with Rose, who had been Seth's wife and Linda's mother. Rose had been dead for many years. The caller hesitated when she was told this, and then said, "Oh, I'm sorry to hear that." She slowly added, "I'm Rose's granddaughter, and I was looking for her."

Neither Seth nor Linda could understand what she was talking about! They mentally sorted through all the grandchildren, but she was not one of them. And yet, she seemed to know a great deal about Rose. Eventually the young woman, named Judith, made it clear that her mother had been placed for adoption by Linda's mother—Seth's wife—and that Judith felt she desperately needed to find this grandmother.

Linda and Seth were confused and disbelieving. Seth asked for Judith's full name and telephone number and said that they would call her back after they had discussed things.

They hung up, turned to one another, and asked, "What was that? Who was she? Was it a lie? Was it a prank?" Several highly disturbed days followed, until Seth decided to call one of his sisters and said to her, "A strange thing happened to me and I just want to talk to someone. I want to know if you know anything about this." He related the story of Judith's call, and his sister said, "Yes. There was a rumor that Rose had a child and placed the baby for adoption many years ago, prior to marrying you."

Seth, who had never been in therapy before, came in with his daughter for our first session. He did not fully understand why she was bringing him to talk about this. But Seth was a remarkable man. At age 84, his mother and all of his siblings were alive; he was self-employed and still worked full time; and he drove his car 30 miles to each of our appointments. His energy and intelligence became a great asset in his therapy.

At our first session, he was very angry and asked, "How could my wife do this to me? It's as if we lived a lie. How could I not have known this about her?" He felt utterly betrayed. Seth asked to be seen alone; it was too difficult for him to talk about all this in front of his daughter.

I often ask clients to bring in photograph albums as a way to talk about the past. Seth eventually brought in old albums and showed them to me. He would ask, "Does she look happy here? Why does she look happy here if she's holding this information? She looks sad here. Shouldn't someone have helped her? Couldn't someone see that she was sad and grieving?" Seth felt distraught because he had not been the one to see any of this and therefore had not been able to help Rose.

I explained what it might have been like to have borne and placed a child for adoption more than 40 years ago and suggested that Rose was probably told to never tell anyone, to keep her child a secret. She probably thought she had been doing the only possible thing, the kindest thing, by never telling anyone. He said, "But I was her husband! I was married to her for all those years."

I asked if he was angry about her having had sex with another man. Seth was appalled by the question. I told him that he didn't have to talk about this, but that in therapy it was often useful to talk about things that may cause shame or guilt. I asked if he had had lovers prior to Rose, and he said, "Yes, but I was never disloyal to Rose."

I added, "The adoption happened before Rose knew you, and she was never disloyal to you. We will never really know what the circumstances are because Rose is not here to tell us."

Eventually Seth's anger dissipated, and he began to experience his sadness. He said many times that Rose should have told him. He could have helped her. He said, "The grave spews up secrets. She should have known that I would find out." He talked about how, after the births of each of their 4 children, Rose was very sad. The doctors all said this was typical, that it was postpartum blues. Slowly, Seth began to see that maybe Rose became depressed because she had lost her first child and that each subsequent birth brought up the guilt, shame, and loss she felt and made her afraid of losing the others.

Something that strongly upset Seth was that 10 years earlier—this was according to the granddaughter, Judith—her own mother, Edith, the very child that Rose had placed for adoption, had telephoned Rose. Edith had searched and discovered where her birth mother was and eventually made the call. But according to Judith, Rose had said, "I can't talk to you. Nobody knows about this, and I really can't talk to you. Please don't call anymore." Edith, Rose's daughter, respected her wishes. She never called again. Seth now felt that not only had his wife not told him in the beginning, but even as little as 10 years ago, she was adding secrecy to secrecy.

It was because Judith knew this story and had seen her mother's anguish about never meeting any of her birth family that she had made her own telephone call to Rose's family. We are finding in our qualitative research that many adopted people do not choose to search for their birth families. However, for those who do not, their children often take on the role of searcher and hold many of the adopted person's issues concerning adoptive identity. Just as with the immigrant family experience in America, in which the second generation simply wants to be "all-American," to lose the old language, customs, and names, and it remains to the following generation, the grandchildren, to revert to custom, to give their grandparents' names to their own children, to visit the old country, so it is with families and adoption.

This is important to note. Patterns caused by loss and an incomplete understanding of adoption are passed down in families and replicate themselves from one generation to the next. When she had made the decision to telephone Rose's family, Judith had been pregnant and not married. She had decided to parent her child. There was a need to tell her birth grandmother, "I am keeping *my* baby even though you gave *yours* (my mother) away." Judith had, in a sense, been given too little choice in the pattern she was entering into—when there are secrets, there is no control of choice-making for those who inherit them.

Seth began to feel better, as if he understood the situation he'd been thrust into. "How long do I have to be in this therapy?" he asked eventually.

I answered, "Well, whenever you feel you're done, Seth, you're done." I explained that with my brief long-term therapy arrangement, he could always come back and visit any time he felt the need.

Seth said, "But wait—there's one last thing I want to do. I want to give my wife a gift. There is something that she did not complete in her life, and I want to complete it for her. I want to meet her daughter, Edith, and her granddaughter, Judith.

I want to do this for Rose, but I want to meet them just once. May I do that here? I don't want them to come to my house, and I don't want to meet at some restaurant or strange place."

I said, "Absolutely."

Edith and Judith were called, and they agreed to come. Seth asked how he should prepare, and I suggested he might have some copies of some of the pictures that he had shown me made for them. He might tell them stories about Rose and her family, and he could give them some medical information. Seth knew he did not want an awkward meeting to occur in the waiting room, so he arranged to come a half-hour earlier with his daughter, Linda, and her husband, David. We were sitting in my office when the receptionist called and said the other family had arrived.

I opened the door to my office. Standing before me was Rose! It was astounding—Edith looked exactly like the pictures I had seen of Rose. And if this was a shock for me, you can imagine how it affected Linda and Seth. Edith, her husband, her son, and Judith with her baby all walked into the office and seated themselves. The entire family had come for this session. Seth told stories about his wife and gave Edith copies of photographs of Rose he had had made.

In the midst of the session, Edith looked over to Seth and asked, "What would you be to me, Seth?"

"Well, I guess I'd sort of be your stepfather," he said.

And she said, with tears in her eyes, "I would have been very proud to have had you for my father."

After this wonderful exchange, Seth explained how he had wanted this moment in time for them all; it was his gift to Rose and to them from Rose. He said he did not feel he wanted a continued relationship, and Edith's family said they understood this.

After the very moving session, there were still unresolved issues. It had been extremely difficult for Linda to see that her half sister looked so much like Rose—almost exactly as she had looked when Linda was a child, as Edith was that much older than Linda. It was an eerie experience for her. It often is. In the world of adoption, we call Linda's status that of the *second first child*. Often this second first child is the sibling who has the hardest time accepting the adopted person. This was true for Linda.

Seth came back for a "50,000-mile checkup" eventually and said, "Well, I'm sleeping and eating and Linda is feeling better now too. I feel that all is at rest for Rose as well. The only one who doesn't know what's happened is my youngest son, but he lives far away with his wife and children—"

I said, "Seth, someone once told me that the grave spews up secrets! What will happen if you have an accident and your son discovers this news after you're gone, and he finds that others knew and he didn't? You can relate to how it might feel, can't you, Seth?"

Seth said, "I *knew* you would say this!" and then agreed to tell his youngest son.

Lessons From Seth's Story

Seth's story underlines the issue of secrecy versus privacy, which I think is an important distinction, especially in adoption. We have seen that secrecy too often has been a corroding aspect of birth parents' lives, as for Rose. Too often, adoption has a great deal of secrecy surrounding it for everyone involved. For adoptive parents who have not been helped to understand that grief over infertility can be a normal part of the adoption process, secrecy concerning these feelings can prevent them from healing. For birth and adoptive children not told the truth about their or their siblings' origins, secrecy can have a profound effect on their ability to trust and form identity.

And yet I feel strongly that secrecy is not usually the fault of the birth or adoptive families but of the system and those professionals in it who do not respect these people enough to feel that they can manage their own lives and stories. Too often it is the system of adoption, with its sealed birth records and its legal fictions (eg, falsified birth certificates) that create an aura of secrecy that lends negatively to something that should be seen as healing and affirming.

Privacy in adoption is a different matter. People need to have boundaries. They need to use discretion in what they talk about and with whom they talk. Secrecy is when things about you are kept from you. Privacy is when you choose with whom you want to share things about yourself.

As we discuss the family situation in adoption, it becomes clear that one thing that should be private is any discussion about the adoption of a particular child. Many children who come in to see me are upset that their parents are discussing their adoption with a stranger or a neighbor in the supermarket. It is the issue of privacy for that child that is being violated when this happens. The family may have many discussions at home about adoption and may tell the story of the adoption of each child nightly. The problem is having many strangers know the story of the child before the child is ready to hear it in full or when the child wants to choose not to have particular people talk about his or her story.

This may happen even more frequently with transracial and international adoptions when parents and child look so obviously different or are speaking different languages. It may be quite obvious that a child is adopted. But the issue of privacy is very important, and the child feels invaded in some ways by having it discussed at a time when it does not feel appropriate or comfortable to him or her.

Humans are inter-relational beings and will always need to have a sense of attachment and connection. We are resilient, especially children, yet we cannot take away too much from any one person, or he or she will suffer emotional cutoff and attachment problems. These can be life-or-death situations, as the previous and following stories illustrate.

Trevor/Ricardo

One of the stories that most touches my heart is that of a young man who was adopted at about age 5 years from an orphanage in Colombia. His adoptive parents went to Colombia and stayed in a hotel while they awaited the processing of papers. They finally were granted custody of their little boy and brought him back to their home. They decided to name him Trevor, a family name.

Trevor did quite well. He adapted and fit in. He had language problems expected for a child of his age that slowed him down in school, and he got extra help for that. He was into sports and was kept very busy and seemed quite happy.

At approximately age 13, he attempted suicide. On his release from the hospital, the family was referred to me for family therapy. I sat in a room with a severely depressed young man and his parents, who were very nervous. I asked them to tell me, first, the story of Trevor's adoption. I then asked what was going on around the time of the attempted suicide. The parents both said, "Nothing; everything seemed fine." I probed some more and Trevor's dad said that they were in the process of having Trevor become a naturalized citizen, but that could not be the problem! I asked the parents to wait outside, and I spent time alone with Trevor.

He was deeply depressed. I asked if we could think together about anything that would make him want to live. Would he want to go back to Colombia? Would he fantasize about what would make him have the will to live? He looked at me candidly and said, "Joyce, you do not understand. I do not live. I died when I was 5 years old. I had another name, another language, another family, and I became this person that I am trying to be. I can't try any longer." I sat and listened.

I asked, "What do you call yourself in your head, when you talk to yourself?"
He said, "Ricardo."

I asked if we could see if his parents would give him back his name and he responded, "You don't understand. I love my parents. I don't want to hurt them." I suggested then that the suicide attempt had hurt them, but that they were probably able to withstand a name change. I asked him what else he would like.

He said, "I'd like to be around people who look like me....I am in a white family and an all-white school and neighborhood, and there is no one like me."

I asked, "What else?"

He said that he didn't want to be a citizen of the United States. "I lost my country, my language, my people, and I don't want to lose anything else. That is all that I have."

I asked if we could invite his parents back in and tell them what we had talked about and he said, "You tell them," and so I did.

When the parents heard about his name, they cried. Mom said, "I wanted you to have a family name so that you would feel that you belonged. I never wanted to make you feel bad." Ricardo then put his arm around his mom's shoulder and told her that it had been hard for him to get used to a new name and he knew she would slip but that it was OK.

We then talked about the citizenship, and his dad explained how important it would be. He suggested that if he got his name back, he could have something from his past and that at age 21, he could choose to be a citizen of anywhere. They extended the discussion.

We then talked about the issue of Ricardo being the only minority in his world. I asked if the parents would consider moving to an area that was more ethnically diverse. The dad said the market was bad—after all, they had a huge property now with stables and all, and why would they want to move? I then suggested that they look into private schools with a commitment to diversity—not just of students, but with faculty and board that would be mirrors for Ricardo as well. I asked Ricardo if this would do. He said, "I guess so."

To make a long story short, Ricardo lived. He went on to high school and had a good experience. He studied and relearned Spanish. He and his dad took a bicycle trip through Colombia when he graduated from high school, and they went back to visit the orphanage and find out if there was any information about his birth family. There was. Ricardo did nothing more on that trip. He went to college and decided to spend his junior year in Colombia—he wanted to be in an American program, but in Colombia. He felt worried that he would not fit in there either.

While in Colombia, Ricardo found his birth family. He found difficult things. There had been violence and death and poverty. This was all true, and Ricardo had felt it and had memories that he felt were just "bad thoughts." He thought he was a "bad person" when in fact he had witnessed violence and had been subjected to it. His finding out this hard information actually freed him to be present. Ricardo then went on to law school and majored in international law and human rights. He is a champion for the children of the world.

Lessons From Trevor/Ricardo's Story

I love to tell Ricardo's story because he is an example of the danger and fragility of moving a child without thinking of long-term consequences. Ricardo felt dead. He was almost dead. He needed to have his past brought back to him to feel that he might have a future.

Ricardo continues to call me at intervals. He likes my brief long-term therapy model. His most recent call was about commitment. He is in love. The woman is white. He feels that he will be repeating his own life in the life of his children. He feels divided loyalty. Should he be with a dark-skinned woman? His identity confusion continues. He feels that he loves her and will probably marry her, but he wonders what this all means. It is critical for all working with families of adoption to realize that identity issues for adopted persons may be accentuated at the time of adult milestones such as marriage and childbirth.

Children's past traumas may pose long-term threats to family stability and well-being. Traumas, severe deprivation, prenatal drug exposure, mental illness—the effects of these are not erased when a child is placed in foster care or adopted. Also, children adopted through the child welfare system are 4 times as likely as other children to have serious mental health problems and receive special education services.

A Poem for Adoptive Parents

You cannot change the truth
these are your children
but they came from somewhere else
and they are the children of those places
and of those people as well

Help them to know all about their past
and all about their present
help them to know that they are from extended families
that they only have one parent or set of parents
but that they have more mothers and fathers
they have grandmothers, godmothers, birth mothers, mother countries, mother earth
they have grandfathers, godfathers, birth fathers, and fatherlands
they have family by birth and by adoption
they have family by choice and by chance

Childhood is short
they are our children to raise
they are our children to love
and then they are citizens of the world
What we do to them creates the world that we live in
Give them life
Give them their truth
Give them love
Give them all that they came with
Give them all that they grow with

Your children do not belong to you
but they belong with you
you cannot keep them from what is theirs
but you can keep loving them
You do not own your children
but they are your own
…With love to adoptive parents

Poem credit: From Joyce Maguire Pavao, EdD, MEd, LCSW, LMFT. All rights reserved, Joyce Maguire Pavao. March 1997.

Resources

For Prospective Birth Parents

Concerned United Birthparents
www.cubirthparents.org

Concerned United Birthparents is a national organization serving those touched by adoption and others who are concerned about adoption issues. Although the primary focus began with birth parents, long the forgotten people of the adoption community, adoptees, adoptive parents, and professionals are welcome.

For Prospective Adoptive Parents

Resolve: The National Infertility Association
www.resolve.org

Resolve is a national organization providing support for those with a history of infertility and discussing a range of family-building options. Local chapters are outlined on the Web site.

Adoption Community of New England
www.adoptioncommunityofne.org

Local adoption communities such as this provide a great deal of helpful information for families affected by adoption (pre- and post-adoption).

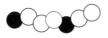

Intercountry Adoption Under the Hague Convention

Nicole Ficere Callahan and Chuck Johnson

According to the US Department of State, the May 29, 1993, Hague Convention on Protection of Children and Co-operation in Respect of Intercountry Adoption establishes "internationally agreed-upon rules and procedures for adoptions between countries that have a treaty relationship under the [convention]." On November 16, 2007, the US Department of State Bureau of Consular Affairs Office of Children's Issues announced that President Bush had signed the US instrument of ratification of the Hague Convention. The United States officially joined the Hague Convention on December 12, 2007, and the convention entered into force in the United States on April 1, 2008.

The goal of the Hague Convention is increased oversight and transparency within the intercountry adoption process to protect children, birth parents, and adoptive parents from exploitation, child trafficking, or adoption fraud. The Hague Convention represents a significant and worthy attempt on the part of many nations to regulate the intercountry adoption process and prevent cases of adoption fraud and wrongdoing.

Under the convention, a central authority in each Hague country will be established to provide one authoritative source of adoption information and set all standards and practices for the intercountry adoption process. In the United States, the central authority is the Department of State. All American adoption agencies that coordinate intercountry adoptions between the United States and a fellow Hague Convention nation must be accredited and approved by organizations or agents authorized by the Department of State.

The Hague Convention outlines precise requirements for accredited intercountry adoption agencies, which must follow Hague guidelines in the United States as well as in the sending countries. The Hague Convention also provides for investigations into any adoption agency suspected of fraudulent activity. Hague agency standards and regulations are intended to provide an additional level of security and protection for adopted children as well as families wishing to adopt internationally.

While US adoptions from non-Hague countries will still be permitted, adoption professionals expect that over time, the convention will help make these non-Hague adoption processes more uniform as well, similar to the Hague adoption process.

The Hague Convention establishes requirements for prospective adoptive parents, who must complete a minimum of 10 hours of pre-adoption training prior to undertaking the intercountry adoption process. This training provides parents with information about the adoption process under the Hague Convention, common challenges encountered in intercountry adoption, child- and country-specific information, and procedural steps the parents are required to complete with the help of their agency, the US Department of State, and US Citizenship and Immigration Services to complete the adoption and cooperate with post-adoption requirements. The adoption agency chosen by the prospective parents will work with them to ensure an appropriate training program is completed.

What Steps Must Parents Complete When Adopting Internationally Under the Hague Convention?

Each sending and receiving country under the Hague Convention, including the United States, has developed its own regulations for the accreditation of adoption service providers. In the United States, accredited adoption agencies must work in compliance with US and Hague adoption policies, assisting state welfare workers in identifying safe, permanent homes for children. The adoption agency chosen by the prospective adoptive parents should possess a thorough knowledge of the adoption procedures in the sending country and can lead parents through the adoption process.

Adoption agencies typically employ a number of individuals "on the ground" within a sending country to act as liaisons between the adoptive parents and local welfare workers, orphanage directors, attorneys, courts, and guides. While the Hague Convention requires an adoption agency to oversee its in-country staff and most agencies work diligently to encourage collaborative working relationships between individuals in each country, it is important to note that an agency's liaisons typically have limited or no legal authority over child referrals, court decisions, laws, delays, or the procedures of the particular country. They are present to aid prospective adoptive parents and help to ensure the smoothest possible adoption experience, but they are limited in their influence and cannot exert control over the sending country's child welfare authorities or significantly hasten the adoption process.

The successful completion of an intercountry adoption relies on the close working relationship between prospective adoptive parents and their chosen adoption agency and the timely submittal of required information and documentation. Once parents have applied to work with a particular adoption agency in the United States, they must submit appropriate forms to the agency and US Citizenship and Immigration

Services. A criminal and child abuse background check is typically performed by the Federal Bureau of Investigation and the prospective adoptive parents' state of residence. Prospective parents must also complete a home study with the help of their adoption agency. To meet Hague requirements for home studies, the country where the planned adoption is to take place must be known and the home study tailored to this country's adoption requirements. After initial clearance is obtained from US Citizenship and Immigration Services, prospective parents must collect and authenticate other forms and information to complete their adoption dossier.

Once the adoption dossier has been completed, parents wait to receive a referral for a child, at which point they may travel to the sending country to meet or retrieve the child. In some adoptions from non-Hague nations, referrals for specific children are not made prior to travel, as the parents are expected to choose a child once they travel to the country. Whenever the official referral takes place, documented proof of the child's identity and his or her legal status as an orphan is required and should be provided to the adoption agency and prospective parents by the sending country's central adoption authority.

Once a child has been identified, parents must obtain documents and follow all designated steps for finalization of the adoption. It is also their responsibility to apply for the child's visa so that he or she can leave the sending country and enter the United States. In the months following the adoption, parents can expect to receive post-placement visits from adoption agency representatives and provide the necessary information for post-placement reports.

When parents in the United States adopt from a Hague Convention country, biographic information about the child must be made available before the adoption can be finalized. Child welfare officials in the sending country will attempt to gather documentation on the child's identity and social and medical background to be provided to the adoption agency and prospective parents. Official information contained in the child's record may include his or her birth certificate, social and medical history, information about the termination of parental rights and proof of his or her orphan status, and reason for institutionalization. Legal custody of the child still belongs to child welfare authorities in the sending country; parents who have received a given child's referral information and accepted the referral still have no legal authority over the child until the adoption has been finalized.

In some rare cases, the adoption of a particular child will unravel at this stage, even after a referral has taken place and been accepted by the adoptive parents. Individuals within the child's country of origin may decide to adopt the child, or the adoptive parents may come to the conclusion that the child is not the best fit for their family after all. In these rare instances, the parents' adoption agency can usually work with the central adoption authority to help them find another child who is eligible for adoption.

What Should Parents Be Aware of When Adopting From Non–Hague Convention Countries?

As mentioned, the Hague Convention on intercountry adoption is designed to promote increased oversight and transparency within the intercountry adoption process for the purpose of protecting children, birth parents, and adoptive parents. But not all countries with intercountry adoption programs will choose to ratify the Hague Convention, and many American families will continue to adopt from these nations. Even if non-Hague adoption procedures become more standardized and streamlined, as American adoption authorities predict, non-Hague nations will still maintain different guidelines and requirements. In some places, there may remain a lack of oversight and regulation in the adoption process.

Some parents wishing to adopt internationally seem to expect a certain level of corruption within the process and are not surprised if asked for goods or sums of money that do not appear to be part of the standard adoption fee. While this may still happen in some places, it is imperative for prospective parents to question any apparent corruption rather than feel pressured to cooperate with it. Adoptive families should endeavor not to agree to any requirement that appears fraudulent or perpetuate any pattern of adoption abuse. This may be more difficult in some countries than others, and there will always be risks involved in attempting intercountry adoption. But the more transparent the intercountry adoption process, the more we can hope for these risks to be identified and minimized to ensure better outcomes for children and families.

Adoptive parents can protect themselves by doing their research, reading extensively about the adoption process within the sending country, and consulting with trusted adoption agency staff and other families who have adopted internationally. The better parents understand the intercountry adoption process and the country from which they are adopting, the less likely they are to become victims of fraud. When working with adoption authorities in the sending country, parents should endeavor to check the credentials of all the people with whom they interact. While a certain degree of flexibility is necessary to pursue a successful intercountry adoption, prospective parents must do all they can not to be taken by surprise by any individual or any point of procedure so that all adoption requirements are completed in a timely, accurate, and ethical manner.

What Can Parents Expect When Traveling to Another Country to Adopt Their Child?

Prospective adoptive parents should do all they can to prepare for international travel so they are informed and know what to do when the time comes to bring their child home. It is recommended that if at all possible, parents enroll in a language class before traveling to the child's country of origin. At the very least, parents should not travel without a good pocket dictionary and local guidebook in case a translator or guide is not always readily available in country. The adoption agency should be able to provide current information on the sending country, its climate, and its culture; another excellent source is the US Department of State Web site (www.state.gov), which lists updates and potential adoption delays for each country. Parents also have the responsibility to learn as much as possible about travel security, passports, visas, customs, and any required medical checkups or immunizations prior to travel. International adoption health clinics may prove especially helpful, as the physicians in these clinics are experts in the field of intercountry adoption and aware of the health risks in a particular country.

When prospective parents arrive in the sending country, whether the purpose of the trip is to finalize the adoption, visit the child, or receive a referral, they should expect a consultation with the foster parents or orphanage as well as the child. It may be necessary to arrange for a translator during these in-country foster home or orphanage visits.

Every country has its own legal system and procedures that dictate how long adoptive parents must remain in country and when and how adoption is finalized and custody formally transferred from the government or orphanage to the adoptive family. In Asian and Latin American countries, for example, parents are usually given custody right away. In Eastern Europe, multiple visits with the child may be required, and often parents are not given custody until the adoption has been finalized

Further delays may occur as the adoption is being finalized within the sending country. Prior to obtaining the US orphan visa, adoptive parents and their agency must be sure to obtain the child's American passport and meet other immigration requirements of the sending country. The documentation requirements of the American consulate abroad will vary depending on the country; however, nearly all consulates require identifying documents for parents and child, as well as appropriate adoption and immigration documents. Photos and an in-country medical evaluation of the child are usually required before the orphan visa can be issued; this process generally takes 1 to 3 days. Following adoption finalization and issuing of the child's visa, parents can return to the United States with their child.

What Should Parents Expect After Bringing Their Child Home?

Adoptive parents should examine their child's passport stamp to determine the type of visa that was issued before leaving the country of origin. The type of visa issued determines when the child can qualify for US citizenship. Registration of the adoption in the United States or re-adoption is the only way to officially rename a child, if this is desired. After registration or re-adoption, the child will be issued a new birth certificate citing the child's birth city and country and listing the adoptive parents as the legal parents. The adoption agency may employ its own legal representative or help parents find an attorney with international adoption experience who can assist during the registration and re-adoption process.

In a majority of cases, children adopted in other countries automatically become citizens of the United States once they enter the country, but in some instances additional documentation may be required. Some countries require that adopted children keep their original nationality until age 18 years; in these cases, the United States recognizes the child's dual citizenship. Many countries will require the adopted child to be registered with their US embassy.

What Is Post-placement Reporting and What Function Does It Serve Under the Hague Convention?

The only way for Hague central authorities to measure the quality of an agency's work and progress of the adopted child is through post-placement reports provided by the agency or adoptive family. Post-adoption reports, which document a child's health, development, and progress in his or her new family, are required by several sending countries that wish to monitor the health and welfare of children adopted internationally. Post-adoption reporting requirements vary from country to country, and the adoption agency should make sure that prospective adoptive parents understand all reporting requirements of their sending country. Parents have a responsibility to fully comply with all post-adoption reporting requirements and procedures, including receiving post-placement visits from an agency representative or social worker and providing the necessary information for post-placement reports.

Post-placement and post-adoption reports are translated and sent abroad to the child-placing entities. The reports may include medical updates, photographs, and school reports. These reports attempt to chart the child's development and progress in every area, as well as the adjustment of the entire adoptive family. If any problems have been identified, including medical or developmental issues, these reports should also include descriptions of the prognosis and treatment. In addition, post-adoption reports provide documented proof that the child is being raised and cared for properly, reassuring adoption authorities abroad and affirming the benefits of intercountry adoption.

Post-placement, post-adoption visits are generally scheduled in accordance with an adoption agency's internal policies as well as the requirements of the child's country of origin. Post-placement visits take place in the family's home and give parents the opportunity to provide updates and other information about the child to the adoption agency and country of origin. Post-placement visits by an agency representative may also help to assist the family with a smooth transition and adjustment.

Most agencies are obligated to include an array of health, developmental, and social information in their reports. Pictures of the child are also requested in many cases, providing further record of the child's growth and development and conveying proof that the child is happy and well cared for in his or her new home. Each post-adoption report is then signed and notarized; a state apostille or other verification may also be required before it is sent to the appropriate authorities.

It is critical for adoptive families to follow through with their commitment to provide timely post-placement reports at the required intervals. Foreign nations and their Hague central authorities expect American adoption agencies and adoptive parents to honor the agreements made prior to and during the adoption process; if these requirements are later ignored, it perpetuates abuses within the intercountry adoption system and can lead to adoption delays and shutdowns.

Conclusion

The Hague Convention on Protection of Children and Co-operation in Respect of Intercountry Adoption represents an important step toward a regulated and more transparent intercountry adoption system, potentially benefiting millions of children worldwide who stand to gain permanency and stability in loving adoptive families. It is imperative to keep in mind the ultimate goal of all intercountry adoption reforms—that children continue to find families through adoption.

Most adoption advocates recommend a holistic approach to intercountry adoption, one that respects adoption as part of the country of origin's overall child welfare program, second in preference to timely domestic adoption but to be preferred over domestic foster care and group or institutional care. As the Hague Convention is implemented around the world, many countries are now taking a similarly holistic look at their adoption and child welfare programs. America's ratification of the Hague Convention presents a great opportunity for expanding intercountry adoption and encouraging best practices in all Hague member states. In the future, we can look for more countries to join the Hague Convention, working alongside other Hague member states to promote a global culture of adoption and child welfare and benefit children and families around the world.

US adoption leaders and advocates hope that America's ratification of the Hague Convention will help to promote the ease with which American families can adopt overseas. But prospective adoptive parents should do all they can to inform themselves of what to expect when adopting internationally and how to do so under Hague Convention requirements so that they reach the decision to pursue an intercountry adoption only after considerable care, serious consideration, and detailed planning. Parents wishing to adopt internationally must be prepared for not only the cost, travel, and extensive requirements involved here and abroad but also the unique risks and rewards of intercountry adoption.

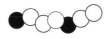

Resources for Foster and Adoptive Parents

The following resources are only a small collection of those available and are provided as an introduction to the adoption process. The inclusion or exclusion of any resources is by no means an endorsement or rejection of any of the organizations involved in adoption. The American Academy of Pediatrics and the authors and editors of this manual do not endorse and are not responsible for any content or information provided by these organizations.

Adoption Nutrition
http://adoptionnutrition.org

Adoptive Families Magazine
Building Your Family: 2013–'14 Donor, Surrogacy, and Adoption Guide
www.adoptivefamilies.com/order/adoption_guide.php

AdoptUSKids
www.adoptuskids.org

American Academy of Adoption Attorneys
www.adoptionattorneys.org

American Academy of Pediatrics
    Council on Foster Care, Adoption, and Kinship Care
    www.aap.org/sections/adoption/index.html

    Healthy Foster Care America
    www.aap.org/fostercare

Centers for Disease Control and Prevention
International Adoption: Health Guidance and the Immigration Process
www.cdc.gov/immigrantrefugeehealth/adoption

Child Welfare League of America
www.cwla.org

The Donaldson Adoption Institute
www.adoptioninstitute.org

Joint Council on International Children's Services
www.jointcouncil.org

National Council for Adoption
www.adoptioncouncil.org

North American Council on Adoptable Children
www.nacac.org

US Department of Health and Human Services
Administration for Children & Families
Child Welfare Information Gateway: Adoption
www.childwelfare.gov/adoption

US Department of State
Bureau of Consular Affairs
Intercountry Adoption
http://adoption.state.gov

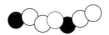

Index

M